RENAL NURSING

To Ken
who suggested I should write a book

RENAL NURSING

Edited by
TONI SMITH MBE RGN
SENIOR NURSE MANAGER, DEPARTMENT OF NEPHROLOGY
LEICESTER GENERAL HOSPITAL TRUST,
LEICESTER, UK

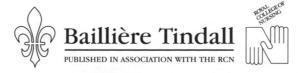

Baillière Tindall
PUBLISHED IN ASSOCIATION WITH THE RCN

London Philadelphia Toronto Sydney Tokyo

Baillière Tindall 24–28 Oval Road
London NW1 7DX

The Curtis Center
Independence Square West
Philadelphia, PA 19106-3399, USA

Harcourt Brace & Company
55 Horner Avenue
Toronto, Ontario, M8Z 4X6, Canada

Harcourt Brace & Company, Australia
30–52 Smidmore Street
Marrickville
NSW 2204, Australia

Harcourt Brace & Company, Japan
Ichibancho Central Building
Chiyoda-ku, Tokyo 102, Japan

A catalogue record for this book is available from the British Library

ISBN 0-7020-2286-1

Typeset by Florencetype Ltd, Stoodleigh, Devon
Printed and bound in The Bath Press, Bath, Avon

CONTENTS

LIST OF CONTRIBUTORS

JULIET AUER CQSW, MPhil, Renal Social Worker, The Renal Unit, The Churchill Hospital Trust, Oxford

ANNE BELL SRN, SCM, formerly Ultrasonographer, University Department of Surgery, Transplant Unit, Leicester General Hospital Trust, Leicester

GEMMA BIRCHER BSc, SRD, Renal Dietetic Manager, Department of Nutrition and Dietetics, Leicester General Hospital Trust, Leicester

JANET E COLEMAN BSc, SRD, Chief Paediatric Renal Dietitian, Department of Nutrition and Dietetics, City Hospital Trust, Nottingham

PATRICIA FRANKLIN BSc(Hons), RGN, Dip Nursing, RCNT, FETC, Adv Dip in Counselling, DMS, Senior Transplant Practitioner and Transplant Manager, The Oxford Transplant Centre, The Churchill Hospital Trust, Oxford

MARIE-CLAIRE HAMILTON MEd, Cert Ed, RGN, Senior Nurse Manager, Renal and Urology Directorate, University Hospital Birmingham NHS Trust, Birmingham

LOUISE HARRIS BSc(Hons), MRPharmS, Dip Hosp Pharm, formerly Renal Pharmacist, Leicester General Hospital Trust, Leicester

JANE HATTERSLEY BSc, Dip Medical Ethics, RGN formerly Research Sister, Department of Nephrology, Leicester General Hospital Trust, Leicester

MAGGIE HICKLIN RGN, RSCN, Clinical Nurse Manager, Paediatrics, Guy's and St Thomas' Hospital Trust, London

ELEANOR MELDRUM RGN, Dip in Training and Development, Nurse Development Practitioner/ENB Renal Course Tutor, Department of Nephrology, Leicester General Hospital Trust, Leicester

MARCELLE DE SOUSA RGN, RSCN, Peritoneal Dialysis Sister (Paediatrics), Guy's and St Thomas' Hospital Trust, London

PHIL SAUNDERS RGN, Dip in HC Studies, Nurse Practitioner, Department of Nephrology, Leicester General Hospital Trust, Leicester

TONI SMITH RGN, Senior Nurse Manager, Department of Nephrology, Leicester General Hospital Trust, Leicester

DAVID SPENCE BSc(Hons), MRPharmS, Research Fellow, formerly Senior Pharmacist, Leicester General Hospital Trust, Leicester

MARIANNE VENNEGOOR SRD, Senior Renal Dietitian, Renal Unit, Guy's and St Thomas' Hospital Trust, London

VICTORIA WARMINGTON BSc(Hons), RGN, G Dip DN, Community PD Specialist Nurse, Wandsworth Community Health Trust, London

SUSAN WHARTON BSc(Hons), RGN, Cert Ed, formerly ENB 136 Renal Course Tutor, Leicester General Hospital Trust, Leicester

JANET WILD RGN, Education Services Manager, Baxter Healthcare Ltd, Renal Training Centre, Springfield Hospital, London

FOREWORD

This book aims to provide a practical guide to caring for renal patients and is therefore a welcome improvement to the previous lack of published books for nephrology staff. It has been written by experts from within the speciality who have extensive knowledge of caring for the renal patient and who address the important current topics and look forward to issues for the future.

In line with current professional thinking, foundations are laid from which professionals can build their own research-based practice. The book will be of value both to those individuals undertaking renal courses and those wishing to update their knowledge and I am confident that all nurses will be able to use the knowledge gained, to develop their skills in patient care. The provision of holistic care requires a multidisciplinary approach and, although this book gives special consideration to nurses, it is designed to be relevant to all health care professions and will help to increase the level of knowledge and skills for all members of the health care team. It will be welcomed by English-speaking health professionals both in the UK and throughout Europe.

ANNE KEOGH
President, European Dialysis and Transplant Nurses Association/
European Renal Care Association (EDTNA/ERCA)
October 1995–October 1996

PREFACE

As the Key Member for the European Dialysis and Transplant Nurses Association/European Renal Care Association (UK) for 3 years (from 1991 to 1993), I had many requests to recommend a book on renal nursing. It is not possible to reply positively to these requests as there was no book available which could provide a guide to cater for all aspects of care pertinent to nursing the renal patient.

Renal nursing has a reputation for being 'highly technical' and this, combined with the lack of nursing information, has led to difficulty in recruitment of nurses into this speciality. Well-trained renal nurses in possession of a post registration qualification in renal nursing have more expertise than junior doctors and are keen and willing to pass on their knowledge. Medical books are too complicated for the new nurse entering the speciality.

Renal nursing is patient centred, and not, as is so often portrayed, machine orientated. It is the intention of this book to encourage nurses into this speciality and to educate them into the realisation that becoming an expert in a specialised field can be both rewarding and give a sense of job satisfaction not recognised in many fields of patient care professions.

The aim of writing the book is to provide a tool for educating nurses, both those entering the field of renal nursing and those already established. It will give a basic insight into renal disease, as well as providing detailed accounts of the various treatments available for patients with renal impairment, and end stage renal failure, including renal transplantation. Psychological aspects of nursing patients and supporting their carers will feature highly, and will include conservative treatment. This is particularly relevant to nursing children and the elderly.

Many units provide the facility for nurses to rotate around the department to gain an overall knowledge in all aspects of renal care. A good reference will be gained for these nurses changing course within the field of renal nursing, giving them confidence and expertise to counsel patients in their care, who may be changing treatment modality, drug regimes or simply teaching patients the technique of dialysis.

Each individual chapter is written by an expert in that particular field and the text is research-based, providing further reading suggestions. Renal is a fast changing field of medicine with new treatments regularly becoming available. The authors have reviewed future trends in this expanding field of medicine.

TONI SMITH
Co-ordinating Editor

ACKNOWLEDGEMENTS

The editor would like to thank the following companies for providing an educational grant to help publication of *Renal Nursing*.

Baxter Healthcare Ltd.
Boehringer Mannheim Pharmaceuticals (UK) Ltd.
Cilag Biotech, a division of Janssen-Cilag Ltd.
Fresenius Medical Care
Gambro Ltd.
Kimal Scientific Products Ltd.

Personal thanks also to Dr John Feehally, Consultant Nephrologist at Leicester, for his ideas, help and support throughout, and Professor John Walls, Professor of Nephrology at Leicester and President of the Renal Association, for his encouragement and advice.

Every effort has been made to check the drug doses given in this book. However, as it is possible that dosage schedules have been revised, the reader is strongly urged to consult the drug companies' literature before administering any of the drugs listed.

INTRODUCTION

Over the last decade, research carried out by nurses has increased in both quality and quantity. Reflections on practice guided by the theory of nursing care has allowed the profession to gain information to introduce new ideas and advance the role of clinical nurse specialists and nurse practitioners in renal units. Nurses themselves have begun to recognize the contribution they make to patient care, and feel valued and willing to contribute to the goals of the multidisciplinary renal team.

Baer (1979) suggested that 'A nephrology nurse is a professional practitioner who possesses sufficient knowledge in delivering health care to individuals with renal failure who may be at any stage of the therapeutic continuum'.

Nursing the renal patient probably started in Roman times, when patients required assistance in the taking of hot baths. In the 1960s, the renal nurse's role was arguably nothing more than an assistant to the doctors and technicians performing the dialysis. Even to do this, nurses were encouraged to learn the principles involved, and with the advent of permanent vascular access came the gradual evolution of the specialist renal nurse. As the treatment became more routine and the skills of the nurse developed, it was no longer necessary for medical staff to be present, and the treatments, though medically prescribed, became nurse managed.

In the early 1960s home haemodialysis was initiated, and this necessitated the need for the nurse to become the teacher of patients and carers in the techniques required to carry out the procedure in the home environment.

When transplantation became available, the nurse was made aware of the need for monitoring and controlling of immunosuppression therapy, and more importantly, the need for counselling and support of patients through the pathways of change. As the duties of the transplant nurse became more diverse, the transplant co-ordinator evolved, who was often a nurse, responsible not only for teaching and liaising with medical teams within such areas as accident and emergency, and intensive therapy units, teaching staff to recognize the suitability of patients for organ donation, but also for co-ordinating both nationally and internationally the matching of the donor organ with the recipient through close liaison with the national networks.

Peritoneal dialysis, once initiated by the doctors for acute treatment, has always been a nurse-led treatment in practice, and with the advent of continuous ambulatory peritoneal dialysis (CAPD) in the mid to late 1970s as an alternative to home dialysis treatment, the skills and knowledge of the nephrology nurse became even more diverse.

Through the evolution of technology, the character and skills of renal nursing have adapted and changed, resulting in the nurse having the autonomy to monitor the progress as well as giving expert advice and psychological support to a caseload of patients.

The result of these changes has enabled the large expansion of facilities which has been born of necessity to cope with the tremendous growth in dialysis programmes throughout the world. These facilities include nurse-led and managed minimal care units for haemodialysis (small units often with no on-site medical cover – often referred to as satellite units), which are under the direction of the larger parent unit, thus taking the dialysis treatment to the location of the patient.

The intensive care setting, and the fast-changing technology together with the continuous long-term intense contact with patients, make this speciality of nursing unique. The nurse's knowledge has become technically sophisticated to give the patient, whose life depends on the expertise, the feeling of safety and quiet efficiency.

The nurse has to deal with physical and psychological problems which accompany nursing the chronically sick. Thus, stress and burnout are common in the renal nurse. The consequences of burnout are potentially very serious (Lewis *et al.*, 1992), leading to absenteeism, low morale and high staff turnover. All of these factors are known to occur in renal nursing, and support and guidance where problems are identified are indeed necessary.

In direct response to the new body of knowledge and skills required by the renal nurse, the Joint Board of Clinical Nursing Studies created the JBCNS 136 course, which in 1985 was replaced by the English National Board (ENB) 136 (Renal Course) and ENB 143 (Urology/Renal Course) and there are growing numbers of modules and courses throughout the UK, and indeed the world, for the renal nurse.

With the growth of scientific knowledge, renal nurses are encouraged to extend and develop the scope of practice, thereby increasing the role and responsibility to the renal patient. The nurse becomes a counsellor, a teacher, a resource, a leader, a technician, and an advocate, as well as the expert practitioner. The role may now include conducting clinics, organizing seminars for patients, heading patient support groups, and pre-admission assessment of patients for routine procedures. These nurse-centred initiatives have resulted in the necessity for referral of the patient to the medical team only when the findings are unusual. Nurses work closely with the renal doctors to monitor the patients during research of treatment initiatives. Assessing patients' treatments through dialysis prescriptions using urea kinetic modelling (UKM) in both CAPD and haemodialysis ensures the optimum treatment is given for the individual patient. Locally set guidelines give the nurse the autonomy to change treatment prescriptions, always keeping the patient at the focus of clinical practice.

Renal community nurses have been responsible, since the early 1980s, in the continuous assessment of patients undergoing treatment for renal disease in the home. This can be invaluable in the early recognition of problems, and timely action may negate the necessity for admission to hospital, or more importantly, prevent failure of dialysis by early initiation of appropriate treatment. Predialysis counselling and evaluation of home circumstances can assist the clinician in prescribing the most appropriate mode of dialysis. A sound knowledge base as well as an understanding of the research and theory behind the practice is essential to enable care and support to be delivered to the patient both in the ward situation and the home environment. The hospital is maintained as the centre of expert knowledge rather than a care centre for the chronically sick.

The recognition of the need for a professional organization for renal nurses to meet and share progress, experiences and developments, came about in the early 1970s. Since the inaugural one-day meeting of 150 nurses of the European Dialysis and Transplant Nurses Association (EDTNA) in Florence in 1972, professional nursing associations for renal care workers have made a significant impact in providing a forum for research and communication not only in Europe, but worldwide. In 1990, the World Council for Renal Care was launched.

These professional associations make a significant impact on the daily practices in renal units, by setting standards for patient care (Van Waeleghem and Edwards, 1994) and by producing a core curriculum for renal nurse training (Kunzle and Thomas, 1994). Implementation of these standards in renal units is worldwide, thus giving continuity where resources allow, leading to improvements and parity in patient care.

It is widely recognized that there is a need to continue to expand and develop renal services, to provide treatment for the increasing number of patients (Walls, 1994). The nurse prescribing and delivering a high standard of individualized care to renal patients, both in the centre and the community, will always continue looking for new horizons in which to practice. Nowhere can the fundamental principles of nursing be better implemented than in the workplace of the renal nurse. The Statement of Strategic Intent by Yvonne Moores, Chief Nursing Officer for the Department of Health, and Director of Nursing, National Health Service Executive, and Ken Jarrold, Director of Human Resources, National Health Service Executive (1994), suggests that nurse education will be patient focused and practice led.

Practitioners are demanding the development necessary to function confidently, competently and with sensitivity, leading to effective use of resources whilst achieving the highest standards.

Research-based practices and evaluation of the delivery of care is focused on the changing health needs as new treatments become available. Renal nurses will continue to work as key members of the multidisciplinary team, to recognise and achieve a common purpose and to create opportunities for shared learning with other associated clinical professions worldwide.

REFERENCES

BAER, C.L. (1979) The growth and development of nephrology nursing practice. *Heart and Lung*, **8**(5): 896–902.

DEPARTMENT OF HEALTH NURSING, MIDWIFERY AND HEALTH VISITING EDUCATION (1994) A statement of strategic intent.

KUNZLE, W. AND THOMAS, N. (1994) EDTNA/ERCA. European Core Curriculum for the post basic course in nephrology nursing document.

LEWIS, S.L., CAMPBELL, M.A., BECKTELL, P.J. *et al.* (1992) Work stress, burnout and sense of coherence among dialysis nurses. *ANNA J.*, **19**: 6.

VAN WAELEGHEM, J.P. AND EDWARDS, P. (1994) EDTNA/ERCA. European standards for nephrology nursing practice document.

WALLS, J. (1994) Consensus on renal dialysis provision seminar, London. Sponsored by Baxter Healthcare Ltd.

FURTHER READING

ATKINSON, A., EVANS, M., DONOVAN, M. AND GATHERCOLE, W. (1987) The role of the Nephrology Nurse. The Royal College of Nursing Dialysis and Transplant Nursing Forum discussion document.

CHAPTER 1

THE HISTORY OF DIALYSIS AND TRANSPLANTATION

INTRODUCTION

The introduction of dialysis as a life-saving treatment for kidney failure was not the result of any large-scale research programme, rather it emerged from the activities of a few pioneering individuals who were able to utilise ideas, materials and methods from a range of developing technologies.

Haemodialysis (HD) as a routine treatment for renal failure was initiated in the 1960s, followed by continuous ambulatory peritoneal dialysis (CAPD) in the 1970s. The recognition of the need for immunosuppression in transplantation in the 1960s enabled this to become the preferred treatment for many patients.

HAEMODIALYSIS

The Beginning

It was the Romans who first used a form of dialysis therapy by giving hot baths to patients to remove urea. The action of the hot water made the patient sweat profusely and this, together with the toxins diffusing through the skin into the bath water, would temporarily relieve symptoms.

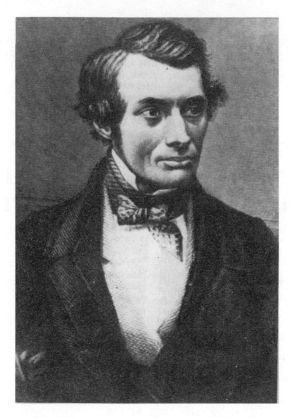

Fig. 1.1 *Thomas Graham 1805–1869. Engraving by C. Cook after photograph by Claudet.*

However, the Romans did not understand why the treatment worked. The effect was to leave the patient fatigued but, as the only hope, this treatment was still used on occasions into the 1950s.

The first time that the term 'dialysis' was used was in 1854 by Thomas Graham (Fig. 1.1), a Scottish chemist (Graham, 1854). He used dialysis to describe the transport of solutes through an ox bladder, and this was the catalyst for other researchers working in a similar field to focus on the membrane.

Membranes were made from a variety of substances including parchment and collodion (Eggerth, 1921). Collodion is a syrupy liquid which dries to form a porous film, and allows the passage of small molecular weight substances, whilst being impermeable to substances with a molecular weight greater than 5000 Da. In 1889, B. W. Richardson referred to the use of collodion membranes in the dialysis of blood. So by this method, living animals were dialysed in experimental conditions (Richardson, 1889), but the limiting factor which prevented the treatment being used in humans at this time, was the lack of suitable materials.

Pre-1920

It was not until 1913 that the first article on the technique of HD, named the 'artificial kidney', was reported. Experimental dialysis was performed on animals, by using variances in the composition of dialysis fluid (Abel *et al.*, 1914) Substances could be added to the solution to avoid their net removal. The main aim of the experiments was the removal of salicylates. The removal of fluid and toxins accumulated due to kidney disease was not, at this time, considered.

In 1914, Hess and McGuigan were experimenting with dialysis in a pharmacology laboratory in Chicago. As a result they were able to transfer sugar from tissue to blood and from the blood across a collodion membrane (Hess and McGuigan, 1914). The design of the dialyser minimised the length of tubing from the patient, and a high blood flow was achieved by connection to the carotid artery in an effort to minimise the necessity to use an anti-coagulant. A single U-shaped collodion tube was inserted into a glass cylinder with a rubber stopper at one end. The blood flow both to and from the dialyser was at one end, with a port for adjusting the pressure inside the tube. These experiments were still only performed on animals. The only anticoagulant available was in the form of an extract obtained from crushed leech heads, called hirudin. This was far from satisfactory, even though leeches were plentiful and readily available from the corner shop for around $25 per 1000.

The 1920s

The first dialysis performed on a human (Fig. 1.2) was carried out by the German physician, Georg Haas, in Giessen in the latter half of the 1920s. He performed six treatments in six patients. Hand-made collodion membranes were used, and clotting was prevented by using hirudin and, later, a crude form of heparin. Haas used multiple dialysers to increase the surface area of blood exposed to the dialysis fluid. This necessitated as many as six dialysers arranged in parallel and he found that the arterial pressure of the blood was insufficient to propel the blood through the entire extracorporeal circuit. He therefore introduced a pump into the circuit (Fig. 1.3). Haas was aware of the lack of support given to him by the hospital and his colleagues and by the late 1920s he gave up and the work was stopped. Georg Haas died in 1971 aged 85 years and was honoured as the pioneer of dialysis.

In spite of these treatments carried out from the 1920s to the 1940s, the uraemic patient suffering from poor appetite and vomiting could be offered nothing more than bed-rest, and a bland salt-free diet composed mainly of vegetables, carbohydrate and fat to reduce protein metabolism. Dialysis was not considered a realistic option and the conservative therapy was only offered as a palliative measure.

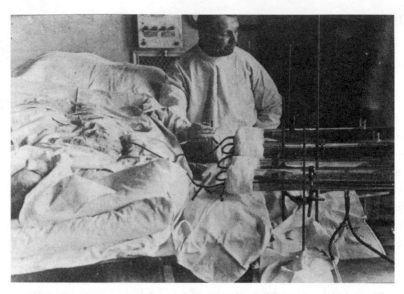

Fig. 1.2 *The first human dialysis – 1923. Reprinted by permission of Kluwer Academic Publishers.*

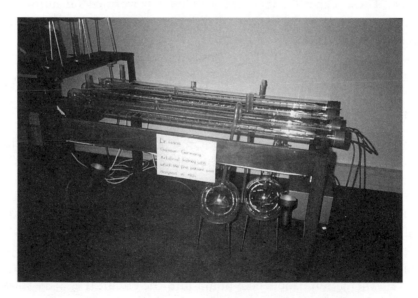

Fig. 1.3 *The equipment used by Georg Haas.*

Heinrich Necheles was the founder of the contemporary dialyser. In 1923, he experimented with the sandwiching of membranes, thus giving an increased surface area without the necessity for multiple dialysers. The membrane used was the peritoneum of a sheep, and because the membrane was prone to expansion, support sheets were placed between the layers of membrane, thus allowing a large surface area of membrane to come into contact with the dialysis fluid. Other features introduced by Necheles were a heater, the priming of the pathway for the blood, and a filter to prevent clots returning to the patient.

The 1930s

The 1920s and 1930s saw great advances in synthetic polymer chemistry, resulting in the availability of cellulose acetate which could be used as a membrane for HD. It was in 1937 that the first synthetic membrane was used by the American scientist William Thalhimer. The material, cellophane – a form of cellulose acetate, which was used extensively in the sausage industry – had potential which was not recognised for some years. In the mid-1930s came the purification of heparin (Thalhimer *et al.*, 1938) which could be used as an anticoagulant and together these two advances gave rise to the next stage of development which took place in 1943 in occupied Holland.

The 1940s and 1950s

Willem Kolff (Fig. 1.4), a physician working in Groningen in Nazi-occupied Holland, had his attention drawn to the work of a colleague who was concentrating plasma by using cellulose acetate as a membrane and immersing it in a weak solution of sugar. Kolff noticed that toxins in the blood were altered by this method (Kolff, 1950). He built a rotating drum dialyser (Figs 1.5 and 1.6) which provided sufficient surface area for his first attempt at human dialysis (Kolff and Berk, 1944). His machine consisted of 30 m of cellophane tube which was wound round a large cylinder. The cylinder was placed in a tank containing a weak solution of salts – the dialysate. The patient's blood was passed through the cellophane tube, the walls acting as a semipermeable membrane. Blood flow was achieved by the addition of a circuit containing a burette which, when filled with blood, could be raised high enough to allow the blood to flow into the dialyser. The burette was then lowered allowing the blood to drain back, and raised again to allow the blood to return to the patient. The slats in the construction of the cylinder were of wood due to the shortage at this time of such materials as aluminum, fortunate in retrospect now the toxicity of aluminium is appreciated. Six hours were required for the treatment, and it is interesting to note that similar efficiency of dialysis could be achieved by this method as with the dialysers in use today: a clearance of 170 ml min^{-1} of urea could be achieved. Fluid could only be removed by increasing the osmotic pressure of the dialysate fluid by the addition of sugar, as an increase in the pressure on the membrane would result in rupture (Kolff, 1965).

The whole procedure was very time consuming and labour intensive, as the operation required attention at all times, to raise and lower the burette

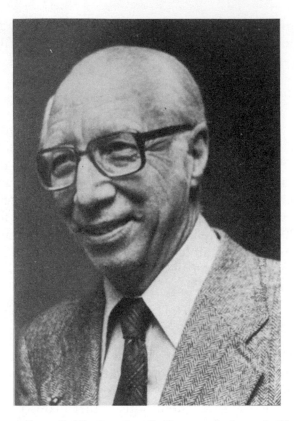

Fig. 1.4 *Willem Johan Kolff. Reprinted by permission of Kluwer Academic Publishers.*

and observe the membrane for frequent ruptures. Repairs to the membrane were carried out by the insertion of a glass tube at the point of rupture. Kolff's first clinical experience was gained on a 29-year-old woman with chronic nephritis. The blood urea was kept stable for 26 days, but after 12 sessions of dialysis, her blood urea began to increase, and she subsequently died.

After the war, in 1945, Kolff's technique was widely used, particularly in Sweden and the USA. The treatment was initially for acute renal failure when kidney function could be expected to return to normal following a short period of dialysis treatment. It was widely used in the Korean war in 1952 to treat trauma-induced renal failure. The group, led by Paul Teschan, trained to use the rotating drum dialyser and saved many lives by lowering the high potassium levels of the victims (Teschan, 1955).

Some of the earliest research carried out on fluid removal from the blood using negative pressure was conducted by M. R. Malinow and W. Korzon at Michael Reese Hospital in Chicago in 1946 (Malinow and Korzon, 1947). The device used was the earliest version of a dialyser with multiple blood

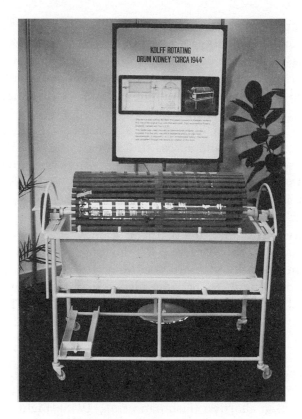

Fig. 1.5 *The Kolff rotating drum.*

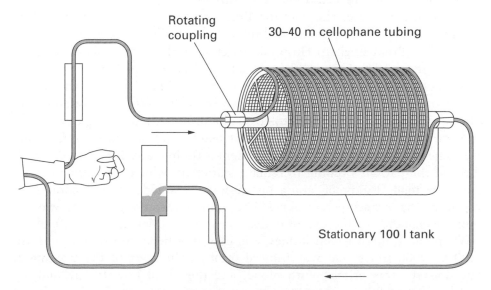

Fig. 1.6 *Diagram of the Kolff rotating drum system.*

paths and negative pressure capacity. It had parallel sections of cellulose acetate tubing and, by adding layers of tubing, the surface area of the device could be increased. The diffusion properties of this device were not considered, as it was intended for removal of water only from the blood. The device required a low priming volume and the circuit included a blood pump.

In the 1940s, interest in dialysis as a treatment for renal failure had spread throughout Europe and across to Canada as the need was becoming widely recognised by the medical profession. After obtaining drawings of the Kolff dialyser, Russell Palmer and a colleague, of Vancouver, Canada, built a replica and dialysed their first patients in September 1947 (Palmer and Rutherford, 1949).

Kolff was invited to take his artificial kidney to New York where he trained physicians in the operation of the life-saving device. There was resistance from hospital staff at the Mount Sinai Hospital, who only permitted the treatment to be administered in the surgical suite after normal surgical schedules were completed for the day. The first patient scheduled for treatment was a victim of mercuric chloride poisoning, but treatment was cancelled when a spontaneous diuresis occurred, caused perhaps by the patient seeing the formidable equipment!

The first successful dialysis in Mount Sinai Hospital was in January 1948, in a female admitted to hospital having inserted mercury tablets into her vagina to induce an abortion (Fishman et al., 1948). Eight hours after the first dialysis using the Kolff machine, the patient diuresed. The treatment had been a success. Victims of drug overdose were then regularly treated by use of the rotating drum dialyser until 1950.

To expand the use, the rotating drum would have to be modified to become easier to use. Kolff enlisted the help of Dr Carl Walter, who worked at the Peter Brent Brigham Hospital. Together with Edward Olson, an associate engineer from Fenwal, they set about designing and building a new version of the Kolff device. Stainless steel was used for the drum, and refinements included a hose for filling the pan with the 100 l of dialysate fluid, which was heated, and a hood to cover the drum. A tensioning device was used on the cellophane membrane as it had a tendency to stretch during use. The split connection for the patient's tubing was introduced which allowed the patient's tubing to remain stationary whilst the drum rotated. This was made leakproof, and a Lucite hood was added to overcome heat loss from the extracorporeal blood. These improvements paved the way for wider acceptance of the use of dialysis treatment (Merrill et al., 1950).

When the Kolff–Brigham kidney was used, the heparin dose ranged from 6000 to 9000 units, and was infused prior to the start of the treatment. The dialyser was primed with blood, and the blood flow to the dialyser was limited to 200 ml at a time to prevent hypotension. To assist blood flow a pump was inserted in the venous circuit rather than the arterial side, to minimise the probability of pressure build-up in the membrane which would cause a rupture.

This version of the Kolff–Brigham dialysis machine was used in 1948, and in all, over 40 machines were built and exported all over the world. Orders for spare parts were still being received as late as 1974, from South America and behind the iron curtain.

The 1950s

The Allis–Chalmers Corporation was one of the first companies to produce dialysis machines commercially. They were prompted into the manufacture when an employee developed renal failure. There was no machine available and so the firm turned its attention to producing a version of the Kolff rotating drum. The resulting machine was commercially available for $5600 and included all the sophistication available at the time. Allis–Chalmers produced 14 of these machines and sold them all over the USA into the early 1950s.

In October 1956, the Kolff system became commercially available, so the unavailability of equipment could no longer be used as an excuse for non-treatment of patients. Centres purchased the complete delivery system for around $1200 and the disposables necessary for the treatment were around $60. The system was still used mainly for reversible acute renal failure drug overdose, and poisoning (Fig. 1.7).

The Development of The Dialyser

Jack Leonards and Leonard Skeggs produced a plate dialyser which would permit a reduction in the priming volume, and allow negative pressure to be used to remove fluid from the patient's system (Skeggs et al., 1949). A modification to this design included a manifold system which allowed variation of the surface area without altering the blood distribution. Larger dialysers followed, which necessitated the introduction of a blood pump.

In the late 1950s Fredrik Kiil of Norway developed a parallel plate dialyser, with a large surface area (1 m²) requiring a low priming volume (Fig. 1.8). A new cellulose membrane, Cuprophan, was used which allowed the passage of larger molecules than other materials available at that time. The Kiil dialyser could be used without a pump. Kiil dialysed the patients using their own arterial pressure. This dialyser was widely used because the disposables were relatively inexpensive when compared with other dialysers around at that time.

A crude version of the capillary-flow dialyser, the parallel dialyser using a new blood pump, and a more advanced version of the Alwall kidney was developed (MacNeill, 1949). However, it was John Guarino who incorporated the important feature of a closed system, a visible blood pathway.

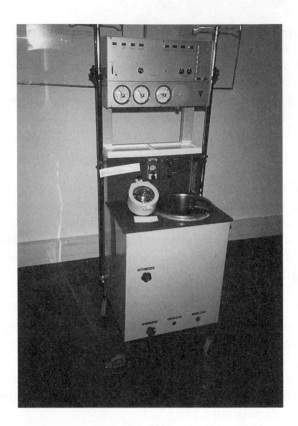

Fig. 1.7 *A typical dialysis machine from the 1950s – Fresenius.*

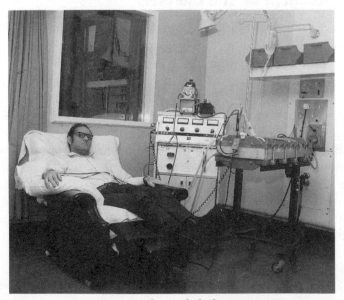

Fig. 1.8 *The Kiil dialyser.*

To reduce the size of the dialyser without reducing the surface area, William Y. Inouye and Joseph Engelberg produced a plastic mesh sleeve to protect the membrane. This reduced the risk of the dialysis fluid coming into contact with the blood. Because this was a closed system, the effluent could be measured to determine the fluid loss of the patient. It is the true predecessor of the positive and negative pressure dialysers used today.

The first commercially available dialyser was manufactured by Baxter and based on the Kolff kidney. It provided a urea clearance of approximately 140 ml min^{-1}, equivalent to today's models, and was based on the coil design. The priming volume was 1200–1800 ml and this was drained into a container at the end of treatment, refrigerated and used for priming for the next treatment. It was commercially available in 1956 at $59.00.

The forerunner of today's capillary-flow dialyser was produced by Richard Stewart in 1960. The criteria for design of this hollow-fibre dialyser were low priming volume and minimal resistance to flow. The improved design contained 11 000 fibres which provided a surface area of 1 m^2.

Future designs for the dialyser will focus on refining the solute and water removal capabilities, as well as reducing the size and priming requirements of the device, thus allowing an even higher level of precise individual care.

The Emergence of Home Haemodialysis

It was Scribner's shunt which provided vascular access, thus leading to the first dialysis unit to be established for chronic patients at the University of Washington Hospital. Belding Scribner also developed a central dialysate delivery system for multiple use and set this up in the chronic care centre, which had 12 beds. These beds were quickly taken and his plan for expansion was rejected. The only alternative then was to send the patients home, and so the patient and family were trained to perform the dialysis and care for the shunts. Home dialysis was strongly promoted by Scribner (Fig. 1.9).

Stanley Shaldon reported in 1961 that a patient dialysing at the Royal Free Hospital in London was able to self care by setting up his own machine, initiate and terminate dialysis; so home HD in the UK was made possible. The shunt was formed in the leg for vascular access, to allow the patient to have both hands free for the procedures. Hence Shaldon was able to report the results of his first patient to be placed on overnight home HD in November 1964. With careful patient selection, the venture was a success. Scribner started to train patients for home at this time, and his first patient was a teenager assisted by her mother. Home dialysis was selected for this patient, so that she would not miss her high school education. The average time on dialysis was 14 h twice weekly. To allow freedom for the patient, overnight dialysis was widely practised. At first, emphasis was on selection of the suitable patient and family, even to the extent of

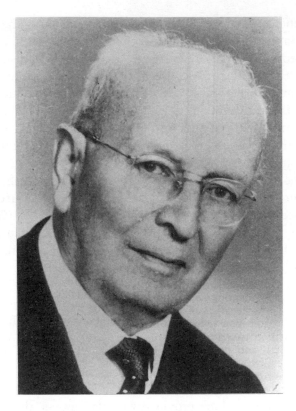

Fig. 1.9 *Belding H. Scribner.*

a stable family relationship, before the patient could be considered for home training (Baillod *et al.*, 1965).

From these beginnings, large home HD programmes developed in the USA and in the UK, thus allowing expansion of the dialysis population without increasing hospital facilities. Many patients could now be considered for home treatment, often with surprisingly good results, as the dialysis could be moulded to the requirements of the individual, rather than the patients conforming to a set pattern. However, with the development in the late 1970s and early 1980s of CAPD as the first choice for home treatment, the use of home HD has steadily dwindled (Fig. 1.10).

Vascular Access for Haemodialysis

It was Sir Christopher Wren, of architectural fame, who in 1657 successfully introduced drugs into the vascular system of a dog. In 1663, Sir Robert Boyle injected successfully into humans. Prison inmates were the subjects and the cannula used was fashioned from a quill. For HD to become a widely accepted form of treatment for renal failure, a way to provide long-

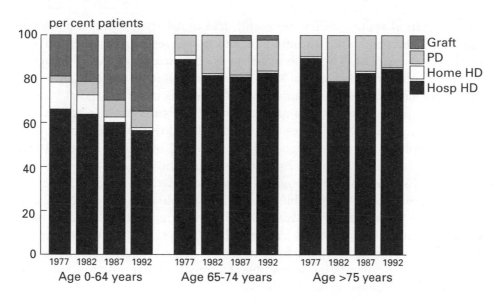

Fig. 1.10 *Mode of therapy 1977–1992 EDTA registry report published 1993. HD, haemodialysis; PD, Peritoneal dialysis. Reprinted by permission of EDTA.*

term access to the patient's vascular system had to be found and until this problem was solved, long-term treatment could not be considered. In order for good access to be established, a tube or cannula had to be inserted into an artery or vein thus giving rise to a good blood flow from the patient. The repeated access for each treatment quickly led to exhaustion of blood vessels for cannulation. The need for a system whereby a sufficiently large bloodflow could be established for dialysis, without destroying a length of blood vessel every time dialysis was required, was imperative.

Teschan, in the 11th Evacuation Hospital in Korea, was responsible in the 1950s for developing a method of heparin lock for continuous access to blood vessels. The cannulae were made from Tygon tubing and stopcocks, and the blood was prevented from clotting by irrigation with heparinised saline. It was not a loop design, as the arterial and venous segments were not joined together.

In 1960 in America, George Quinton, an engineer, and Belding Scribner, a physician, made use of two new synthetic polymers – teflon and silastic – and by using the tubing to form the connection between a vein and an artery, were able to re-route the blood outside the body (usually in the leg). This was known as the arteriovenous shunt. The tubing was disconnected at a union joint in the centre, and each tube then connected to the lines of the dialysis machine. At the end of treatment, the two ends were then reconnected, establishing a blood flow from the artery to the vein outside the body. In this way, repeat dialysis was made possible without further trauma to the vascular system.

This external shunt, whilst successful, had drawbacks. It was a potential source of infection, often thrombosed and had a restrictive effect on the activity of the patient. This form of access is still occasionally used for acute treatment, although the patient's potential requirements for chronic treatment must be considered when the choice of vessels is made, so that vessels to be used in the formation of an arteriovenous fistula are not scarred. In 1966, Michael Brescia and James Cimino developed the subcutaneous radial artery-to-cephalic vein arteriovenous (AV) fistula (Cimino and Brescia, 1962) – Cimino's colleague Kenneth Appel performing the surgery.

The AV fistula avoided the need for anticoagulation, reduced infection risk and gave access to the blood stream without danger of shunt disconnection. Subsequently, a number of synthetic materials have been introduced to create internal AV fistulas. These are useful when the patient's veins are not suitable to form a conventional AV fistula: in severe obesity, loss of superficial veins due to repeated cannulation, or self-inflicted loss of veins in drug addicts.

Percutaneous access by way of cannulation of the femoral or subclavian veins has now largely replaced the shunt for emergency dialysis. A 'single needle' device is used which alternately allows arterial pull and venous return through the same catheter. Alternatively, double lumen subclavian catheters are now available, allowing a continuous flow of blood. Vessels later required for more permanent access are not used and this type of access is conveniently gained using an aseptic technique in the ward area so that immediate dialysis is possible.

The Present

Monitoring and total control of the patient's treatment became more important as the treatment became widespread, and so equipment development continued. Sophisticated machines incorporated temperature monitoring, positive pressure gauges and flow meters. Negative pressure monitoring followed, as did a wide range of dialysers with varying surface areas, ultrafiltration capabilities and clearance values. Automatic mixing and delivery of the dialysate and water supply to the machine greatly increased the margin of safety for the procedure, and made the operation much easier to manage. The single patient system now evolved provides a machine that monitors all parameters of dialysis through the use of microprocessors, allowing the practitioner to programme a patient's requirements – in terms of factors such as blood flow and duration – so that the resulting treatment is a prescription for the individual's needs. Average dialysis time is reduced to 4 h three times weekly, or less if a high flux (high performance) dialyser is used. With the use of a simple formula, urea kinetic modelling can be introduced, allowing the provider to deliver a quality of treatment which is measurable. This is explained fully in the chapter on HD.

The early 1970s saw the number of patients increase due to the increased awareness brought about by the availability of treatment. Free-standing units for the sole use of kidney dialysis came into being, leading to dialysis becoming a full-time business. Committees for patient selection were disbanded, and the problems concerned with inadequate financial resources came to the fore. The 1990s has seen the setting of standards for treatment quality. Attempts continue to reduce duration of treatment, to enhance the patient's quality of life. Dialysis facilities are demanded within easy reach of patients' homes, and this expectation has led to the emergence of small satellite units, managed and monitored by larger units, as a popular alternative to home HD treatment.

PERITONEAL DIALYSIS

Continuous ambulatory peritoneal dialysis (CAPD) as a form of treatment for renal failure has been brought about by a climax of the innovative efforts and tenacity of many pioneers over the past two centuries. It was probably the early Egyptian morticians who first recognised the peritoneum and peritoneal cavity as they embalmed the remains of their influential countrymen for eternity. The peritoneal cavity was described in 3000 BC in the Ebers papyrus, as a cavity in which the viscera were somehow suspended. In Greek times, Galen, a physician, made detailed observations of the abdomen whilst treating the injuries of gladiators.

The earliest reference to what may be interpreted as peritoneal dialysis (PD) was in the 1740s when Christopher Warrick reported to the Royal Society in London that a 50-year-old woman suffering from ascites was treated by infusing Bristol water and claret wine into the abdomen through a leather pipe (Warrick, 1744). The patient reacted violently to the procedure which was stopped after three treatments. The patient is reported to have recovered, being able to walk 7 miles a day without difficulty. A modification of this was subsequently tried by Stephen Hale of Teddington, England, by using two trocars – one on each side of the abdomen – allowing the fluid to flow in and out of the peritoneal cavity during an operation to remove ascites (Hale, 1744).

Subsequent experiments on the peritoneum (Wegner, 1877) determined the rate of absorption of various solutions, the capacity for fluid removal (Starling and Tubby, 1894) and evidence that protein could pass through the peritoneum. It was also noted that the fluid in the peritoneal cavity contained the same amount of urea that is found in the blood, indicating that urea could be removed by PD (Rosenberg, 1916). This was followed by Tracy Putnam suggesting that the peritoneum might be used to correct physiological problems, when he observed that under certain circumstances fluids in the peritoneal cavity can equilibrate with the plasma and that the rate of diffusion was dependent on the size of the molecules. Research also suggested at this time that the clearance of solutes was proportional to their molecular size and solution pH, and that a high flow rate maximised the transfer of solutes, which also depended on peritoneal surface area and blood flow (Putman, 1923).

George Ganter was looking for a method of dialysis which did not require the use of an anticoagulant (Ganter, 1923). He prepared a dialysate solution containing normal values of electrolytes and added dextrose for fluid removal. Bottles were boiled for sterilisation and filled with the solution, which was then infused into the patient's abdomen through a hollow needle.

The first treatment was carried out on a woman who was suffering acute renal failure following childbirth. Between 1 and 3 l of fluid was infused at a time, and the dwell time was 30 min to 3 h. The blood chemistry came within acceptable limits. The patient was sent home, but unfortunately died as it was not realised that it was necessary to continue the treatment in order to keep the patient alive.

Ganter recognised the importance of good access to the peritoneum, as it was noted that it was easier to instil the fluid than it was to attain a good return volume. He was also aware of the complication of infection, and indeed it was the most frequent complication that he encountered. Ganter identified four principles, which are still regarded as important today:

- adequate access to the peritoneum;
- sterile solutions to reduce infection;
- altering glucose content of the dialysate to remove greater volumes of fluid;
- varying dwell times and fluid volume infused to determine the efficiency of the dialysis.

There are reports of 101 patients treated with PD in the 1920s (Abbott and Shea, 1946; Odel et al., 1950). Of these, 63 had reversible causes, 32 irreversible and in two the diagnosis was unknown. There was recovery in 32 of 63 cases of reversible renal failure. Deaths were due to uraemia, pulmonary oedema and peritonitis.

Stephen Rosenak, working in Europe, developed a metal catheter for peritoneal access, but was discouraged by the results because of the high incidence of peritonitis. In Holland, P.S.M. Kop, who was an associate of Kolff during the mid 1940s, created a system of PD by using materials for the components that could easily be sterilised: porcelain containers for the fluid, latex rubber for the tubing, and a glass catheter to infuse the fluid into the patient's abdomen. Kop treated 21 patients and met with success in 10.

Morton Maxwell, in Los Angeles, in the latter part of the 1950s, had been involved with HD, and it was his opinion that HD was too complicated for regular use. Aware of the problems with infection, he designed a system for PD with as few connections as possible. Together with a local manufacturer, he formulated a peritoneal solution, and customised a container and plastic tubing set and a single polyethylene catheter. The procedure used was to instil 2 l of fluid into the peritoneum, leave to dwell for 30 min, and return the fluid into the original bottles. This would be repeated until the blood chemistry was normal. This technique was carried out successfully on many patients and the highly regarded results were published in 1959. This became known as the 'Maxwell Technique (Maxwell *et al.*, 1959). This simple form of dialysis recognised it was no longer necessary to have expensive equipment with highly specialised staff in a large hospital to initiate dialysis. All that was required was an understanding of the procedure and available supplies.

The Catheter

Up to the 1970s, PD was used primarily for patients who were not good candidates for HD, or who were seeking a more gentle form of treatment. Continuous flow using two catheters (Legrain and Merrill, 1953) was still sometimes used, but the single catheter technique was favoured because of lower infections rates.

The polyethylene catheter was chosen by Paul Doolan (Doolan *et al.*, 1959) at the Naval Hospital in San Francisco when he developed a procedure for the treatment to use under battlefield conditions in the Korean war. Because of the flexibility of the catheter, it was considered for long-term treatment. A young physician called Richard Ruban decided to try this procedure, known as the 'Doolan Technique' (Ruben *et al.*, 1960) on a female patient who improved dramatically, but deteriorated after a few days without treatment. The patient was therefore dialysed repeatedly at weekends, and allowed home during the week, with the catheter remaining in place. This was the first reported chronic treatment using a permanent indwelling catheter.

Catheters were made from tubings available on the hospital ward and included gall-bladder trocars, rubber catheters, whistle-tip catheters and stainless steel sump drains. However, as with the polyethylene plastic tubes, the main trouble was kinking and blockage. Maxwell described a nylon catheter with perforations at the curved distal end and this was the catheter to become commercially available. Advances in the manufacture of the silicone peritoneal catheter by Palmer (Palmer *et al.*, 1964) and Gutch (Gutch, 1964) included the introduction of perforations at the distal end and later Tenckhoff included the design of a shorter catheter, a straight catheter and a curled catheter. He also added the Dacron cuff, either single or double, to help to seal the openings through the peritoneum (Tenckhoff and Schechter, 1968). He was also responsible for the introduction of the trocar which gave easy placement of the catheter. Dimitrios Orepoulos, a Greek physician, was introduced to PD in Belfast, Northern Ireland, during his training and he noted the difficulties encountered with the catheters there. He had been shown a simple technique for inserting the catheter by Norman Dean from New York City, which allowed the access to be used over and over again.

Peritoneal Dialysis at Home

In 1960, Scribner and Boen (Boen, 1959) set up a PD programme that would allow patients to be treated at home. An automated unit was developed which could operate unattended overnight. The system used 40 l containers that were filled and sterilised at the University of Washington. The bottles were then delivered to the patient's home, and returned after use. The machine was able to measure the fluid in and out of the patient by a solenoid device. An indwelling tube was permanently implanted into the patient's abdomen, through which a tube was inserted for each dialysis treatment. The system was open, and therefore was vulnerable to peritonitis. A new method was then used, whereby a new catheter was inserted into the abdomen for each treatment, and removed after the treatment ended. This was still carried out in the home, when a physician would attend the patient at home for insertion of the catheter, leaving once the treatment had begun. The carer was trained to discontinue the treatment and remove the catheter. The wound would be covered by a dressing, and the patient would be free of dialysis until the next week. This treatment was carried out by Tenckhoff *et al.* (1965) in a patient for 3 years, entailing 380 catheter punctures.

The large 40 l bottles of dialysate were difficult to handle and delivery to the home and sterilisation were not easy. Tenckhoff, at the University of Washington, installed a water still into the patient's home, thus providing a sterile water supply. The water was mixed with sterile concentrate to provide the correct solution, but this method was not satisfactory as it remained cumbersome and dangerous due to the high pressure in the still. Various refinements were tried using this method, including a reverse osmosis unit, and this was widely used later for HD treatment.

Lasker, in 1961, realised the potential of this type of treatment and concentrated on the idea of a simple version by instilling 2 l of fluid by a gravity-fed system. This proved to be cheaper to maintain but was labour intensive. Later that year, he was approached by Ira Gottscho, a businessman who had lost a daughter through kidney problems, and together they designed the first peritoneal cycler machine. The refinements included the ability to measure the fluid in and out, and the ability to warm the fluid before the fill cycle. Patients were sent home using the automated cycler treatment as early as 1970, even though there was a bias for HD at that time.

In 1969, Oreopoulos accepted a position at the Toronto Western Hospital, and together with Stanley Fenton, they decided to use the Tenchkoff catheter for long-term treatment. Because of the lack of space and facilities at the hospital, it was necessary to send the patients home on intermittent PD. He reviewed the Lasker cycler machine and ordered a supply, and by 1974 was managing over 70 patients on this treatment at home. Similar programmes were managed in Georgetown University and also in the Austin Diagnostic Clinic in the USA.

The Beginning of Continuous Ambulatory Peritoneal Dialysis

It was in 1975, following an unsuccessful attempt to haemodialyse a patient at the Austin Diagnostic Clinic, that an engineer, Robert Popovich, and Jack Moncrief became involved in working out the kinetics of 'long dwell equilibrated dialysis' for this patient. It was determined that five exchanges each of 2 l per day would achieve the appropriate blood chemistry, and that the removal of 1–2 l of fluid from the patient was needed per day. Thus came the evolution of CAPD (Popovich et al., 1976).

The treatment was so successful that the Austin Group were given a grant to allow them to continue dialysing patients with CAPD. Strangely, their first description and account of this clinical experience was rejected by the American Society for Artificial Internal Organs. At this time the treatment was called 'a portable/wearable equilibrium dialysis technique'. The stated advantages compared to HD included:

- good steady-state biochemical control;
- more liberal diet and fluid intake;
- improvement in anaemia.

The main problems were protein loss (Popovich et al., 1978) and infection. It was recognised that the source of infection was almost certainly related to the use of the bottles. Oreopoulos found that collapsible polyvinyl-chloride (PVC) containers for the solution were available in Canada. Once the fluid was instilled, the bag could then be rolled up and concealed under the clothing. The fluid could be returned into the bag during draining by gravity, without a disconnection taking place (Oreopoulos et al., 1978). New spike connections were produced for access to the bag of fluid, and a luer connection for fitting to the catheter, and together with tubing devised for HD, greatly reduced the chances of infection. The patients treated on an intermittent basis (intermittent peritoneal dialysis – IPD) were rapidly converted to CAPD and evaluation of the new treatment was rapid, due to the large numbers being treated. Following approval by the Food and Drug Administration, many centres were then able to develop CAPD programmes.

The first complete CAPD system was released on to the market in 1979, giving a choice of three strengths of dextrose solution. Included in this system were an administration line, and sterile items packed together to form a preparation kit, to be used at each bag change in an attempt to keep infection at bay. The regime proposed by Robert Popovich and Jack Moncrief entailed four exchanges over a 24 h period, three dwell times of approximately 4 h in the daytime, and one dwell overnight of 8 h. This regime is the one mainly used today.

The systems are continually being improved, with connectors moving from spike to luer to eliminate as far as possible the accidental disconnection of the bag from the line. A titanium connector was found to be the superior form of adaptor for connection of the transfer set to the catheter, and probably led to reduced infection rate for peritonitis. A disadvantage of this technique is the flow of fresh fluid down the transfer set along the area of disconnection, thus encouraging any bacteria from the disconnection to be instilled into the abdomen. The development of the 'Y' system in the mid-1980s in Italy resulted in a further decrease in peritonitis.

Automated Peritoneal Dialysis

Automated PD in the form of continuous cyclic peritoneal dialysis (CCPD) was further developed by Diaz-Buxo in the early 1980s to enable patients who were unable to perform exchanges in the day to be treated with PD overnight (Fig. 1.11).

Advances in Peritoneal Dialysis for Special Needs

Recent advances in CAPD treatment include a dialysate which not only provides dialysis, but which contains 1.1% amino acid, to be administered to malnourished patients. This may be particularly useful for the elderly CAPD patient, in whom poor nutrition is a well-recognised complication.

Diabetic patients initially were not considered for treatment, because of the complications of the disease. Carl Kjellstrand, at the University of Minnesota, suggested that insulin could be administered to the diabetic patient by adding it to the PD fluid (Crossley and Kjellstrand, 1971). However, when this suggestion was first put forward, it was not adopted because the 30-min dwell did not give time for the drug to be absorbed into the patient. It became viable later, when the long dwell dialysis was initiated, and this gave the advantage of slow absorption, resulting in a steady state of blood sugar in the normal range, thus alleviating the need for painful injections (Flynn and Nanson, 1979).

Realisation that patients are individuals, bringing their own problems associated with training, brought many exchange aid devices on to the market to assist the patient in the exchange procedure. These exchange

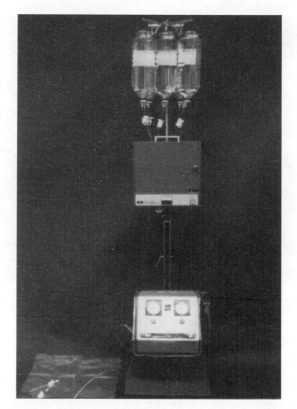

Fig. 1.11 *The American Medical Products (AMP) continuous cyclic peritoneal dialysis (CCPD) machine 1980.*

devices were mainly used to assist such disabilities as blindness, arthritis (particularly of the hands) and patients prone to repeated episodes of peritonitis (Fig. 1.12).

The Future

PD is a first choice of treatment for end-stage renal disease in many countries, and because of lack of facilities for in-centre HD, will remain so. New ideas and techniques will continue to improve the systems, born of chance and design, and in many instances, proposed by patients themselves.

TRANSPLANTATION

In The Beginning

Kidney transplantation as a therapeutic and practical option for renal replacement therapy was first reported in published literature at the turn

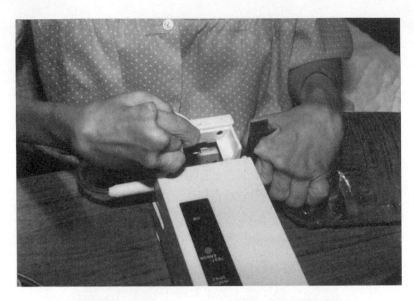

Fig. 1.12 *The Baxter Ultraviolet (UV) exchange device.*

of the century. The first steps were small and so insignificant that they were overlooked or condemned.

The first known attempts at renal transplantation on humans were made without immunosuppression between 1906 and 1923 using pig, sheep, goat, and subhuman primate donors (Elkington 1964). These first efforts were conducted in France and Germany but others followed. None of the kidneys functioned for long, if indeed at all, and the recipients all died within a period of a few hours to 9 days later.

Of all the workers at this time, the contribution made by Alixis Carrel (1873–1944) remains the most famous. His early work in Lyons, France and in Chicago involved the transplantation of an artery from one dog to another. This work became invaluable later in the transplantation of organs. In 1906, Carrel and Guthrie, working in the Hull Laboratory in Chicago, reported the successful transplantation of both kidneys in cats and later a double nephrectomy on dogs, re-implanting only one of the kidneys. He found that the secretion of urine remained normal and the animal remained in good health, despite having only one kidney (Carrel, 1908). Carrel was awarded the Nobel Prize in 1912 for his work on vascular and related surgery.

Whilst at this stage there was no clear understanding of the problem, some principles were clearly learned. Vascular suture techniques were reviewed and the possibility of using pelvic implantation sites was investigated and practised. No further renal heterotransplantations (animal to man) were tried until 1963 when experiments using kidneys from chimpanzee (Reemtsma *et al.*, 1964) and baboon were tried, with eventual death of the patients. This ended all trials using animal donation.

The first human-to-human kidney transplant was reported in 1936 by the Russian Voronoy, when he implanted a kidney from a cadaver donor of B-positive blood type into a recipient of O-positive blood type, a mismatch that would not be attempted today. The donor had died 6 h prior to the operation and the recipient died 6 h later without making urine. The following 20 years saw further efforts in kidney transplantation, all without effective immunosuppression (Groth, 1972). The extraperitoneal technique developed by French surgeons Dubost and Servelle became today's standard procedure.

The First Successes

The first examples of survival success of a renal transplant can probably be attributed to Lawer or Hume. Hume placed the transplanted kidney into the thigh of the patient, with function for 5 months. Then at the Peter Bent Brigham Hospital in Boston, USA, in December 1954, the first successful identical twin transplant was performed by the surgeon Joseph E. Murray in collaboration with the nephrologist John P. Merrill (Hume *et al.*, 1955). The recipient survived for more that two decades. The idea of using identical twins was proposed when it had been noted by David C. Miller of the Public Health Service Hospital, Boston, that skin grafts between identical twins were not rejected (Brown, 1937). The application of this information resulted in rigorous matching, including skin grafting, prior to effective immunosuppression.

Over the period between 1951 and 1976 there were 29 transplants performed between identical twins, and the survival rate for 20 years was 50%. Studies of two successfully transplanted patients, who were given kidneys from their non-identical twins were also reported (Merrill *et al.*, 1960). The first survived 20 years (died of heart disease) and the second, 26 years (died of carcinoma of the bladder). Immunosuppression used in these cases was irradiation.

Immunosuppression

It was Sir Peter Medawar who appreciated that rejection is an immuno-logical phenomenon (Medawar, 1944), and this led to research into weakening the immune system of the recipients to reduce the rejection. In animals, corticosteriods, total body irradiation and cytotoxic drug therapy were used. Experiments in animals were still far from successful, as were similar techniques when used in humans. It was concluded that the required degree of immunosuppression would lead to destruction of the immune system and finally result in terminal infections.

A few patients were transplanted between 1960 and 1961 in Paris and Boston, using drug regimes involving 6-mercaptopurine or azathioprine with or without irradiation. They all died within 18 months. Post-mortem examination of kidney grafts failed showed marked changes in the renal histology, which at first were thought unlikely to be due to immunological rejection, but later it was convincingly shown that this was indeed the underlying process.

In the early days of kidney transplantation, the kidney was removed from either a living related donor or a cadaver donor and immediately transferred to the donor after first flushing the kidney with cold electrolyte solution such as Hartman's solution. In 1967, Belzer and his colleagues developed a technique for continuous perfusion of the kidney using oxygenated cryoprecipitated plasma, which allowed the kidney to be kept up to 72 h before transplantation. This machine perfusion required constant supervision, and it was found that the flushing of the kidney with an electrolyte solution and storage at $0°C$ in ice saline allowed the kidney to be preserved for up to 24 h or more (Marshall *et al.*, 1988). This was a major development in transplantation techniques.

During the 1950s it was recognised that many of the survivors of the Hiroshima atomic bomb in 1945 suffered impairment to their immune system. It was concluded that radiation could therefore induce immunosuppression, and clinical total body irradiation was used to prolong the survival of renal transplants in Boston in 1958. This did improve the survival of some transplants; however, the overall outcomes were poor. There was clearly a need for a more effective form of immunosuppression than irradiation.

A breakthrough in immunosuppressive therapy occurred in 1962 in the University of Colorado, when it was discovered that the combination of azathioprine and prednisone allowed the prevention and in some cases reversal of rejection (Starzl *et al.*, 1963). Transplantation could at last expand. A conference sponsored by the National Research Council and National Academy of Sciences in 1963 in Washington resulted in the first registry report, which enabled the tracing of all the early non-twin kidney recipients. In 1970 work commenced on the development of cyclosporin by Sandoz in Basle, Swizerland, following recognition of the potential (Borel *et al.*, 1976). Clinical trials carried out in Cambridge, UK (Calne *et al.*, 1979), showed that outcomes on renal transplantation were greatly improved, both with graft and with patient survival. Cyclosporin revolutionised immunosuppression treatment for transplant patients, even though it is itself nephrotoxic and its use needs close monitoring.

Tissue typing is a complex procedure and, as yet, is far from perfection. The use of the united networks for organ sharing has increased the efforts of matching donor and recipient, and data available from these sources show a significant gain in survival of well-matched versus mismatched cadaver kidneys. Cross-matching remains as important today as it was 25 years ago at its conception. None of the immunosuppressive measures available today can prevent the immediate destruction of the transplanted organ by humoral antibodies in the hyperacute rejection phase. This was recognised as early as 1965 (Kissmeyer-Neilsen *et al.*, 1966), and it may be that this phenomenon holds the key to the future of successful heterotransplantation.

Blood Transfusions

It was observed in the late 1960s that patients who had received multiple blood transfusions before organ transplantation did not have a poorer graft survival than those who had not been transfused. In 1974, Opelz and Terasaki observed that patients who had received no transfusions whatsoever were more likely to reject the transplant. It became evident, therefore, that a small number of blood transfusions resulted in an improved organ survival and so the transfusion policies for non-transfused recipients were changed throughout the world. This 'transfusion effect' is of much less importance with the cyclosporin era.

Present

Renal transplantation has been a dramatic success over the past 30 years with patient survival rates between 90 and 100% at 1 year after transplantation for both living related and cadaver transplants. Although short-term survival for the graft is good (75–85% expectation of survival of the graft at 1 year), cadaveric graft survival at 5 years of around 60% leaves considerable room for improvement.

The Future

There is no doubt that renal transplantation is the treatment of choice for many patients requiring renal replacement therapy giving, in general, a better quality of life than dialysis. A change in the law may result in more kidneys becoming available for transplantation, by allowing easier access to donors or removing the need for relatives' consent, but until a significant breakthrough is achieved there will continue to be a waiting list for transplantation and the need to continue to improve the techniques of dialysis will be necessary.

SUMMARY

A consensus statement in the UK in 1994 suggested that facilities for the treatment of end-stage renal failure in the UK are cost effective but still are of variable quality and limited. Acceptance rates in some areas are lower than requirements indicate (Figs 1.13 and 1.14). Therefore, both

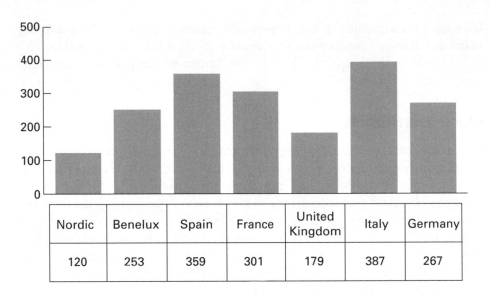

Nordic	Benelux	Spain	France	United Kingdom	Italy	Germany
120	253	359	301	179	387	267

Fig. 1.13 *Patients per million population receiving renal replacement therapy (RRT) 1992 European Dialysis and Transplant Association (EDTA) report. Reprinted by permission of EDTA.*

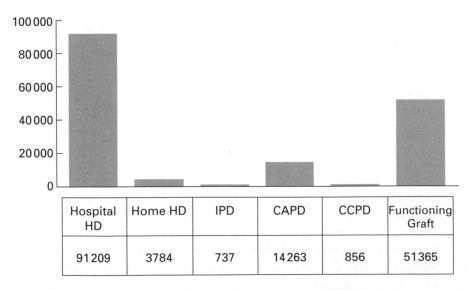

Hospital HD	Home HD	IPD	CAPD	CCPD	Functioning Graft
91 209	3784	737	14 263	856	51 365

Fig. 1.14 *European Dialysis and Transplant Association (EDTA) registry report for 1992 – mode of therapy. HD, haemodialysis; CAPD, continuous ambulatory peritoneal dialysis; CCPD, continuous cyclic peritoneal dialysis; IPD, intermittent peritoneal dialysis. Reprinted by permission of EDTA.*

hospital- and community-based services need to be expanded to enable patients to have a choice of treatment, and the standard of treatment given to these patients should be monitored. The medical profession should be made aware of the outcomes such as quality of life. Funding for treatments and the provision of highly trained staff are required to achieve these objectives.

Dialysis has come a long way from the small beginnings of the hot baths in Rome. Refinements and improvements continue, most recently with the emergence of erythropoeitin in the late 1980s to correct the major complication of anaemia in these patients.

Improvements in access for both HD and PD will emerge. The challenge of adequate dialysis for all who need treatment remains.

Transplantation is still not available for all those who are eligible, and changes in the law may help with availability of donor organs.

The multidisciplinary teams will continue to strive to give patients the best possible quality of treatments available until a revolutionary breakthrough in prevention of renal failure emerges.

REFERENCES

ABBOTT, W.E. AND SHEA, P. (1946) Treatment of temporary renal insufficiency (uraemia) by peritoneal lavage. *Am. J. Med. Sci.*, **211**: 312.

ABEL, J.J., ROWNTREE, L.G. AND TURNER, B.B. (1914) The removal of diffusable substances from the circulating blood of living animals by dialysis. *J. Pharmacol. Exp. Ther.*, **5**: 275–316.

BAILLOD, R.A., COMTY, C., ILAHI, M. *et al.* (1965) *Proceedings of the European Dialysis and Transplant Assn. 2.* Excerpta Medica, Amsterdam p.99.

BOEN, S.T. (1959) *Peritoneal Dialysis.* Van Gorcum & Comp N.V., Amsterdam, p.26.

BOREL, J.F., FEURER, C., GUBLER, H.U. *et al.* (1976) Biological effects of cyclosporin A. A new antilymphocytic agent. *Agents Actions*, **6**: 468–75.

BROWN, J.B. (1937) Homografting of the skin. With report of success in identical twins. *Surgery*, **1**: 558–63.

CALNE, R.Y., ROLLES, K., WHITE, D.J.G. *et al.* (1979) Cyclosporin A initially as the only immunosuppressant in 34 recipients of cadaveric organs: 32 kidneys, 2 pancreases, and 2 livers. *Lancet*, **1**: 1033–6.

CARREL, A. (1908) Results of the transplantation of blood vessels, organs and limbs. *JAMA* **51**: 1662–67. (Reprinted in 1983 in JAMA, **250**: 994–53).

CIMINO, J.E. AND BRESCIA, M.J. (1962) Simple venepuncture for haemodialysis. *N. Engl. J. Med.*, **267**(12): 608–9.

CROSSLEY, K. AND KJELLSTRAND, C.M. (1971) Intraperitoneal insulin for control of blood sugar in diabetic patients during peritoneal dialysis. *Br. Med. J.*, **1**: 269–90.

DOOLAN, P.D., MURPHY, Jr, W.P., WIGGINS, R.A. *et al.* (1959) An evaluation of intermittent peritoneal lavage. *Am. J. Med.*, **26**: 831–44.

EGGERTH, A.H. (1921) The preparation and standardization of collodion membranes. *J. Biol. Chem.*, **48**(1): 203–21.

ELKINGTON, J.R. (1964) Moral problems in the use of borrowed organs artificial and transplanted. *Ann. Intern. Med.*, **60**: 309–13.

FISHMAN, A.P., KROOP, I.G., LEITER, H.E. *et al.* (1948) Management of anuria in acute mercurial intoxication. *NY. State J. Med.*, **48**: 2393–6.

FLYNN, C.T. AND NANSON, J.A. (1979) Intraperitoneal insulin with CAPD – an artificial pancreas. *Trans. Am. Soc. Artif. Intern. Organs.*, **25**: 114–7.

GANTER, G. (1923) About the elimination of poisonous substances from the blood by dialysis. *Munch. Med. Wchnschr.*, **70**: 1478–80.

GRAHAM, T. (1854) The Bakerian lecture – On osmotic force. *Phil. Trans. R. Soc. Lond.*, **144**: 177–228.

GROTH, C.G. (1972) Landmarks in clinical renal transplantation. *Surg. Gynecol. Obstet.*, **134**: 323–8.

GUTCH, C.F. (1964) Peritoneal dialysis. *Trans. Am. Soc. Artif. Int. Organs.*, **10**: 406–7.

HALE, S. (1744) A method of conveying liquors into the abdomen during the operation of tapping. *Phil. Trans. Royal Soc.*, **43**: 20–21.

HESS, C.L.V. AND McGUIGAN, H. (1914) The condition of the sugar in the blood. *J. Pharmacol. Exp. Ther.*, **6**: 45–55.

HUME, D.M., MERRILL, J.P., MILLER, B.F. *et al.* (1955) Experience with renal homotransplantation in the human. Report of nine cases. *J. Clin. Invest.*, **34**: 327–82.

KISSMEYER-NEILSEN, F., OLSEN, S., PETERSON, V.P. *et al.* (1966) Hyperacute rejection of kidney allografts, associated with pre-existing humoral antibodies against donor cells. *Lancet*, **2**: 662–5.

KOLFF, W.J. (1950) Artificial kidney – treatment of acute and chronic uraemia. *Cleveland Clin. Q.*, **17**: 216–28.

KOLFF, W.J. (1965) First clinical experience with the artificial kidney. *Ann. Intern. Med.*, **62**(3): 608–19.

KOLFF, W.J. AND BERK, H.T. (1944) The artificial kidney : A dialyser with a great area. *Acta Med. Scand.*, **117**: 121–34.

LEGRAIN, M. AND MERRILL, J.P. (1953) Short term continuous transperitoneal dialysis. *N. Eng. J. Med.*, **248**: 125–9.

MacNEILL, A.E. (1949) Some possible uses of blood dialysers. Surgeons practice meeting. *New England Surgical Soc.* Sept 23 1949, Bretton Woods, NH, p.3.

MALINOW, M.R. AND KORZON, W. (1947) Experimental method for obtaining an ultrafiltrate of the blood. *J. Lab. Clin. Med.*, **31**: 461–71.

MARSHALL, V.C., JABLONSKI, P. AND SCOTT, D.F. (1988) Renal preservation. In *Kidney Transplantation: Principles and Practice*, 3rd edn (ed, P.J. Morris). W.B. Saunders, Philadelphia, pp.151–82.

MAXWELL, M.H., ROCKNEY, R.E. and KLEEMAN, C.R. (1959) Peritoneal dialysis, techniques and application. *JAMA*, **170**: 917–24.

MEDAWAR, P.B. (1944) The behaviour and fate of skin autografts and skin homografts in rabbits. *J. Anat.*, **78**: 176–99.

MERRILL, J.P., THORN, G.W., WALTER, C.W. *et al.* (1950) The use of an artificial kidney. 1. Technique. *J. Clin. Invest.*, **29**(4): 412–24.

MERRILL, J.P., MURRAY, J.E., HARRISON, J.H. *et al.* (1960) Succesful homotransplantation of the kidney between non-identical twins. *N. Eng. J. Med.*, **262**: 1251–60.

ODEL, H.M., FERRIS, D.O. AND POWER, H. (1950) Peritoneal lavage as an effective means of extrarenal excretion. *Am. J. Med.*, **9**: 63–77.

OPELZ, G. AND TERASAKI, P.I. (1974) Poor kidney transplant surival in recipients with frozen-blood transfusions or no transfusions. *Lancet*, **2**: 696–8.

OREOPOULOS, D.G., ROBSON, M., IZATT, S., CLAYTON, S. AND DE VEBER, G.A. (1978) A simple and safe technique for continuous ambulatory peritoneal dialysis. *Trans. Am. Soc. Artif. Organs.*, **24**: 484–9.

PALMER, R.A. AND RUTHERFORD, P.S. (1949) Kidney substitutes in uraemia: the use of Kolff's dialyser in two cases. *Can. Med. Assc. J.*, **60**: 261–6.

PALMER, R.A., QUINTON, W.E. AND GRAY, J.F. (1964) Prolonged peritoneal dialysis for chronic renal failure. *Lancet*, **1**: 700–2.

POPOVICH, R.P., MONCRIEF, J.F., DECHERD, J.F., BOMAR, J.B. AND PYLE, W.K. (1976) The definition of a novel portable/wearable equilibrium peritoneal dialysis technique. *Abstract. Trans. Am. Soc. Artif. Organs.*, **5**: 64.

POPOVICH, R.P., MONCRIEF, J.W., NOLPH, K.D. *et al.* (1978) Continuous Ambulatory Peritoneal Dialysis. *Ann. Inter. Med.*, **88**: 449–56.

PUTMAN, J. (1923) The living peritoneum as a dialysing membrane. *Am. J. Physiol.*, **63**: 548–55.

REEMTSMA, K., McCRACKEN, B.H., SCHLEGEL, J.U. *et al.* (1964) Renal heterotransplantation in man. *Ann. Surg.*, **160**: 384–410.

RICHARDSON, B.W. (1889) Practical studies in animal dialysis. *Asclepiad (London)*, **6**: 331–2.

ROSENBERG, M. (1916) Nitrogenous retention of substances in the blood and in other body fluids in the core of the kidneys. *J. Ber. Klin. Wochenshr.*, **53**: 1314–16.

RUBEN, R.E., LEWIS, A.E. AND HASSID, E. (1960) The use of peritoneal dialysis in a patient with chronic renal insufficiency. Unpublished paper.

SKEGGS, L.T., JR, LEONARDS, J.R. AND HEISLER, C.R. (1949) Artificial kidney: 11. Construction and operation of an improved continuous dialyser. *Proc. Soc. Exp. Biol. Med.*, **72**(3): 539–43.

STARLING, E.H. AND TUBBY, A.H. (1894) On the paths of absorption from the peritoneal cavity. *J. Physiol.*, **16**: 140.

STARZL, T.E., MARCHIORO, T.L. AND WADDELL, W.R. (1963) The reversal of rejection in human renal homografts with subsequent development of homograft tolerance. *Surg. Gynecol. Obstet.*, **117**: 385–95.

TENCKHOFF, H., SHILIPETAR, G. AND BOEN, S.T. (1965) One year experience with home peritoneal dialysis. *Tran. Am. Soc. Artif. Int. Organs.*, **11**: 11–14.

TENCKHOFF, H. AND SCHECHTER, H. (1968) A bacteriologically safe peritoneal access device. *Trans. Am. Soc. Artif. Int. Organs.*, **14**: 181–6.

TESCHAN, P.E. (1955) Haemodialysis in military casualties. *Trans. Am. Soc. Artif. Intern. Organs.*, **2**: 52–4.

THALHIMER, W., SOLANDT, D.Y. AND BEST, C.H. (1938) Experimental exchange transfusion using purified heparin. *Lancet*, **11**: 554–5.

WARRICK, C. (1744) An improvement in the practice of tapping, whereby that operation instead for the relief of symptoms, became an absolute cure for ascites, exemplified in the case of Jane Roman. *Phil. Trans. Royal Soc.*, **43**: 12–19.

WEGNER, G. (1877) Surgical comments on peritoneal cavity with special emphasis on ovariotomy. *Arch. f. Klin. Chir.*, **20**: 53–145.

CHAPTER 2

APPLIED ANATOMY AND PHYSIOLOGY

INTRODUCTION

This chapter is aimed at the student who has a special interest in renal nursing, particularly those who wish to make their career in this speciality or are studying for a postregistration award. With this in mind, this chapter provides the reader with a detailed discussion on all aspects of renal physiology, together with its relationship to important pathophysiological processes in renal disease and some brief discussion on related nursing observations. The main text covers the normal renal anatomy and physiology and is divided into many small sections for ease of reading and for easy location of the required knowledge. The reader will also find many clear diagrams to assist in their understanding of the text. At appropriate points in the text are boxes containing information on related pathophysiology and nursing observations which the reader can then compare to the normal physiology in the main text. It is hoped that this layout will help the student's understanding of the relationship between physiology and pathology.

Functions of the Kidney

The main functions of the kidney are to rid the body of the end-products of metabolism and to regulate the electrolytes found in the body fluids. A more detailed list of the functions of the kidney can be found in Table 2.1. These vital functions are achieved through the production of that extraordinary fluid we call urine. Before looking at how the kidney achieves its functions there follows a discussion on the impressive versatility of urine.

Table 2.1 *The functions of the kidney*

Excretory
- excretion of metabolic waste products e.g. urea and creatinine

Regulatory
Regulation of:
- body water volume
- body water osmolality
- electrolyte balance
- acid–base balance

Metabolic
- 'activation' of vitamin D
- production of renin
- production of erythropoietin

The Versatility of Urine

When one considers the immense variability in the qualities of urine that we can produce in order to control our internal environment, one cannot fail to be impressed by the complexities of the workings of the kidney. Broadly speaking, there are three parameters that can be varied in order to maintain the constancy of our bodily fluids: urinary volume, urinary concentration and urinary content.

Urinary Volume

In a healthy person, the volume of urine produced per day can vary from as little as 300 ml, if no water is ingested or there is excessive water loss from the body (as in diarrhoea), up to a maximum of 23 l in cases of excessive fluid ingestion (Lote, 1987). In health, urine output cannot drop below 300 ml day^{-1} because this is the absolute minimum water volume required to excrete the daily load of toxic waste products. If the amount of waste products to be removed by the kidney rises, then the minimum urine volume must also rise. However, the average urine output per day is approximately 1500 ml. The kidneys' ability to vary the volume of daily urine output over such a wide range is essential if we are to maintain a constant body fluid volume in the face of such adverse factors such as excessive heat, which causes sweating; colonic infections causing diarrhoea; or excessive thirst and water ingestion, as seen in the condition psychogenic polydipsia (see Table 2.2).

Table 2.2 *Normal fluid inputs and outputs*

Inputs (ml)		Outputs (ml)		
Water	1500	Urine*		1500
Food	500	Insensible } lungs		400
		loss } skin**		400
Water of metabolism	400	Faeces***		100
Total	2400			2400

* Urinary volume is the only factor that can be regulated by the body to balance fluid inputs.
** This insensible loss of fluid through the skin is by simple evaporation (not sweat). Sweat is called 'sensible loss' and may reach up to $5\,l\,h^{-1}$, for example, when a person is excessively exercising.
*** Loss of fluid with the faeces can be as high as several litres per day in the presence of severe colonic infections such as cholera.

Urinary Concentration

Though the volume of urine can vary over a wide range, the amount of solutes to be excreted by the kidney each day is much less variable. Thus, in order to excrete a fairly fixed volume of solutes each day in a very variable volume of water, the kidney must have the ability to concentrate or dilute the urine. We have all noticed how on a hot summer's day when we have drunk very little, our urine is dark in colour and small in volume, whereas, if we consume liberal amounts of beer at a party we pass large volumes of watery urine all evening! This ability to excrete all the body's excess solutes in varying amounts of water by concentrating or diluting the urine is essential for maintaining a constant body osmolality (Table 2.3). The mechanism in the kidney that controls the concentration or dilution of the urine is often affected early on in renal disease, making it difficult for the individual to control both body fluid volume and osmolality in response to changes in fluid inputs and outputs. This can result in the individual tipping back and forth from states of dehydration to fluid overload.

Table 2.3 Concept of body osmolality

- Water can move between the different body fluid compartments by the process of osmosis (see Fig. 2.8b)
- Osmosis is driven by changes in the solute concentration in one of the body's fluid compartments
- Any solute in solution that can cause the movement of water across a membrane is said to be 'osmotically active'
- The osmotic activity of substances in solution is dependent on:
  (a) the NUMBER of dissolved molecules in the solution and *not* their size or valency
  (b) the biological membrane being non-permeable to the solute (i.e. the solute cannot diffuse out of the fluid compartment that is exerting the osmotic effect)
- Osmotically active particles in solution are measured by the unit called the *Osmole*
- 1 Osmol is equivalent to 1 mole of osmotically active particles dissolved in solution (i.e. represents the molecular weight of the substance in grams)
- 1 Osmol of a substance therefore contains 6.061×10^{23} molecules (Avagadro's number)
- 1 Osmol is equal to 1000 mOsmol (mosmoles)
- Osmolality is measured in mosmoles kg^{-1} H_2O and is a measure of the potential osmotic activity of dissolved solutes in solution
- *Normal body fluid osmolality* is 285 mOsmol kg^{-1} H_2O

Urinary Content

The range of substances that can be constituents of urine is varied and includes:

- *ions*: sodium, potassium, calcium, magnesium, chloride, bicarbonate, phosphate and ammonium;
- *metabolic waste*: urea, creatinine and uric acid;
- *drug metabolites*: most metabolites of pharmacological agents are eventually excreted from the body through the kidneys, many being detoxified in the liver first;
- *other products of normal metabolism*: e.g. metabolites of hormones can be detected in the urine by appropriate assays and may be a diagnostic aid, for example the appearance of human chorionic gonadotrophin (hcg) in the urine in the early stages of pregnancy forms the basis of the pregnancy test.

Normal urine is clear in appearance, though it may vary in colour from a pale straw colour to a dark amber colour, depending on its concentration. It has no unpleasant odour, though urine that has been standing a long time may develop a strong ammonium smell. Finally, normal urine has a pH that is slightly acidic, around pH 6, though urine can have a pH in the range 4.0–8.0 in cases of severe acidosis or alkalosis respectively.

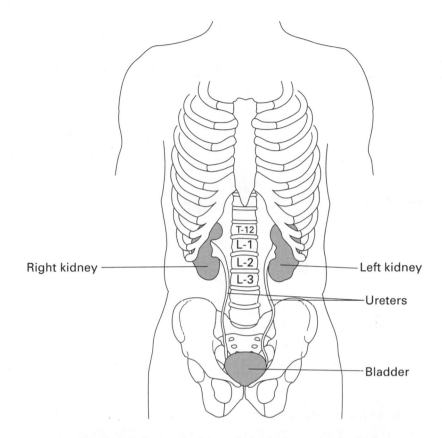

Fig. 2.1 *Relative position of the kidneys in the body.*

STRUCTURE OF THE KIDNEY

The kidneys are paired organs lying behind the peritoneum, either side of the vertebral column. The upper pole of the kidney is at the spinal level of T12 and the lower pole at approximately L3. The right kidney is a little lower due to the presence of the liver on that side. Usually, the kidneys are oriented with the concave surface facing the spine. However, due to developmental aberrations, other orientations of the kidney may occasionally exist (e.g. lying in the pelvis) but these do not usually affect function. Each kidney is approximately 11 cm long and weighs about 150 g (Fig. 2.1)

On the concave surface of the kidney lies the hilus, from which the ureter and the main blood vessels and nerves access the kidney. The cut surface of the kidney reveals two distinct regions: a dark outer region, the cortex, and a pale inner region called the medulla. The outer cortex is covered by a fibrous capsule and the whole kidney is surrounded by a pad of fat that offers some protection against injury. Broadly speaking, the cortex contains the filtering and reabsorptive components of the nephrons, whilst

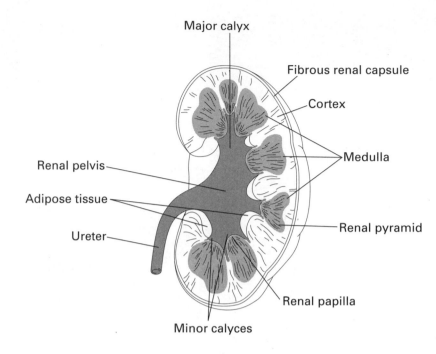

Fig. 2.2 *The kidney cut in longitudinal section.*

the medulla contains the concentrating and diluting components of the nephrons and a system of collection ducts which funnel the urine into the pelvis at the heart of the medulla from where it moves down the ureter into the bladder (see Fig. 2.2).

The Nephron

The nephron is the functional unit of the kidney and each kidney contains approximately 1 million nephrons (see Fig. 2.3). The unique structure of the nephron is critically related to its complex functions and contains five distinct components, each performing a distinct process:

- the Bowman's capsule – forming a blind ending capsule around a knot of capillaries called the glomerulus (the site of filtration);
- the proximal convoluted tubule (the site of 'bulk phase' reabsorption and some secretion);
- the loop of Henle (where the concentration and dilution of urine mainly occurs);
- the distal convoluted tubule (the site of 'fine tuning' reabsorption and more secretion);
- the collecting duct (also important for the concentration of urine and for carrying urine into the renal pelvis).

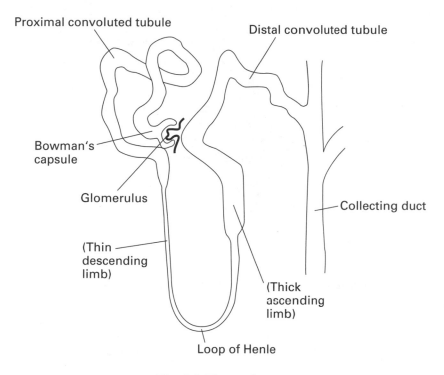

Fig. 2.3 The nephron.

These processes do not occur in isolation but are interdependent and intimately related to each other by the shape of the nephron. The importance of this fact will become clear when the renal processes are discussed in more detail.

There are broadly two types of nephron found in the kidney (Fig. 2.4). Approximately 85% of nephrons are cortical nephrons, which have short loops of Henle that are contained in the cortex of the kidney. The other 15% of nephrons are called juxtamedullary nephrons and they have long loops of Henle which extend deep into the medulla of the kidney (Lote, 1987). It is the loops of Henle, together with the collecting ducts which also pass through the medulla that give the pyramids of the medulla a striated appearance (Fig. 2.4).

BASIC RENAL PROCESSES

Glomerular Filtration

This is a process of filtration of plasma across the glomerular basement membrane from the glomerulus into the Bowman's capsule (Fig. 2.5). The glomerular filtration surface is a unique structure composed of three layers (Fig. 2.6):

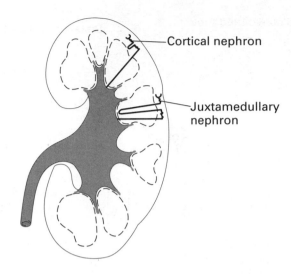

Fig. 2.4 *The position of the nephrons in the kidney.*

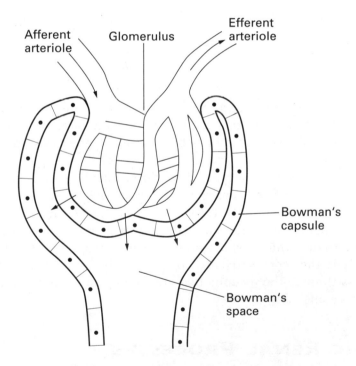

Fig. 2.5 *The glomerulus and Bowman's capsule.*

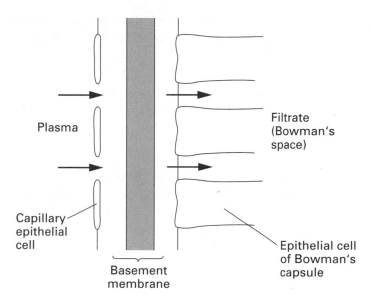

Plasma

Filtrate
(Bowman's
space)

Capillary
epithelial
cell

Epithelial cell
of Bowman's
capsule

Basement
membrane

Fig. 2.6 *The glomerular filtration membrane.*

- the endothelial lining of the glomerular capillaries;
- the basement membrane;
- the epithelial cells of the Bowman's capsule.

These three layers are fused together and act as a barrier to the filtration of large molecular weight molecules such as proteins.

Blood enters the glomerulus from a series of branches of the renal artery ending in the afferent arteriole. Blood then leaves the glomerulus through the efferent arteriole before entering a second capillary bed called the peritubular and vasa recta capillaries, which surround the tubules and loop of Henle. Blood then leaves the kidney through a series of larger converging veins ending in the renal vein which returns the blood to the vena cava.

This unusual arrangement of two capillary beds in tandem enables a pressure gradient to exist within the nephron, with high pressure in the glomerulus, favouring filtration, and a relatively low pressure in the peritubular capillaries, favouring reabsorption.

The formation of a filtrate from plasma flowing through the glomerulus occurs due to Starling's forces. These are the same forces that cause the filtration and reabsorption of tissue fluid in other capillary beds in the body, but with some important adaptations. In the glomerulus, fluid is forced across the glomerular basement membrane because of the high hydrostatic pressure of blood flowing through the afferent arteriole. This pressure is greater than the oncotic pressure opposing it. In an ordinary capillary bed, this filtrate would be almost entirely reabsorbed back into the capillary at the venule end because the hydrostatic pressure would have fallen to below the oncotic pressure of the capillary, which would then pull the fluid back in by osmosis. However, in the glomerulus, because blood leaving enters another arteriole (the efferent arteriole) rather than a venule, a high hydrostatic pressure is maintained and oncotic pressure is insufficient to draw fluid back into the capillary. This situation is obviously desirable so that large amounts of filtrate can be made. All of the filtrate formed in the glomerulus passes into the Bowman's capsule and is often referred to as tubular urine (Fig. 2.7).

Amount and composition of glomerular filtrate

The amount of glomerular filtrate formed per minute is referred to as the glomerular filtration rate (GFR), and in the average healthy person is approximately 125 ml min^{-1}. This volume is the sum amount from all 2 million nephrons in the kidneys and thus the amount from each nephron is relatively small. A quick calculation tells us that at a GFR of 125 ml min^{-1}, the total amount of filtrate formed per day is 180 l, approximately 60 times our circulating plasma volume! Obviously, the majority of this must be reabsorbed if we are not to become prunes.

The 'average' GFR quoted is generally only average for a young adult. Children have a lower GFR than this because their nephrons are still increasing in size (all nephrons are present at birth). After the age of about 30 years the number of functioning nephrons starts to decrease because of the ageing process, thus the GFR decreases proportionately. However, this only becomes significant to health when the GFR falls to around 5 ml min^{-1} – a situation that only occurs in a diseased kidney (see Box 2.1). The GFR can be calculated clinically by measuring the creatinine clearance rate. This requires a 24-h urine sample and blood sample from the patient. The principles of this test are described in Chapter 6.

The composition of the initial glomerular filtrate is that of a plasma ultrafiltration; that is, without proteins. The main determinant of what can pass through the glomerular basement membrane is molecular size, although the molecular shape and charge are also important. The passage of strongly negatively charged molecules such as albumen tends to be retarded because of the presence of fixed negative charges in the basement membrane which repel their movement (Lote, 1987). The molecular weight cut-off point in the filter is about 70 000 Da. Albumen, a small protein, has a molecular weight of 69 000 Da and thus only crosses the filter in minute quantities (also hindered by its negative charges). Only molecules with molecular weights under 7000 Da are freely permeable (Lote, 1987). It is because of this free permeability of small molecules that the composition of the initial glomerular filtrate is the same as that of the plasma for small molecules, and will include the major ions sodium, potassium, chloride, bicarbonate, calcium and phosphate; glucose; amino acids; and the toxic waste products of urea and creatinine. Any albumen filtered is

(a)

Arteriole end
Outward pressure:

Capillary hydrostatic
pressure = 35 mmHg

Inward pressure:

Protein oncotic
pressure = 25 mmHg

Net outward pressure
= 10 mmHg

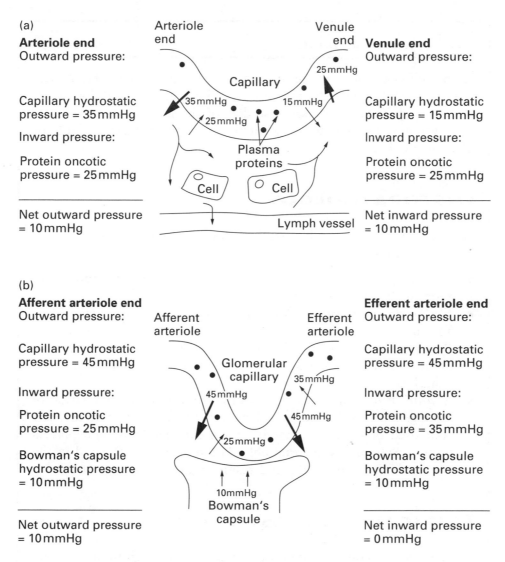

Venule end
Outward pressure:

Capillary hydrostatic
pressure = 15 mmHg

Inward pressure:

Protein oncotic
pressure = 25 mmHg

Net inward pressure
= 10 mmHg

(b)

Afferent arteriole end
Outward pressure:

Capillary hydrostatic
pressure = 45 mmHg

Inward pressure:

Protein oncotic
pressure = 25 mmHg

Bowman's capsule
hydrostatic pressure
= 10 mmHg

Net outward pressure
= 10 mmHg

Efferent arteriole end
Outward pressure:

Capillary hydrostatic
pressure = 45 mmHg

Inward pressure:

Protein oncotic
pressure = 35 mmHg

Bowman's capsule
hydrostatic pressure
= 10 mmHg

Net inward pressure
= 0 mmHg

Fig. 2.7 *Comparison of Starling's forces between muscle capillaries and glomerular capillaries. (a) Starling's forces operating in muscle capillaries – resulting in the formation and reabsorption of tissue fluid. (b) Starling's forces operating in glomerular capillaries – resulting in the formation of glomerular filtrate.*

reabsorbed through the proximal tubule into the renal lymph system and returned to the blood stream.

Selective Reabsorption

Reabsorption is a process that involves the movement of water and dissolved substances from the tubular fluid back into the blood stream. The term *selective* infers a regulatory function to this process as indeed

Box 2.1 Glomerular disease.

Glomerulonephritis is the term used to describe a variety of disorders that principally affect the glomeruli in the kidney. Such glomerulopathies may arise as primary disorders of the glomerulus, or as part of a systemic disorder such as systemic lupus erythematosus (SLE) or diabetes mellitus.

HISTOPATHOLOGY

Glomerular damage may be manifest as one or more of the following tissue reactions:

- *Cellular proliferation* – leading to an increase in the number of cells in the glomerular tufts.
- *Leukocyte infiltration of inflammatory cells* – mainly neutrophils and monocytes.
- *Basement membrane thickening* – as occurs in diabetes mellitus, or this may be a response caused by precipitated immune complexes.
- *Hyalinisation and sclerosis* – hyalinisation is the accumulation of homogenous, amorphous substance in the glomerular tuft composed of mesangial matrix, basement membrane and plasma protein. Sclerosis is the total obliteration of structural detail in the glomerular tuft and is the end result of glomerular damage.

CLINICAL MANIFESTATIONS

Clinical presentation of glomerular disease may range from an acute onset of disease with a reversible outcome, to a chronic insidious onset that eventually leads to renal failure after several decades. A number of syndromes of glomerular disease are defined:

- *Proteinuria* – occurs if the glomerular basement membranes are damaged so that they leak protein.
- *Nephrotic syndrome* – occurs if the basement membranes are damaged more severely and increase the protein leak to greater than 3.5 g proteinuria 24 h^{-1}. This in turn induces a low serum albumen and generalised oedema. Hyperlipidaemia usually also occurs.
- *Haematuria* – occurs if capillary walls are disrupted, allowing red

cells to pass into the urine. This may be microscopic or macroscopic. However, most forms of haematuria are non-glomerular in origin.

- *Nephritic syndrome* – occurs when basement membrane damage and red blood cell leakage are present together leading to proteinuria and haematuria, accompanied by generalised oedema and mild hypertension.

- *Renal failure (acute or chronic)* – occurs when damage to the glomeruli is severe enough to impair the normal filtering function of the glomerulus, resulting in an accumulation in the blood of substances such as urea, creatinine and potassium.

SOME SPECIFIC NURSING OBSERVATIONS

Parameter	Rationale
Temperature	Patients with nephrotic syndrome are prone to infection which exacerbates the disease if not detected and treated promptly
Blood pressure	Hyper or hypotension may be present, dependent on the patient's fluid and cardiac status. One should also monitor for a postural drop
Respiration	Rapid, shallow breaths may indicate pulmonary oedema. Severely acidotic patients may develop Kussmaul's respirations (deep, sighing hyperventilation)
Daily weight	Serial measurements of the patient's weight (at the same time each day) give the clearest indication of changes in fluid status
Urinalysis	The urine should be tested for protein and blood as indicators of glomerular disease. Urinary volume should also be monitored, and the urine sent for culture if infection is suspected
Skin	The skin should be observed for: oedema, dehydration, pruritis, flaking and dryness, pressure sores and rashes. A skin rash may indicate a systemic disease such as SLE, vasculitis or Henoch-schönlein purpura

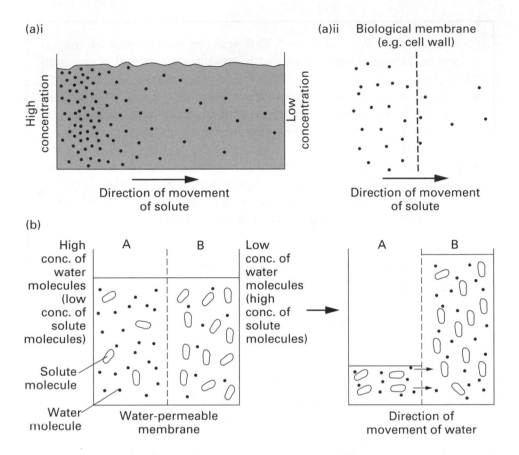

Fig. 2.8 *The principle of passive diffusion. (a) Passive diffusion of solutes. (i) The movement of a solute from an area of high concentration of that solute to an area of low concentration of that solute, until the solute is in equilibrium. (ii) Solutes can diffuse across biological membranes (e.g. cell walls) providing that the membrane is permeable to the solute. (b) Passive diffusion of water (osmosis). The movement of water molecules across a water-permeable membrane from an area of high concentration of water (or low concentration of solute) to an area of low concentration of water (or high concentration of solute), until an equilibrium is reached.*

not all of the filtered substances are returned to the blood. Any substances not reabsorbed will pass with the urine into the bladder to be excreted from the body. The main sites for reabsorption in the nephron are the proximal and distal convoluted tubules.

Mechanisms of reabsorption

Broadly speaking, there are two mechanisms in the nephron for the reabsorption of substances: passive diffusion and active transport (see Figs 2.8 and 2.9 for an outline of the principles of each of these mechanisms).

Active transport is an energy-requiring process that consumes large amounts of oxygen. This large oxygen demand is readily met because of

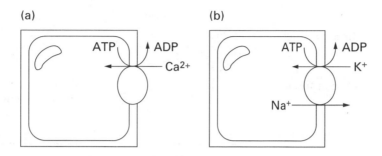

Fig. 2.9 *The principle of active transport. In many physiological systems it is necessary for solutes to move across biological membranes against their concentration gradient, i.e. from an area of low concentration to an area of high concentration. Since this requirement is counter to the process of passive diffusion (see Fig. 2.8), energy must be inputted into the system to drive the reaction. The input of energy to drive the uphill movement of solutes across cell membranes is called active transport. The 'energy' source used to drive the process is adenosine triphosphate (ATP), which is the end-product of glucose metabolism in the cell. (a) Conceptually, active transport is visualised as operating like a pump in the cell membrane, pumping specific solutes, either into or out of the cell. The movement of the solute across the membrane is coupled to the hydrolysis (splitting) of the ATP molecule. In the kidney tubules, active transport 'pumps' exist for sodium and potassium (sodium–potassium pump), calcium and hydrogen. (b) The sodium–potassium pump. As sodium is pumped out of the cell, potassium is pumped into it. ADP, adenosine diphosphate.*

the very high proportion of blood that flows to the kidney (21% of cardiac output). The epithelial cells that line the renal tubules also need to be very specialised to cope with the high levels of active transport required of them. For example, in the proximal tubule cells, where the majority of reabsorption is by active transport, the cells are packed with mitochondria. Mitochondria are cell organelles which are the site for the manufacture of the 'energy' component of active transport – adenosine triphosphate or ATP. Proximal tubule cells also have a large brush border on their luminal surface (the surface facing into the tubule) to increase their surface area for reabsorption. In contrast, cells lining the descending loop of Henle are comparatively thin, have no brush border, and have relatively few mitochondria. This suggests that these cells are not very metabolically active and are adapted for reabsorption by passive diffusion. The epithelial cells of the distal tubule are similar to those of the proximal tubule but with a less well defined brush border and fewer mitochondria. This suggests that these cells are capable of active transport of substances but in much lesser quantities than in the proximal tubule. This again illustrates how each segment of the nephron is anatomically adapted to carry out its unique functions. The different cell types lining the tubules are illustrated in Fig. 2.10.

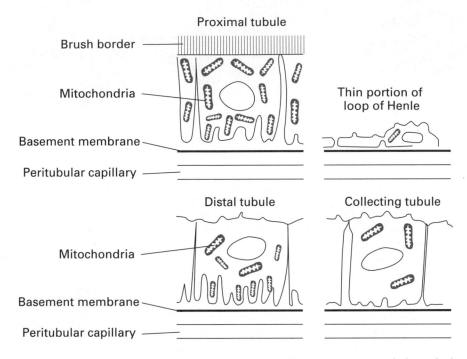

Fig. 2.10 *Characteristics of epithelial cells in different segments of the tubules.*

Reabsorption in the proximal convoluted tubule – the site of bulk phase reabsorption

Approximately 65% of all reabsorption occurs in the proximal tubule (hence the term 'bulk phase') and is obligatory rather than regulatory. Most substances here are reabsorbed by active transport mechanisms, including sodium, chloride, potassium, glucose, amino acids, phosphate and bicarbonate. Urea is absorbed by passive diffusion and water is reabsorbed by osmosis. Some substances are reabsorbed almost entirely in the proximal tubule such as glucose and amino acids, which do not appear in the urine, whereas others have only between 60 and 70% reabsorption, such as sodium, water and potassium. Approximately 50% of urea is reabsorbed here but creatinine is not reabsorbed at all. However, for all substances that are reabsorbed, the proximal tubule is the site where the bulk of this reabsorption occurs.

Reabsorption in the distal convoluted tubule – the site of fine tuning reabsorption

This is the site where more specific regulation of substances occurs according to the needs of the body. In order for the distal tubule to be aware of precisely what the body's reabsorptive needs are, there needs to be some method of communication between the cells of the distal tubule and the

Components of a negative feedback system:

a. *Sensor* e.g. osmoreceptors, thermoreceptors, baroreceptors, stretch receptors.
b. *Communication pathway* e.g. nervous system, hormones via the circulatory system.
c. *Effector* i.e. the cell(s) or organ(s) effecting the response.

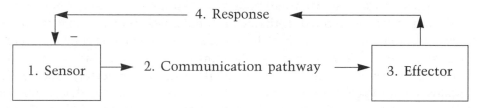

Step 1: The sensor detects a disturbance in the system, e.g. fall in blood pressure or rise in plasma osmolality.
Step 2: A 'message' is sent via the appropriate communication pathway to the effector cells or organ.
Step 3: The effector responds to the stimulus to correct the disturbance, e.g. vasoconstriction or reabsorption of water in the kidney tubules.
Step 4: Once the system returns to normal, the sensor reduces or stops the stimulus (negative feedback).

See Figs 2.14, 2.15 and 2.16 for specific negative feedback examples.

Fig. 2.11 *Model of a negative feedback system.*

rest of the body. This communication system is via a range of hormones which form part of a negative feedback system for the homeostatic control of ions and water. For example, sodium and water reabsorption are under the control of aldosterone and antidiuretic hormone (ADH) respectively. Potassium reabsorption is also controlled by aldosterone, whereas calcium and phosphate are controlled by parathyroid hormone (PTH). All negative feedback systems function in a similar way, and the basic model is outlined in Fig. 2.11. The precise mechanisms for controlling the electrolytes outlined above will be dealt with in later sections in this chapter.

Secretion

The process of secretion occurs in both the proximal and distal tubules and involves the movement of substances from blood flowing through the peritubular capillaries, through the tubule wall cells, into the tubular fluid.

In this respect, secretion is the opposite process to reabsorption. Substances that are secreted into the tubules are excreted in the urine. Though creatinine is freely filtered at the glomerulus, total creatinine excretion is increased by 20% by the process of secretion (Guyton, 1991). Important ions that are transported into the tubules by secretion are hydrogen, which is secreted in both the proximal and distal tubules and is important in acid–base control, and potassium, which is secreted in the distal tubule under the control of aldosterone. In fact, potassium and hydrogen ions actually compete to be secreted in the distal tubule, which means that if excess potassium ions need to be secreted, then fewer hydrogen ions can be secreted and vice versa. Clinically, this phenomenon results in an association between metabolic acidosis and hyperkalaemia (or conversely, metabolic alkalosis and hypokalaemia), since in the acidotic patient the distal tubules will increase the rate of hydrogen ion secretion (to prevent a fall in plasma pH) by reducing the rate of potassium ion secretion, resulting in the retention of potassium ions in the blood, leading to hyperkalaemia.

Excretion of drugs and drug metabolites

Many drugs and their metabolites are finally excreted from the body through the kidneys by the processes of glomerular filtration and secretion. Like other filtered substances, the rate of filtration of drugs will depend on their molecular size and charge, smaller molecules being filtered more rapidly than larger ones. Drugs that bind to plasma proteins are filtered very slowly because of the size of the complex. Some drugs are cleared from the blood purely by glomerular filtration and thus the rate of clearance cannot exceed the GFR of 125 ml min^{-1}, whereas other drugs are excreted by a combination of filtration and secretion, such as benzylpenicillin, which achieves a total clearance rate of 480 ml min^{-1} (Laurence and Bennett, 1987).

Concentration and Dilution of Urine

The components of the nephron that are involved in the concentration and dilution of the urine are the loop of Henle and the collecting ducts. The concentration of urine is measured in units of osmolality (mosmoles kg^{-1} water). The most dilute urine that humans can produce is approximately 60 mosmoles kg^{-1} water (Lote, 1987) but this situation only occurs in the pathological condition of diabetes insipidus in which the pituitary gland fails to produce ADH. The most concentrated urine that can be produced is approximately 1400 mosmoles kg^{-1} water (Lote, 1987), which is more than four times more concentrated than plasma (plasma osmolality = 285 mosmoles kg^{-1} water) and requires maximum ADH secretion. The average range of urine osmolality in people with normal kidneys is between 300 and 500 mosmoles kg^{-1} water.

Counter-current mechanism of urinary concentration

The counter-current mechanism is a complex physiological process which will not be discussed in great detail in this chapter. Only the basic principles of the mechanism will be outlined.

In order to concentrate the urine the following factors are required:

- The creation and maintenance of a local environment in the kidney that allows large quantities of water to be reabsorbed by osmosis from the collecting duct back into the blood.
- A mechanism that can influence the opening and closing of water channels in the collecting ducts in order to control the exact amount of water reabsorbed.

Creation of the local environment (see Fig. 2.12)   This local environment consists of an increasing hyperosmotic medullary interstitium as one moves towards the tip of the loops of Henle. In other words, the tissue spaces between the loops of Henle in the medulla of the kidney must be made hyperosmotic compared to the fluid in the collecting duct. As the collecting ducts pass through the medulla on their way to the renal pelvis, water can be pulled out by osmosis, resulting in less water entering the urine.

This hyperosmotic environment is created by the active and passive transport of ions (mainly sodium and chloride) out of the tubular fluid as it passes through the loop of Henle into the medullary interstitium. The build-up of ions here gradually increases and becomes more concentrated as the loop of Henle descends into the medulla. The tip of the medulla can reach osmolalities of up to 1400 mosmoles kg^{-1} water. Water does not follow the transport of ions into the medullary interstitium by osmosis because the thick ascending limb of the loop of Henle is impermeable to water. Urea also makes an important contribution to the creation of the hyperosmotic environment. Urea can diffuse passively through the walls of the tubules at most points along the nephron, but urea diffusion is greatly enhanced across the collecting tubule wall in the presence of even small amounts of ADH. Thus large amounts of urea become concentrated in the medullary interstitium.

Maintenance of the local environment: the counter-current mechanism   One may think that as fast as the hyperosmotic environment is created it will be washed out by processes of diffusion and reabsorption back into the blood. However, the environment is maintained because of the unique arrangement of the looped vasa recta capillaries around the loops of Henle (Fig. 2.13). The vasa recta are only supplied with 1–2% of the blood entering the kidneys, so there is very little blood flow for ions to be reabsorbed back into. In addition, the vasa recta lie with their ascending and descending limbs in very close proximity. This close proximity allows for rapid

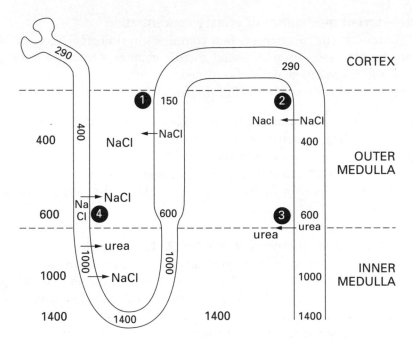

Fig. 2.12 *Creation of the hyperosmotic environment in the medullary interstitium. (1) Active transport of chloride and passive diffusion of sodium out of the thick ascending limb of the loop of Henle into the medullary interstitium. (2) Active transport of sodium and passive diffusion of chloride out of the collecting duct into the medullary interstitium. (3) Passive diffusion of urea out of the collecting duct in the presence of antidiuretic hormone (ADH). (4) Passive diffusion of sodium chloride into the medullary interstitium from the thin descending limb of the loop of Henle. The figures show the osmolality of the tubular and interstitial fluids at different points of the tubule.*

exchange of water and solutes between the two limbs. So as blood flows down the descending limb of the vasa recta, the high concentration of ions in the medullary interstitium enables ions to diffuse into the vasa recta (markedly increasing their concentration), and water to move out by osmosis, but as the blood moves into the ascending limb of the vasa recta, the high concentration of ions in the blood then enables ions to diffuse back out into the medullary interstitium (and water back into the blood), maintaining the hyperosmotic environment.

Opening and closing of water channels in the collecting duct   The opening and closing of water channels in the collecting duct is controlled by the hormone ADH. The more ADH that is circulating in the blood the more water channels will be open in the walls of the collecting duct and thus the more water that will be reabsorbed by osmosis into the medullary interstitium (and eventually into the circulation). ADH is secreted from the

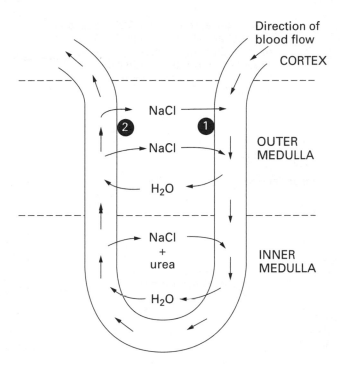

Fig. 2.13 *Maintenance of the hyperosmotic environment. (1) As blood flows down the descending limb of the vasa recta, the high concentration of sodium chloride and urea in the medullary interstitium causes passive diffusion of these ions into the blood, whilst water diffuses out of the blood by osmosis. (2) As blood enters the ascending limb, the high concentration of sodium chloride and urea that has accumulated in the tip of the vasa recta then diffuses back out into the interstitium, whilst water is osmotically attracted back into the blood, thus maintaining the hyperosmotic environment in the medullary interstitium. The net result of this process is that solutes circulate around in the vasa recta but are not washed out into the main circulation.*

posterior pituitary gland in response the osmolality of the plasma. Osmoreceptors in the hypothalamus detect small fluctuations in the plasma osmolality and send signals to the pituitary gland to secrete more or less ADH into the circulation (Fig. 2.14). If the plasma becomes too concentrated more ADH is secreted so that more water is reabsorbed in the kidney to dilute the plasma and return it to normal osmolality. If the plasma is too dilute then less ADH is secreted, resulting in less water reabsorption and the production of a more dilute urine.

The concentrating and diluting abilities of the kidney are severely affected by diseases that affect the renal tubules. See Box 2.2 for a discussion on tubulo-intersitial diseases.

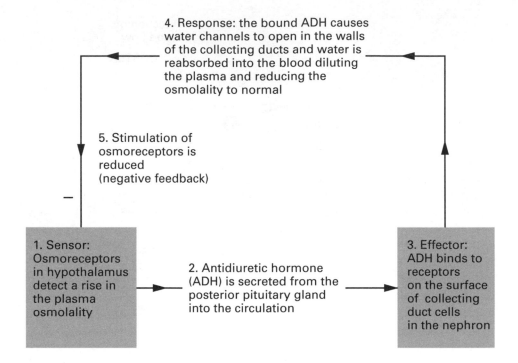

Fig. 2.14 *Negative feedback loop for antidiuretic hormone (ADH) release and control of plasma osmolality.*

Box 2.2 Tubulo-interstitial disease.

Tubulo-interstitial disease is the term used to describe a range of disorders that damage the renal tubules and invariably involve the interstitial tissue between the renal tubules. Glomerular abnormalities may be present but are usually mild or occur in the late stages of the disease. Tubulo-interstitial disease can be divided into two broad groups: *acute tubular necrosis* (the commonest cause of acute renal failure), and *tubulo-interstitial nephritis* which can be acute or chronic.

HISTOPATHOLOGY

Acute Tubular Necrosis (ATN)

Tubular damage may be of ischaemic or toxic origin. In the ischaemic type, the necrosis of the tubules is patchy with the proximal tubules and ascending limb of Henle most vulnerable. In the toxic type, the necrotic damage is more extensive, particularly in the proximal tubule. In both types casts are found in the distal tubules and the collecting ducts.

Tubulo-Interstitial Nephritis (TIN)

Acute TIN is histologically characterised by interstitial oedema and leukocyte infiltration with focal tubular necrosis. In chronic interstitial nephritis there is infiltration with mononuclear cells, interstitial fibrosis and widespread tubular atrophy. The causes of TIN are very varied and include infections, toxins, metabolic diseases (e.g. urate nephropathy), chronic urinary tract obstruction, myeloma, immunologic reactions (e.g. transplant rejection) and vascular diseases.

CLINICAL MANIFESTATIONS

TIN presents with defects of tubular function. A number of syndromes may be distinguished:

- *Acute renal failure* – with oliguria (not always present), and a rising blood urea level.
- *Failure of reabsorption and regulation* – with salt wasting and volume depletion, polyuria due to impaired ability to concentrate urine, hypokalaemia, renal tubular acidosis and renal bone disease. Some or all of these features may be present.
- *Loin pain* – due to ureteric obstruction with stones or detached renal papillae.
- *Chronic renal failure.*

Other clinical findings may be apparent specific to the cause of the TIN but are beyond the scope of this box.

SPECIFIC NURSING OBSERVATIONS

Parameter	Rationale
Blood pressure	Hypotension may be severe in some patients if there is significant volume depletion. Postural drop should be monitored
Respiration	Kussmaul's respirations may indicate development of a serious metabolic acidosis

Urinary volume	Should be monitored regularly as an aid to calculating fluid replacement regimes, and for progress of the disease
Urinalysis	Urine specimens may be required for culture (if infection is suspected), urea, electrolytes and osmolarity (to test for concentrating ability of kidney), and microscopy (to detect casts, cells or crystals)
Skin	Some causes of TIN may be associated with a skin rash. Loss of skin turgor and dehydration should also be observed for
Temperature	Fever may be present in pyelonephritis or acute interstitial nephritis

Control of Sodium and Potassium Balance

Sodium and potassium ions are handled in very similar ways by the kidney. Both are cations that are freely filtered at the glomerulus, and both have approximately 65% reabsorption in the proximal tubule. Finally, the body fluid concentrations of both these ions arc ultimately controlled by the distal tubules under the influence of the hormone aldosterone. However, this is where the similarity between sodium and potassium ends.

Sodium and the control of extracellular fluid volume

Sodium is the main extracellular cation and together with its associated anion chloride, contributes approximately 95% of the extracellular fluid osmolality (Lote, 1987). Since plasma osmolality is intimately related to plasma volume (through the ADH negative feedback system – Fig. 2.14), it follows that extracellular sodium content must also be intimately related to extracellular fluid volume. Thus, an increase in body sodium content would lead to an increase in extracellular fluid volume leading to hypertension and oedema; and a decrease in body sodium content would lead to a decrease in extracellular fluid volume leading to hypotension and dehydration. Thus, it is vitally important that body sodium content is kept at a constant level if body fluid volume is to remain constant.

Body sodium content is influenced by the action of the hormone aldosterone on the distal tubule in the nephron. The more aldosterone that is circulating the more sodium will be reabsorbed (Fig. 2.15). Increases in sodium reabsorption lead to an increase in the plasma osmolality and this triggers the ADH negative feedback system discussed above. Thus, increases in circulating aldosterone tend to be paralleled by increases in circulating

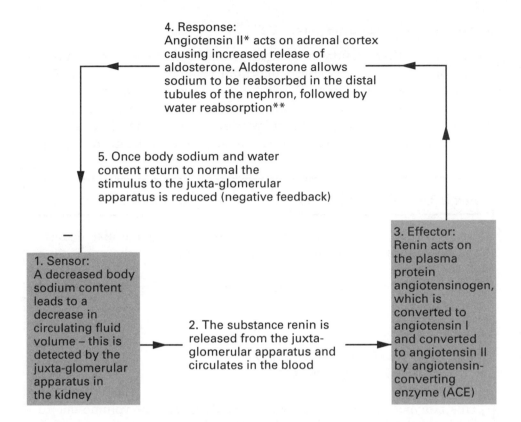

Fig. 2.15 *Negative feedback loop for aldosterone release and control of body sodium content. *, Angiotensin II also exerts other effects which help to restore normal sodium and water balance: vasocontriction (to restore blood pressure), directly increases proximal tubular sodium reabsorption and causes thirst; **, water reabsorption is a function of the parallel rise in antidiuretic hormone secretion caused by the rise in plasma osmolality as sodium is reabsorbed (Fig. 2.14).*

ADH. However, one must not overstate the importance of aldosterone in the regulation of sodium balance since conditions in which there is excess aldosterone production do not lead to excessive sodium and water retention (Lote, 1987). This suggests that other factors are also important in the regulation of sodium and extracellular fluid volume. For example, when there is excess sodium and water retention leading to an expansion in the extracellular fluid volume, a hormone called atrial natriuretic peptide (ANP) is released from cardiac atrial cells in response to an increased atrial stretch. This peptide has five known major effects:

- inhibition of aldosterone secretion by the adrenal cortex;
- reduction of renin release from the kidney;
- reduction of ADH release from the posterior pituitary;
- vasodilatation;

- natriuresis and diuresis (Lote, 1987).

All of these effects result in the excretion of sodium and water through the kidney, reducing the extracellular fluid volume back to normal. Other factors that may be important in sodium regulation are renal prostaglandins, kinins and the renal nerves. Failure to regulate the extra-cellular fluid volume occurs commonly in people with renal disease and leads to hypertension. Hypertension in renal disease is discussed in detail in Box 2.3.

Box 2.3 Hypertension in renal disease.

Hypertension is a common sign, particularly in glomerular disease, the severity of the hypertension often increasing with the progression of the disease.

Two distinct types of hypertension can be identified in the renal patient:

1. VOLUME-DEPENDENT HYPERTENSION

This is hypertension caused by an expanding vascular volume due to failure of the kidney to filter adequate amounts of sodium and water through the glomerulus. This type of hypertension is extremely common in chronic renal failure and particularly end-stage renal failure (ESRF). Patients on haemodialysis often arrive for dialysis with elevated blood pressure due to fluid retention and leave with a lowered blood pressure once fluid has been removed by the treatment. Patients with acute glomerulonephritis also exhibit a mild volume dependent hypertension.

2. RENIN-DEPENDENT HYPERTENSION

In a minority of renal patients, despite correction of sodium and water balance, hypertension still persists. It is presumed in these patients that hypertension is due to an abnormality in the renin–angiotensin system. Renin is a peptide molecule released from specialised cells in the walls of the afferent and efferent arterioles. These specialised cells come into contact with other cells called the macula densa which are found in the wall of the distal tubule as it passes in the angle between

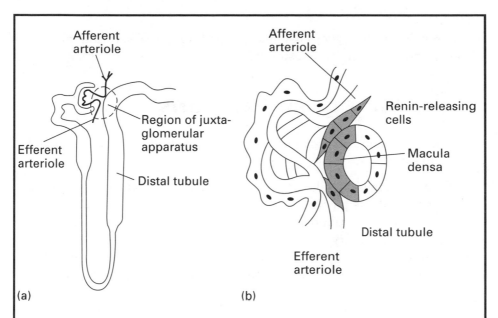

Afferent arteriole

Region of juxta-glomerular apparatus

Efferent arteriole

Distal tubule

Afferent arteriole

Renin-releasing cells

Macula densa

Distal tubule

Efferent arteriole

(a)   (b)

Diagram 1(a) *Nephron showing how the juxta-glomerular apparatus is positioned in the angle between the afferent and efferent arterioles and the distal tubule. (b) The juxta-glomerular apparatus.*

the afferent and efferent arterioles (see Diagrams 1a and 1b). The macula densa and the renin-releasing cells are collectively called the juxta-glomerular apparatus or complex.

The juxta-glomerular apparatus is responsible for maintaining a constant blood flow through the glomerulus and thus a constant GFR despite fluctuations in arterial pressure. This is achieved through a tubulo feedback mechanism in which a fall in GFR results in a fall in the chloride ion concentration in the distal tubule. This stimulates the macula densa cells which send 'signals' to the renin secreting cells to release renin. Renin acts via the renin–angiotensin system (see Fig. 2.15) to produce both local vasoconstriction of the efferent arteriole (increasing the GFR) and peripheral vasoconstriction to increase arterial blood pressure. In addition salt and water retention increase due to the effects of aldosterone.

In renal patients with either renal artery stenosis or disease of small renal arteries, impaired renal blood flow may chronically stimulate the release of renin by affected nephrons. This circulating renin will then exert its effects on 'normal' unaffected nephrons causing the GFR to rise by efferent arteriole vasoconstriction and for their salt and water retention to increase, causing arterial pressure to rise above normal. Thus, this renin-dependent hypertension is often accompanied by a volume dependent hypertension as salt and water reabsorption increase under the influence of aldosterone.

NURSING CONSIDERATIONS

When measuring a patient's blood pressure the following points should be considered:

- The patient is as relaxed and comfortable as possible and is in a sitting or lying position.
- The correct-sized cuff is used and the inflation bag is placed over the brachial artery.
- Readings are taken from the same arm each time – systolic pressure can vary by up to 10 mmHg between right and left brachial arteries.

REMEMBER

- There is diurnal variation in blood pressure, the pressure being greater in the day than at night.
- Standing usually causes a slight drop (< 20 mmHg) in systolic pressure and a slight rise (< 10 mmHg) in diastolic pressure. However, postural hypotension causes a large fall in both pressures and is accompanied by dizziness.
- Blood pressure may be variable if the patient has an irregular heart rhythm.
- Blood pressure recordings should be considered together with fluctuations in the patient's weight and presence or absence of oedema.

Aldosterone and the control of body potassium content

Potassium is the main intracellular cation. Only about 2% of the total body potassium content is extracellular. This unequal distribution of potassium across cell membranes is essential for normal nerve and muscle conduction. Disturbances in potassium balance show their effects in abnormal nerve and muscle function and may be life threatening. For example, in hypokalaemia there is a reduction in the excitability of nerve and muscle conduction which in severe cases can lead to a flaccid paralysis. Hyperkalaemia, on the other hand, tends to lead to an increase in the excitability of nerve and muscle cells leading to cardiac arrhythmias and even cardiac arrest. It may even lead to paralysis in skeletal muscles by making it impossible for the muscles to relax after a contraction. Thus potassium content needs to be controlled precisely to prevent sudden fluctuations in the extracellular fluid concentration.

Unlike sodium regulation, where aldosterone is just one factor in the regulation of sodium content, aldosterone is the only hormone involved in the control of potassium content and thus has a very important regulatory role. Small increases in extracellular potassium concentration directly stimulate aldosterone secretion from the adrenal cortex. The effect of aldosterone in the distal tubule of the nephron is to increase the secretion of potassium into the urine. The release of aldosterone stimulated by rises in extracellular potassium concentration are strongly controlled by a negative feedback system. Once the potassium concentration returns to normal the stimulus to secrete aldosterone is quickly switched off.

Control of Calcium and Phosphate Balance

Calcium and phosphate are the main mineral constituents of bone and thus the majority of calcium and phosphate in the body is found in the skeleton. However, small amounts of both these ions are found in the extracellular fluid. Calcium exists in the plasma in two forms. Approximately 50% exists in the free ionised form (1.25 mmol l^{-1}), and the other 50% in a bound form, mainly bound to protein, particularly albumen (1.25 mmol l^{-1}). Usually when serum calcium levels are measured, the total calcium concentration is measured (2.5 mmol l^{-1}). Calcium has an important role in the extracellular fluid in controlling nerve and muscle conduction. It is the ionised form of the calcium that is important in this role and thus any condition that leads to a fall in the ionised calcium concentration (even if total calcium remains normal), will lead to the classic symptoms of hypocalcaemia – tetany, muscle cramps and even convulsions. In situations of hypercalcaemia, the main effects seen are extraskeletal calcification, renal calculi, peptic ulceration and changes in mental function such as depression.

Inorganic phosphate has a normal plasma range of 0.8–1.3 mmol l^{-1}. Phosphate is important in buffer systems to maintain the plasma pH and exists in equilibrium with calcium.

Renal handling of calcium and phosphate

Both calcium and phosphate are freely filtered at the glomerulus. When the plasma phosphate level is below 1 mmol l^{-1}, all of the filtered phosphate is reabsorbed in the early proximal tubule. However, once the plasma phosphate level rises above 1 mmol l^{-1} the amount of phosphate excreted in the urine rises in proportion to the plasma concentration. Further excretion of phosphate in the distal tubule (by secretion) can occur in response to the rise in the circulating level of PTH. Calcium reabsorption is very similar to that of sodium, in that approximately 65% occurs in the proximal tubule, a further 20–25% in the ascending limb of the loop of Henle, leaving around 10–12% of filtered calcium being delivered to the distal tubule. How much more calcium is reabsorbed in the distal tubule depends on the levels of circulating PTH. When PTH levels rise this results in calcium reabsorption and phosphate excretion in the distal tubule, helping to control both calcium and phosphate levels in the plasma.

Homeostatic control of calcium and phosphate balance

Calcium and phosphate balance in the plasma is achieved when inputs of these two ions into the plasma equal outputs from the plasma. Calcium and phosphate can enter the plasma from either the gut (through ingestion – enhanced by the presence of vitamin D), or from the bone (by the influence of PTH). It can leave the plasma either by renal excretion or by being redeposited in the bone (influenced by calcitonin). The most important factors controlling calcium and phosphate balance are vitamin D and PTH. Though calcitonin plays a part in reducing a high plasma calcium level, its role is short lived and of only minor importance in the overall controlling process.

Vitamin D is a steroid that enters the body either through dietary intake or by the effect of sunlight on the skin. However, this is an inactive form of vitamin D called cholecalciferol. To become activated it needs to undergo two metabolic conversions – one in the liver (where hydroxylase enzyme converts it to 25, hydroxycholecalcifcrol); and one in the kidney (where a second hydroxylase enzyme converts it to 1,25 dihydroxycholecalciferol). This active form of the vitamin is then able to enhance the absorption of calcium and phosphate from the gut. This activated vitamin D also decreases the rate of excretion of calcium and phosphate from the kidney, and in the presence of PTH releases calcium and phosphate from the bone. However, its most important effect is on the gut. Vitamin D, therefore, has the overall effect of increasing the plasma concentration of both calcium and phosphate.

PTH is secreted from the four parathyroid glands embedded in the thyroid gland in the neck. PTH secretion is stimulated by a fall in the ionised plasma calcium concentration. The main effects of PTH are: increased bone resorption, enhancement of the second metabolic conversion of vitamin D in the kidney thereby enhancing calcium reabsorption in the gut, and an increased reabsorption of calcium in the distal tubules of the kidney (and increased excretion of phosphate).

The effects of both vitamin D and PTH are to increase the plasma calcium concentration. However, these effects are carefully controlled by a negative feedback system which prevents the calcium level rising to high. The negative feedback system is outlined in Fig. 2.16. Only if calcium levels suddenly rise high (as after a high calcium meal) is calcitonin stimulated to be released from the 'C' cells of the thyroid gland, causing calcium to

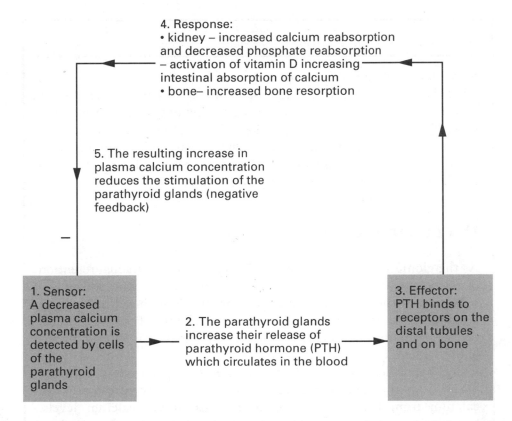

Fig. 2.16 *Negative feedback loop for parathyroid hormone release and calcium and phosphate control.*

be redeposited in the bone. This is a rapid and relatively short-acting effect. The control of calcium and phosphate levels is essential for the maintenance of normal bone. In renal disease this finely tuned negative feedback control system is disturbed, leading to the complication of renal bone disease. Renal bone disease is discussed in Box 2.4.

Acid–Base Control

Acid–base balance is about maintaining the constancy of the pH of the body's fluids. The pH scale is a logarithmic scale (range 1–14) that measures the concentration of free hydrogen ions in a fluid. In fact the scale is reciprocal, which means that as the pH becomes lower the hydrogen ion concentration gets increasingly greater. Thus at acidic pHs (below 7), the hydrogen ion concentration of the fluid is very high relative to that at basic pHs (above 7). In fact, for each point on the scale there is a 10-fold difference in the hydrogen ion concentration. When we consider that the normal pH range of our bodily fluids is between 7.35 and 7.45 this appears very

Box 2.4 Renal bone disease.

Some degree of bone disease accompanies virtually all cases of chronic renal failure and starts to develop relatively early in the disease process. A range of symptoms can occur including bone pain, joint pain, skeletal deformities, pathological fractures, bone cysts and extraskeletal calcifications. Renal bone disease, also termed renal osteodystrophy, is a mix of two disorders: osteomalacia (rickets in children) and secondary hyperparathyroidism.

PATHOGENESIS

As the glomerular filtration rate (GFR) falls there is a gradual retention of phosphate in the plasma. As the kidney mass declines there is a reduction in the amount of activated vitamin D produced resulting in a reduction in the intestinal absorption of calcium. Thus, the typical picture seen in patients with chronic renal failure is one of hyperphosphataemia and hypocalcaemia.

The hypocalcaemia stimulates the release of parathyroid hormone (PTH) from the parathyroid glands which causes the reabsorption of calcium from bone in an attempt to raise serum calcium levels. However, due to the low levels of active vitamin D and high phosphate levels, the calcium level rarely returns to normal, thus the parathyroid glands become chronically stimulated and serum PTH levels remain high. The net effect of this cycle of activity is to demineralise the bone causing the classical mixed picture of osteomalacia and secondary hyperparathyroidism.

In very advanced, long-term renal failure the parathyroid glands may undergo hypertrophy in response to their chronic stimulation. These enlarged glands may then function autonomously secreting PTH at very high doses. This is called tertiary hyperparathyroidism, and may only be detected when the patient's serum calcium level is returned to normal either by calcium or vitamin D supplementation, or by renal transplantation. In tertiary hyperparathyroidism the parathyroid glands no longer respond to the negative feedback signal from serum calcium levels; thus, even when calcium levels have been corrected they continue to produce PTH. The result of this is an acceleration of the renal bone disease, together with the development of hypercalcaemia and extraskeletal calcification.

EXACERBATING FACTORS

- *Chronic metabolic acidosis* – hydrogen ions enter the bone to be buffered in exchange for calcium ions which leach out of the bone.
- *Aluminium retention* – overuse of aluminium-based phosphate binding agents and/or long-term dialysis against inadequately purified water containing aluminium can lead to excessive retention of aluminium in the plasma. One of the effects of aluminium toxicity is to exacerbate renal bone disease causing severe bone pain, fractures and proximal muscle weakness.
- *Chronic overuse of heparin in haemodialysis* – this can lead to the development of osteoporosis with spontaneous fractures including vertebral fractures.
- *β_2-microglobulin amyloidosis* – this condition is unique to patients on long-term haemodialysis and results from a failure of cupraphan dialysis membranes to effectively filter out β_2-microglobulin from the patient's blood. The accumulated β_2-microglobulin deposits as amyloid in the synovium, joints and tendon sheaths leading to the classical symptoms of carpal tunnel syndrome and joint pain seen in this group of patients.

TREATMENT

Treatment is designed to prevent serious bone disease from developing by correcting the primary defect in the calcium–phosphate balance:

- Serum phosphate levels are lowered by the administration of phosphate-binding agents such as Calcichew™. These work by binding phosphate in the gut to prevent its absorption. Dietary restriction of phosphate is also required.
- Serum calcium levels are raised by the administration of oral calcium supplements and/or by the administration of an active vitamin D preparation such as one-Alpha™ to improve intestinal absorption of calcium. NB: patients with tertiary hyperparathyroidism who are treated with Calcichew™ or one-Alpha™ may become hypercalcaemic and may need to be dialysed with calcium-free dialysate to help control serum calcium levels.
- When tertiary hyperparathyroidism is revealed in a patient and is severe, the treatment of choice is usually parathyroidectomy.

SPECIFIC NURSING CONSIDERATIONS

The prevention of serious bone disease in patients with chronic renal failure requires a multidisciplinary approach. The doctor, nurse, pharmacist, dietician and psychologist all play a role in the education, support, treatment and monitoring of the patient. The nurse's specific role is three-fold:

- Reinforcement of patient education regarding dietary advice and drug regimes.
- Monitoring of patient compliance and recognition of potential or actual non-compliant behaviour, with subsequent counselling, support or referral to psychologist.
- Minimising exacerbating factors for bone disease by:

    (a) close monitoring of heparin use during haemodialysis, including considering alternative anticoagulants;
    (b) considering use of synthetic dialysis membranes in patients with symptoms of β_2-microglobulin amyloidosis as these are more effective at clearing β_2-microglobulin.

narrow but actually represents over a 20% difference in the hydrogen ion concentration! It is doubtful we would tolerate a 20% change in our sodium ion concentration with such ease.

So what are acids and bases? Simply put, acids are molecules that in the right environmental conditions will give up or 'donate' a hydrogen ion to the solution it is in, and a base is a molecule that mops up or 'accepts' free hydrogen ions from the solution. Thus, in order to maintain a constant hydrogen ion concentration (and hence constant pH) both acids and bases need to be present in the solution to donate or accept free hydrogen ions as required. Acids and bases working together in this way to minimise changes in pH are called buffers.

Though there are several buffering systems in the body, including haemoglobin, plasma proteins, organic and inorganic phosphates, the most important one physiologically is the bicarbonate buffering system and it is this one that shall be described.

Bicarbonate buffering system

To understand the bicarbonate buffering system one first needs to consider the following reaction sequence:

$$CO_2 + H_2O \leftrightarrow H_2CO_3 \leftrightarrow H^+ + HCO_3^-$$

Basically, this equation explains how the components of the buffering system are generated in the plasma. Carbon dioxide is generated by cells as an end-product of metabolism and diffuses into the plasma. The CO_2 dissolves in water to form carbonic acid (H_2CO_3), which is the acid component of the buffering system. The carbonic acid, in turn, is in equilibrium with the hydrogen (H^+) and bicarbonate ions (HCO_3^-). This forms the basic component of the buffering system. This reaction sequence can run in either direction, thus if there is a build-up of CO_2 in the plasma then more carbonic acid will be formed and the reaction will be driven to the right in order that more bicarbonate ions can be formed to minimise changes in the pH. However, if an excess of hydrogen ions builds up (from metabolic processes) then the reaction will be driven to the left, resulting in CO_2 and water forming. The excess CO_2 can then be blown off in the lungs. Since this reaction sequence constantly runs backwards and forwards to maintain a constant pH, then it follows that pH must be dependent on the relative proportions of CO_2 to bicarbonate ions. This can be shown in the following equation:

$$pH \propto \frac{HCO_3^-}{pCO_2}$$

Both components of this equation can be controlled by the body. The bicarbonate ion concentration is carefully controlled by the kidneys, whereas the pCO_2 is controlled by the lungs. Thus the lungs and the kidneys are the two main organs that together control the acid–base balance of the body.

Control of bicarbonate ion concentration by the kidney

Bicarbonate ions are freely filtered in the glomerulus. When the plasma bicarbonate concentration is normal (25 mmol l^{-1}) then all of the filtered bicarbonate is reabsorbed, 90% reabsorption occurring in the proximal tubule and 10% in the distal tubule. However, if plasma bicarbonate concentration is higher than normal then this excess bicarbonate is lost in the urine.

The reabsorption of bicarbonate ions in the nephron is not a straightforward transport of ions from the tubular fluid into the plasma as with other ions but involves various chemical reactions inside the tubular wall cells. The filtered bicarbonate in the tubule undergoes the whole reaction sequence identified above for the bicarbonate buffering system so that CO_2 and water are formed. This is catalysed by the enzyme carbonic anhydrase which is found in the brush border of the proximal tubular cells. The resulting CO_2 then diffuses into the tubular cell where it undergoes the same reaction sequence again to reform the bicarbonate ion plus a hydrogen ion. The hydrogen ion is secreted into the tubule to be excreted and the

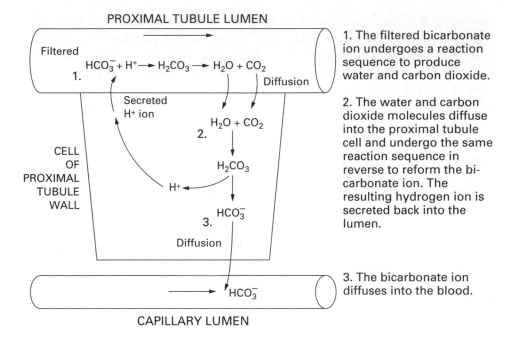

PROXIMAL TUBULE LUMEN

Filtered

$$HCO_3^- + H^+ \longrightarrow H_2CO_3 \longrightarrow H_2O + CO_2$$

1.

Diffusion

Secreted
H+ ion

$$H_2O + CO_2$$

2.

$$H_2CO_3$$

H+

$$HCO_3^-$$

3.

CELL
OF
PROXIMAL
TUBULE
WALL

Diffusion

$$HCO_3^-$$

CAPILLARY LUMEN

1. The filtered bicarbonate ion undergoes a reaction sequence to produce water and carbon dioxide.

2. The water and carbon dioxide molecules diffuse into the proximal tubule cell and undergo the same reaction sequence in reverse to reform the bicarbonate ion. The resulting hydrogen ion is secreted back into the lumen.

3. The bicarbonate ion diffuses into the blood.

Fig. 2.17 *Bicarbonate reabsorption in the kidney tubules.*

bicarbonate ion diffuses into the plasma. This process is sometimes referred to as bicarbonate 'trapping' (Fig. 2.17).

The secreted hydrogen ions do not pass as free ions into the urine but combine with inorganic phosphates or ammonia in the tubules; that is, the urine itself also has a system of buffers. The binding of a hydrogen ion to alkaline phosphate converts it to acid phosphate which is then excreted in the urine. The binding of hydrogen to ammonia converts it to ammonium which again is excreted into the urine. The intracellular production of hydrogen ions for secretion results in the production of new bicarbonate ions for diffusion back into the plasma. This process is sometimes referred to as bicarbonate 'generation'. Hydrogen ion secretion is necessary for both the reabsorption of filtered bicarbonate and the generation of new bicarbonate.

Correcting acid–base fluctuations in the healthy individual

Fall in plasma pH   This is a condition called acidaemia or more commonly acidosis. This problem arises when there are excess hydrogen ions in the body fluids. In the absence of respiratory or renal disease, the initial response to control pH is for the excess hydrogen ions to drive the bicarbonate reaction sequence to the left to produce CO_2 and water. The lungs can then deal with this excess CO_2 by increasing the respiratory rate to 'blow off' the CO_2. This process gives a quick short-term compensation to the problem but not long-term correction. The rise in hydrogen ion concentration is then corrected by the kidneys secreting the excess hydrogen into the urine and in the process generating further bicarbonate for reabsorption into the plasma.

Rise in plasma pH   This condition is called alkalaemia or alkalosis, and arises when there is a reduction in the hydrogen ion concentration of the body fluids. The kidney plays the main role in correcting this problem by reducing the amount of hydrogen ion secretion. However, because hydrogen ion secretion and bicarbonate reabsorption are coupled together, this also results in a reduction in the plasma bicarbonate level. The plasma bicarbonate concentration is then corrected by a reduction in ventilation rate by the lungs which leads to a build-up of CO_2, which drives the reaction sequence to the right to generate more bicarbonate ions.

Though the above compensatory and correction processes buffer the small fluctuations that occur in the acid–base balance in the healthy individual, larger fluctuations in acid–base balance tend to occur when there is either respiratory or metabolic disease. This is because the normal correction mechanisms are blocked. For example, in disorders of ventilation a respiratory acidosis or rarely alkalosis may develop, whereas in disorders of metabolism (including renal disease) a metabolic acidosis or alkalosis may develop. Descriptions of these disorders are beyond this chapter, but the reader is referred to Box 2. 5 for a brief discussion on the metabolic acidosis of renal failure.

Erythropoietin Production by the Kidney

The final important role that the kidney has is the production of the hormone erythropoietin. Erythropoietin is a glycoprotein that promotes the proliferation and differentiation of erythrocyte precursors in the bone marrow. Thus, erythropoietin is necessary for the maintenance of a normal red cell count and prevention of anaemia. The erythropoietin-producing cells of the kidney have been identified as being peritubular cells, most likely endothelial cells of the cortex and outer medulla (Lacombe *et al.*, 1991). Erythropoietin production is stimulated by hypoxia and inhibited when the hypoxia is corrected, thus its production is controlled by the negative feedback principle. The kidney is not the only site of erythropoietin production. Approximately 20% of erythropoietin is produced at extrarenal sites, thought mainly to be the liver. However, in the presence of severe renal disease, this extrarenal production of erythropoietin is insufficient to maintain the red cell count at normal levels, achieving only one-third to one-half the normal level (Guyton, 1991). Box 2.6 outlines the contributing factors to the anaemia of renal failure.

Box 2.5 Metabolic acidosis in renal failure.

Metabolic acidosis accompanies all forms of renal insufficiency, the severity correlating with the number of affected nephrons. Thus, patients with mild chronic renal failure may have a mild asymptomatic acidosis, whereas patients presenting with complete anuria will have severe, life-threatening acidosis with Kussmaul's breathing and depressed consciousness.

CAUSES

The causes of the metabolic acidosis is postulated to be due to:

- reduced renal excretion of fixed acids (fixed acids are produced from the hepatic metabolism of dietary protein), and acids produced during normal cell metabolism;
- reduced renal reabsorption of bicarbonate.

BIOCHEMICAL MARKERS

- Rise in plasma hydrogen ion concentration (and therefore a fall in the plasma pH below 7.4).
- Fall in plasma bicarbonate concentration.
- Increased anion gap.

Anion Gap

The anion gap is the difference between the concentration in the plasma of the cations sodium and potassium and the anions chloride and bicarbonate. The sum of the cations normally exceeds the anions by 10–18 mmol l⁻¹. This anion gap is made up by negatively charged proteins, phosphates and organic acids. The increase in the anion gap in uraemic metabolic acidosis to around 30 mmol l⁻¹ is postulated to be due to the accumulation of fixed acids.

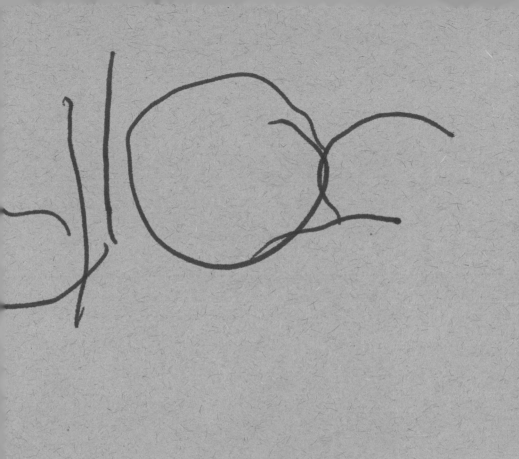

CLINICAL EFFECTS OF ACIDOSIS

Acute and Severe Acidosis, for Example as in Acute Renal Failure or Untreated End-Stage Renal Failure (ESRF):

- contributes to hyperkalaemia by causing a shift of cellular potassium into the extracellular fluid. This may cause fatal cardiac arrhythmias and is a medical emergency;
- leads to respiratory compensation by hyperventilation producing the classical Kussmaul's breathing;
- depresses the central nervous system causing coma;
- depresses the myocardium causing bradycardia and hypotension.

Treatment

Immediate dialysis with bicarbonate dialysate; emergency treatment of hyperkalaemia.

Chronic Acidosis, for Example as in Chronic Renal Failure:

- Excess hydrogen ions are buffered in the bone in exchange for calcium ions. This buffering process may be occurring long before a systemic acidosis is detectable, contributing to the development of renal bone disease.

Treatment

Restricted protein intake to reduce generation of fixed acids.

SPECIFIC NURSING ACTIONS

Severe acidosis is a medical emergency. The nurse must recognise the urgency of the situation and react calmly and promptly in the preparation and administration of prescribed medical treatment including the treatment of hyperkalaemia, the establishment of vascular access for dialysis and the administration of acute haemodialysis treatment.

Box 2.6 Anaemia of renal failure.

Anaemia is virtually a universal problem in patients with chronic and end-stage renal failure (ESRF). The only group of patients that may escape it or have a milder form are those with polycystic kidney disease. The severity of the anaemia is proportional to the severity of the renal failure and it is common to find patients with serum haemoglobin levels <8 g dl^{-1} (normal range 11.5–16.5 g dl^{-1}). The type of anaemia present is generally normachromic and normocytic but may be accompanied by iron deficiency leading to a hypochromic, microcytic picture.

CAUSES

Primary Cause

A reduction in the production of erythropoietin by the kidney, the reduction being proportional to the loss of kidney mass.

Contributing Causes

- Uraemic toxins – the presence of uraemic toxins reduces both red cell survival and the process of erythropoiesis.
- Nutritional deficiencies – iron, folate and vitamin B12 are needed for normal red cell production.
- Increased blood losses:

  (a) platelet dysfunction leads to an increased bleeding tendency;
  (b) some women may experience an increased menstrual loss;
  (c) small blood losses are inevitable on haemodialysis treatment;
  (d) repeated blood sampling.

TREATMENT

- Erythropoietin replacement therapy – regular injections (subcutaneous or intravenous) of human recombinant erythropoietin.
- Blood transfusions – given only when absolutely necessary as they expose the patient to several risks: viral transmission (hepatitis B or C, human immunodeficiency virus (HIV), cytomegalovirus (CMV), transfusion reactions and cytotoxic antibody production

(which may reduce the patient's chance of having a successful kidney transplant in the future).

- Iron and vitamin supplementation.
- Minimisation of blood loss.
- Reduction of uraemia by adequate dialysis.

SPECIFIC NURSING CONSIDERATIONS

The nurse can help reduce a patient's anaemia in the following ways:

- Patient education, including:

    (a) promoting the importance of taking a nutritional diet;
    (b) importance of compliance with vitamin supplementation;
    (c) providing an erythropoietin training programme.

- Dialysis:

    (a) ensure patient receives adequate dialysis to control uraemia;
    (b) minimise blood losses during haemodialysis treatment, e.g. through adequate washback, avoidance of dialysis accidents, e.g. disconnected lines, dislodged needles, etc.
    (c) avoidance of unnecessary blood sampling;
    (d) avoidance of over anticoagulation by accurate and regular measurements of clotting times.

SUMMARY

This chapter has attempted to unravel the complexities of this important organ. Having understood the many and varied functions of the kidney, the reader will appreciate the central importance of this organ to health. Since the normal functioning of the kidney has implications for every organ system in our bodies, then also its diseased state will have implications for every organ system in our bodies. Thus, renal failure cannot be considered to be purely a disease of the kidney, but a disease of our whole being, affecting us physically, mentally and socially. The following chapters in this book deal in detail with the ramifications of renal failure: its causes, presentation, care and treatment.

REFERENCES

GUYTON, A.C. (1991) *Textbook of Medical Physiology, 8th edn.* Philadelphia: W.B. Saunders Company.

LACOMBE, C., DA SILVA, J.L., BRENEVAL, P. *et al.* (1991) Erythropoietin: sites of synthesis and regulation of secretion. *American Journal of Kidney Diseases*, **18**(4 Suppl. 1): 14–19.

LAURENCE, D.R. AND BENNETT, P.N. (1987) *Clinical Pharmacology, 6th edn.* Edinburgh: Churchill Livingstone.

LOTE, C.J. (1987) *Principles of Renal Physiology, 2nd edn.* London: Croom Helm.

FURTHER READING

APBI Data Sheet Compendium 1994–1995 Datapharm Publications Ltd.

COTRAN, R.S., KUMAR, V. AND ROBBINS, S.L. (1994) *Robbins Pathological Basis of Disease 5th edn.* Philadelphia: W.B. Saunders Company.

GRAY, M. (1992) *Genitourinary Disorders.* St Louis: Mosby's Clinical Nursing Series.

GUYTON, A.C. (1991) *Textbook of Medical Physiology 8th edn.* Philadelphia: W.B. Saunders Company.

KUMAR, P.J. AND CLARK, M.L. (1987) *Clinical Medicine.* Eastbourne: Baillière Tindall.

LAURENCE, D.R. AND BENNETT, P.N. (1987) *Clinical Pharmacology 6th edn.* Edinburgh: Churchill Livingstone.

LEVINE, D.Z. (1991) *Care of the Renal Patient 2nd edn.* Philadelphia: W.B. Saunders Company.

LOTE, C.J. (1987) *Principles of Renal Physiology 2nd edn.* London: Croom Helm.

McGEE, J.O'D., ISAACSON, P.G. AND WRIGHT, N.A. (1992) *Oxford Textbook of Pathology – volume 2a Pathology of Systems.* Oxford: Oxford University Press.

SMITH, E. AND KINSEY, M. (1987) *Renal Disease – a Conceptual Approach.* New York: Churchill Livingstone.

WILLATS, S.M. (1984) *Lecture Notes on Fluid and Electrolyte Balance.* Oxford: Blackwell Scientific Publications.

CHAPTER 3

PSYCHOLOGICAL PERSPECTIVES

INTRODUCTION

Ever since dialysis and renal transplantation were introduced in the USA in the late 1950s and early 1960s, and in the UK in the mid-1960s, psychologists and psychiatrists have been involved in studying the impact of living on a life-support machine or with a donor kidney, and with the problems encountered by patients, their families and also the staff who support them over years of survival against the odds (Kaplan de Nour and Czackes, 1968; Abram, 1969; Abram, 1970; Abram *et al.*, 1971; Shambaugh and Kanter, 1969).

Much research has been done into psychological aspects of dialysis and the quality of life of these patients and numerous studies have been published by those most active in this field over the past 20 years, particularly Atara Kaplan de Nour, Roberta Simmons, Norman Levy, Howard Burton, Nancy Kutner and Roger Evans. As dialysis came to be offered to a wider age range in the 1980s, the adjustment of elderly patients has been studied by Westlie *et al.* (1984), Neu and Kjellstrand (1986), and Kline *et al.*, (1986) in North America, and by Auer (1986) and Quarello *et al.* (1992)

in Europe, concluding that there is no reason why there should be any age limit to treatment, and that many patients in their eighth and even ninth decade achieve good quality of life. In the past 10 years, as concern has grown over the seemingly limitless demands of the health-care budget, a number of studies have focused on cost–benefit aspects of quality of life on dialysis, and the need to ration resources (Williams, 1985; Gudex, 1986; Loomes and McKenzie, 1989). In the view of the health economist, dialysis is an expensive way to prolong a life that may lack quality by objective measures, such as vocational rehabilitation and functional capacity. These conclusions, however, raise questions about the validity of *objective* measures in an area that may be better approached from a *subjective* stance; that is, does the patient see his or her life on dialysis as worthwhile?

In the present chapter, a brief overview of some of the important findings is given, but chiefly attention is drawn to some of the everyday experiences of patients, gathered largely from working in a busy dialysis and transplant unit over a 15-year period. This may allow staff to recognise some of the patients' reactions and the reasons for them, and provide a practical insight useful to those working with patients and families.

Every aspect of life is affected by renal failure and its treatment, and the effects spread to all those closely involved with the patient. Greater understanding of the day-to-day stresses and concerns of patients allows staff in renal units to respond with appropriate support. This needs to begin as early as possible, to prevent problems, whether practical (as in employment or finances), or emotional (as in relationship problems and unnecessary fears about prognosis or treatment) (Bradley and McGee, 1994).

THE PREDIALYSIS PATIENT

Unfortunately, only about half of the patients who enter renal replacement programmes are followed in a predialysis clinic during the decline of their renal function towards end stage. The remaining patients present acutely in end-stage renal failure (ESRF), or in acute on chronic renal failure, previously undiagnosed, which progresses rapidly to end stage. Elderly patients (> 70 years) with acute renal failure are less likely to regain function than those < 70 years. Those patients who have time to adjust over a period of months, or even years, to the fact that dialysis and/or transplantation will become necessary, seem to adjust more smoothly to treatment.

Increasingly, units are using this time to good effect, by preparing patients for the transition from chronic renal failure to end-stage renal failure and the need for dialysis, not only medically but also psychologically and socially. Such predialysis education may even delay the need for dialysis (Binik *et al.*, 1993), perhaps as a result of promoting better compliance with antihypertensive medication.

The subjects that need to be addressed vary according to age and circumstances, but may include:

- the importance and purpose of *drugs* and *diet*;
- choosing the *treatment* best suited to the patient's social situation and lifestyle;
- problems with *employment* and *finances* due to the illness;
- problems with *housing*, taking treatment needs into consideration;
- *role changes* within relationships and *effects on family members/carers*;
- difficulties in *sexual and affectionate relationships* (Stout *et al.*, 1985);
- effect of ESRF on *leisure activities* and *holidays*.

In the case of younger patients, the effects can be far-reaching and devastating to contemplate, involving disruption of the overall life plan, including career prospects, marriage and having children. Older patients usually face less fundamental losses.

Predialysis and Pretransplant Groups

With few exceptions, the more information and preparation that can be provided, the better the patient is able to adjust (Bradley and McGee, 1994). This preparation also benefits the spouse or carer, who is often more worried than the patient, having not always had the benefit of talking to the doctor on clinic visits. Spouses are affected by the effects of the illness on the patient. These may include:

- lethargy and tiredness;
- inability to concentrate;
- irritability;
- apathy/depression or anxiety;
- reduced ability to show affection or sexual interest;
- withdrawal and lack of communication;
- constant complaints about symptoms such as itching, loss of appetite or breathlessness.

Spouses have frequently expressed frustration that symptoms are minimised or not reported to the medical team on clinic visits. Patients who are trying to come to terms with their own feelings often find it hard to spare extra energy to cope with the feelings of those close to them. They also feel guilty that the illness is affecting others, making it hard to relate to those they are 'letting down'. As a result, many spouses, who are facing the same worries about the future as the patient, feel unsupported and unappreciated.

Some units run predialysis and pretransplantation groups to assist both patients and their families during this period. In the author's renal unit, predialysis counselling was undertaken on an individual basis by the dietitian, social worker and nurses until the mid-1980s. This always included a visit to the patient's home by the social worker to assess which type of treatment was most likely to suit the individual's requirements. A social report was then prepared for medical and nursing staff, assessing the housing, way of life, employment, social supports, financial position and any particular strengths and weaknesses inherent in the patient's situation. Such factors are far better explored away from the hospital in the patient's own environment. Ideally, this would still be the practice in most cases, but the increase in workload in renal units, certainly in the UK, has made it impractical to visit all patients at home before the need for dialysis treatment.

The solution chosen in an increasing number of units is to invite patients and families to attend sessions where as much information and teaching as possible can be given, to the greatest number, in the most time- and cost-effective way. In some hospitals these groups are run by nursing staff, in others by the social worker. The most effective groups seem to be run on a multidisciplinary basis, with input from medical, nursing, dietetic and social work staff, and include teaching from established dialysis and transplant patients themselves (Bradley and McGee, 1994).

There are a number of different agendas and types of communication that can be used in an information group:

- *Straightforward teaching;* that is, information about the causes and effects of renal failure, and the methods of treatment – drugs, diet, and dialysis/transplantation.
- *Group support.*
- *Reassurance* – the dispelling of myths about renal failure and treatment, ensuring that the patient's concerns are realistic, focusing on the real problems rather than rumours or hearsay (e.g. a number of patients have asked whether it is true that one can only survive a short period on dialysis and can expect to die unless transplanted quickly).
- *Encouraging active participation in treatment*, by establishing a climate of co-operative interaction between patients and staff, rather than passive acceptance.
- *Introducing topics and encouraging questions*, especially on subjects that many patients feel inappropriate to raise with busy medical staff at clinic appointments. This gives validity to a number of concerns that patients and relatives may consider outside the scope of the unit, for example:

  (a) depression
  (b) anxiety
  (c) relationship difficulties
  (d) body image
  (e) sexuality.

Once these are placed on the agenda, patients feel able to approach staff for individual discussion if necessary.

In order to fulfil a number of these criteria at once, patients are taught partly by staff and partly by other patients, thus giving the role of 'patient' both status and an active and positive connotation. It also means that the information given has greater credibility, since it comes from someone who has first-hand experience. Questions to 'patient teachers' are often more freely expressed and wider ranging than those put to staff. The overall impression created is one of teamwork, with the patient as part of the team rather than the passive object of attention.

A continuous ambulatory peritoneal dialysis (CAPD) exchange may be demonstrated by a patient, using a minimum of special equipment (i.e. no special work surface, bag warmer or hospital drip stand), allowing a brief overview of what is involved from a technical point of view. This demonstration gives a clear message that the treatment is portable, flexible and does not require either a clinical setting or the 'safety' of home. It is also shown to be something that can be done without embarrassment in front of others. All these messages are relayed without even needing to be mentioned. Most of the demonstrators used are middle aged (50s plus), and are in employment, at least part time – again giving a positive image of the treatment. The demonstrator is often asked whether they 'skip a treatment from time to time' or break the rules – and they usually give a truthful answer in the affirmative, in spite of the presence of staff – again helping to set the atmosphere for honest and realistic interaction with members of the team.

The teaching session includes a visit to the haemodialysis unit, where predialysis patients and relatives are encouraged to talk to patients on dialysis. Many have not previously entered the unit, and most are relieved and pleasantly surprised to find that the treatment is neither painful nor terrifying. The message conveyed by seeing patients eating, reading, dozing, knitting or watching television during treatment is a powerful one, emphasising the normality that is possible under these circumstances rather than the clinical procedure itself. It is also reassuring for the predialysis patients to be told that only a small amount of blood is outside the body at any one time. They see a number of different types of dialysis access and haemodialysis machines, and can be introduced to patients preparing for home treatment. There is often animated discussion with those on treatment, and many practical questions are asked, diverting thoughts from the general dread of needing a life-support treatment towards the reality of coping effectively with the situation.

By presenting the options for treatment, patients feel involved in the choice of dialysis modality. In some cases there are strong medical arguments for the choice of one or other type of dialysis but patients should, nevertheless, feel that they have been presented with as much choice and information as possible. It is also empowering to patients to be given some control over a situation which has, in many ways, removed their options and self-determination – there can be few more limiting experiences than dependence on a life-support system. The patients who appear most successful, in the sense of making the most of a life that is being sustained against the odds, are those who maintain a sense of control over their treatment rather than being at the mercy of their situation. There is increase in confidence in patients encouraged to perform self-monitoring of weight and blood pressure rather than relying on staff. A sense of control over the situation should include the knowledge and ability to 'bend the rules' within safe limits from time to time, for example missing an occasional CAPD exchange in order to attend a special event or knowing how to over-step the dietary restrictions for a special occasion without risking hyperkalaemia or serious fluid overload. These well-considered events should not be considered as non-compliant behaviour; rather, as the exceptions that prove the rule. It can be hard for staff to encourage flexibility, fearing abuse of any latitude allowed; yet, as in parenting, it is important to encourage an attitude of sensible and responsible independence. Slavish adherence to limiting regimes is probably responsible for more problems and unhappiness than occasional, well-judged 'lapses'.

How much information?

The information presented at this type of meeting needs to cater for a mythical 'average' patient, neither giving unrealistically high expectations by presenting an exceptionally fit, active and well-adjusted patient as an example, nor offering the point of view of a very depressed and disabled patient.

It is useful for the predialysis patient to hear from somebody who has experienced problems with one type of dialysis and has subsequently done well on another. It is also beneficial to introduce a transplant patient who has experienced the failure of a first graft and has later had a successful one.

Honesty is an important part of the contract between the patient and the team, and for this reason the possible complications of treatments, such as CAPD peritonitis, hernias, leaks, need for resiting catheters, failure of a fistula to develop, or the side-effects of immunosuppression post-transplant, need to be openly discussed where appropriate. Staff are not helping or respecting patients if they are overprotective or overoptimistic about what they have to offer. Staff may use denial when interacting with patients – indeed the patient is likely to feel a 'failure' if staff present an idealised picture and he or she does not 'achieve' in line with expectations (Kaplan de Nour, 1983). It is, however, possible to be honest without being unduly negative, and to present a balanced picture of possible benefits and drawbacks.

The philosophy behind information groups is therefore to present a realistic but not over-detailed picture, which sets the scene for a co-operative and interactive relationship with the team. It is always stated that individual problems and questions can be discussed on a one-to-one basis with an appropriate member of staff following the session or in clinic. The timing of sessions is quite important, since an adjustment period of at least 6 months is desirable. This allows time for considerations such as:

- negotiating with employers to arrange changes in hours or duties that will fit the future demands of treatment;
- making adaptations to housing or moving house – this is especially important for elderly patients, who may wish to apply for sheltered accommodation or for a transfer to a bungalow or ground-floor flat (letters from the hospital can often expedite such arrangements in the UK);
- early application for relevant Social Security benefits (e.g. Disability Living Allowance) to minimise financial problems.

Although there is no hard and fast rule, it is usually appropriate to invite those with a creatinine of 400–500 μmol l^{-1}, and whose renal function is declining, to attend information groups.

Access Surgery

The reality of approaching dependence on dialysis is brought home to the patient by the creation of access. The anxious response to this admission for surgery can therefore seem out of proportion to the procedures themselves, which are comparatively trivial. Access is the medical preparation for imminent treatment. It is also therefore the appropriate time for final psychological preparation. During admission for access the patient can be given literature and information, talk to the dietitian about current and future nutrition and to the social worker or nurse counsellor about feelings, psychosocial, housing, employment, family or financial concerns. It is also a good time to discuss future leisure activities and holidays, because the patient is usually most aware of contracting horizons and limitations at this point, and needs to be reminded that the object of dialysis is to enable life to be lived and to provide life that is worth living, not simply to keep the patient alive to be dialysed.

To provide good psychological support and preparation involves spending time with patients and however good one's communication skills and intentions, there is seldom the chance to do all that one would like. In this situation there is sometimes the temptation to abandon even the attempt to talk to patients about their concerns, on the grounds that if it cannot be done 'properly' it is not worth doing at all. This is very far from the case. Excellent and sensitive counselling can often be given with two minutes of listening and responding to a particular worry, provided one remains aware of needs and fears, and able to pick up the cues provided. The creation of haemodialysis access is often a disfiguring experience for patients. Staff become so used to seeing neck lines, permcaths, shunts and fistulae that they can forget that these cause turned heads and curious glances outside the hospital. Women in particular are sensitive to the appearance of access sites, not because of greater vanity, but because their normal clothing is less likely to cover the arms, shoulders and neck than a man's shirt and jacket. Most patients will have seen the well-developed fistulae of long-standing haemodialysis patients at clinic visits, and these can be off-putting. Staff, particularly nursing staff, need to recognise the patient's feelings, advise on clothing, and help to make the lines and dressings as unobtrusive as possible.

Most haemodialysis access surgery is performed under local anaesthetic, and can take a long time. In spite of adequate premedication it can be an anxious and uncomfortable time for the patient, who may benefit from the presence of a familiar nurse to talk to during the procedure.

The Tenckhoff catheter in preparation for CAPD is less noticeable to the outside world but arouses many private concerns, mostly involving body-image and the reaction of the spouse or partner. Many patients fear that they will no longer be attractive to their partner, partly because of the catheter itself and partly because of abdominal distension which changes the figure. Some patients, aware of the problems of colostomies and ileostomies, fear that the catheter will have a detectable smell. Before the patient leaves hospital it is useful for the nurse to make sure that the partner has seen the exit site and understands about the dressing and taping of the catheter securely to the side, whether or not they will be involved in assisting with treatment. It should be possible to explain to the couple at this stage that CAPD need not interfere with sexual relations. Some nurses feel comfortable with addressing this subject, while others do not, particularly if the couple are old enough to be the nurse's parents. If possible, discussions touching on sexuality should be left to someone who is at ease with the topic, since reluctance or embarrassment is hard to disguise and easily transmitted to the patient.

THE PSYCHOLOGICAL IMPACT OF TREATMENT

Haemodialysis

From the earliest days of haemodialysis, it was noted that patients go through a recognizable series of stages following the start of treatment (Abram, 1970). These may overlap, or fluctuate, as with the stages of bereavement (Kubler Ross, 1970), but can usually be identified both by staff and the patients themselves.

First phase – euphoria

Initially there is usually a sense of relief, for several reasons. First, after months or years of waiting in a kind of limbo, the hurdle of dialysis has been reached and cleared. Second, the patient may feel the benefit of treatment immediately, especially if uraemia was symptomatic causing nausea and itching or if breathlessness from pulmonary oedema was a problem. Third, the experience of haemodialysis is usually less traumatic than the patient had expected.

Second phase – depressive reaction

The second stage follows fairly quickly. The novelty of treatment wears off, the limitations, frustrations and the time involved begin to take their toll and the realisation that this situation will continue indefinitely starts to sap the patient's reserves of endurance. In addition, although no longer frankly uraemic, the patient is aware that dialysis cannot make him or her feel fully well. Tiredness, lack of energy and enthusiasm for life, irritability, poor sleep and low-grade depression make life on dialysis hard to tolerate, especially for those who expected to feel 'miraculously' better. The partner and family are also likely to feel the strain and relationships may suffer. The effort of trying to continue with work while under these pressures may seem to be too much, and the patient doubts whether employment will be possible, and fears the financial and family consequences if work has to be abandoned. Those who had been full of determination not to let dialysis affect or interfere with their lives, have to concede defeat – it is not possible to remain unaffected. This stage may last weeks or months, and needs to be handled with tolerance and understanding by all staff.

Third phase – realistic adjustment

If adjustment goes to plan, the patient gradually accepts the inevitable limitations, while making the most of the remaining possibilities. Hobbies, habits and roles at home may have to change. Alternative sources of satisfaction and enjoyment need to be discovered and exploited, but all this takes time and may need to be actively encouraged by staff. In the interim, support and consistency from the team provide the framework within which the patient learns to come to terms with a changed lifestyle.

It is not surprising that during this period of adjustment the patient may be low in mood, irritable, quick to take offence and sometimes uncompliant. It is easy for staff to find this unattractive and 'ungrateful', especially when dialysis is a scarce and expensive resource, and staff are themselves highly pressurised and doing their best. Most patients do not find the dialysis itself a difficult ordeal, unless there are persistent problems with access or cramps, or frequent battles over excessive interdialytic weight gain. The factors most likely to produce irritation are delays, especially caused by the transport system or machines not being ready, changes of schedule due to pressures on dialysis places, and the unpredictability of minor setbacks such as access problems. The time involved in the whole process becomes a central focus for many patients, who resent the amount of their life now dedicated to dialysis, in spite of the fact that it is dialysis that is making life possible at all. Some frustration is directed at staff, but patients are usually anxious not to alienate those who are caring for them, and to be 'good'. As a result, the spouse and family may take the brunt of the negative feelings and often lament that the patient claims that all is well on hospital visits, yet complains of numerous physical problems at home (Auer, 1990b).

This pattern of reaction in the early months of haemodialysis applies to all age groups, but the negative effects are undoubtedly felt more by younger patients, who find the constraints more burdensome. It is normal for people in their twenties and thirties to be fully occupied with jobs, courtship and marriage, families and the fulfilment of ambitions. For the young renal patient, life had lain ahead of them, and that life plan has been brutally altered without the provision of an acceptable alternative. The only chance of re-establishing the course of events lies in the uncertain hope of receiving a good transplant. Sadly, this is not a planned event with a time scale within which to work (unless a living related donor is contemplated). Life for most of the young patients is therefore perceived as being 'on hold', and the longer the wait for a transplant the more frustrated and down-hearted they can become.

The young patient   Many young patients find it hard to make relationships with the opposite sex, feeling that they have little to offer a prospective partner, and those who have a boy or girlfriend often find their fears justified, when relationships break up under the strain of the situation. Research such as the Oxford–Manchester study (Auer, 1990a) suggests that the younger patient and particularly the young male, finds dependence on dialysis particularly frustrating, perhaps because society expects the male to be more active, aggressive and ambitious in forging a role in life. It is certainly evident to those working in renal units that young male patients express more dissatisfaction, and are more likely to show this in non-compliant, self-destructive and despairing behaviour.

The middle-aged patient   Middle-aged patients have usually established a role for themselves, and have achieved a number of their goals, such as marriage, family, a career and a home. From this base they are often, but not always, better able to adjust to limitations. For them, however, there is the fear of losing what has been achieved, and being unable to carry out responsibilities to those who depend on them. Role changes within the family threaten the identity, pride and self-image of the patient, who does not wish to become a burden or liability. It is, however, comparatively rare for well-established relationships to break up in these circumstances. There is a taboo against leaving a sick partner that holds many couples together even in the most difficult situations. Marriages are, however, put under pressure, especially when sexual contact becomes diminished or non-existent.

The elderly patient   Reasonably fit elderly patients are in some ways the most satisfied group (Westlie et al., 1984; Auer, 1986). The attitude of many elderly patients is that they have already 'had a good life' and have reached an age when death would not be unlikely in any case. They have not been cheated of a normal lifespan by their illness. To be given the chance of a further few years due to dialysis is a bonus to those who still have an appetite for life. Those in their seventies and eighties probably do not want to pursue very strenuous activities, preferring a little gardening, cooking and the company of friends and family. Those who live alone and feel isolated regard the trips to the hospital for treatment as a welcome social activity. A number who have never had help with daily living – home adaptations and home help or meals from Social Services – receive this for the first time following contact with the hospital.

Withdrawal from Dialysis

Other elderly patients, however, may be very poorly adjusted to life on treatment, sometimes due to depression following bereavement or experiencing additional medical problems such as stroke, malignancies, amputations and ischaemic heart disease, which further restrict their quality of life. Such patients may wish to withdraw from dialysis, a subject that needs sympathetic exploration. If found to be a considered and serious wish rather than an expression of frustration or an oblique request for a particular problem to be recognised, such requests to withdraw from treatment should be supported and respected. Dialysis may prove to be an intolerable burden to those who have other reasons to feel that life no longer offers any opportunities and satisfactions. Some bitterly resent the limitations of the ageing process, cannot adjust to being a 'spectator' and wish only to turn back the clock. In a minority of cases, it is overwhelmingly the *fear of dying rather than a wish to live* that makes the patient continue with dialysis, making it hard to achieve any real life satisfaction.

It is common for renal unit staff to feel that the treatment of very frail elderly people, especially those with multiple medical problems, by means of a scarce and expensive resource such as hospital haemodialysis, is unjustified. If little or no subjective quality of life results, it would be hard to disagree. It is very important that we explore the attitudes of elderly patients, and do not carry on with treatment which is giving no quality of life, remembering, however, that quality of life is a subjective matter, and only the person concerned can tell whether life is worth living. One can be surprised both by the apparently full life which is unacceptable to one patient, and by the apparently burdensome life which is regarded as worthwhile by another. Respecting these views can be difficult, especially in the case of the patient who seems to have a good life, yet wishes to discontinue treatment. Kaplan De Nour concludes that the answer to the question 'Is it all worth the effort – is machine-dependent life worth living?' lies in the psychological condition of the patient rather than any objective quality of life (Kaplan De Nour, 1995).

Home Haemodialysis

A number of patients, especially those for whom an early transplant is unlikely and who wish to continue full-time work, opt to perform haemodialysis at home. Although the numbers entering home haemodialysis programmes are declining overall, this is still a good option for those who have strong motivation and good reasons for wanting the flexibility of this type of dialysis. It is rarely the best treatment for very frail elderly patients, especially if assisted by an elderly spouse who may find the treatment stressful to learn and to supervise. From the psychological point of view, it is essential to offer good back-up to home patients, including respite treatment in hospital to give the spouse or assistant a break from time to time. It is also advisable, wherever possible, to ensure that at least two home assistants are available in case one is ill or wishes to be away at a certain time. As was stated earlier, patients may be far more negative and demanding towards family members than is evident in the unit, and one should not therefore underestimate the burden that the spouse may be carrying.

CAPD

The individual and the intensive training needed to prepare a patient to perform CAPD safely at home allows the formation of a strong supportive bond with the nurse, probably a closer relationship than that formed in the haemodialysis unit. In a recent survey of 65 patients (33 on CAPD and 32 on haemodialysis (HD) who started treatment in the last year in the author's unit, the question 'Do you feel that you receive enough information about your treatment?' received a 'Yes' from 94% of CAPD patients and 69% of HD patients. Similarly, the question 'Do you feel you receive enough support?' received a 'Yes' from 85% of CAPD patients and only 63% of HD patients. This probably reflects good initial contacts with CAPD staff, and a sense of continued support via phone calls to the unit whenever required. This 'accessibility' of the CAPD nurse is important, because patients discharged home on CAPD might otherwise feel more isolated and unsupported by the unit than those attending for regular HD. Visits from a home CAPD nurse are a regular procedure in some units, and are much appreciated by patients and spouses. At the very least, a visit to the patient's home is desirable before CAPD treatment starts. The equipment takes up a lot of space, and it may be impossible to store a month's supply of fluids at a time. Such initial assessment visits should ideally be made by the social worker, occupational therapist, and a CAPD nurse or community renal nurse together, so that advice can be given on performing exchanges, possible adaptions to the home if needed and any community support that may be available.

CAPD training

The greatest dilemma in teaching the techniques of CAPD is to strike a balance between promoting a consistent, safe and meticulous technique, while encouraging enough flexibility and latitude to enable the patient to explore the potential for freedom that the treatment allows. Younger patients who opt for CAPD in order to carry on with full-time employment are likely to use the possibilities fully, after a short period of 'feeling their way'. Most take holidays away from home, go away for weekends, and can tell stories of unlikely places in which they have successfully performed an exchange. It is harder to encourage elderly patients to do the same. Many feel that it is unsafe to attempt an exchange in unfamiliar surroundings and develop an almost superstitious fear of altering the circumstances of the exchange in any way. Some say that performing the four daily exchanges has become a way of life in itself rather than a means to an end. Patients who are doing well on CAPD and making the treatment work for them, may show this by devising compact travelling exchange kits, with ingenious ways of warming and hanging the bags, and portable surfaces that can be kept clean, such as a large plastic table mat. Such patients will be proud to show staff how they have found ways of solving problems. They also display confidence in the way they dress, finding flattering but convenient clothing, and taking trouble with grooming. In contrast, the patient who is doing less well and may benefit from advice and counselling takes little pride in appearance, seldom or never travels with the treatment, and becomes house bound and isolated. Extrovert characteristics seem to be a great benefit, since such patients are not too shy or inhibited to perform exchanges in places where they may be seen by others. A few patients are so shy that they would rather not be seen dialysing even by family members, particularly children and grandchildren. Because they regard the exchange as an excretory function (which is, in many respects, true) they feel that it should be performed in private. (The HD patient does not see the treatment as excretory, even though the same process of waste removal is taking place.) The CAPD nurse who is

sensitive to signs of good or poor adjustment to treatment is able to reinforce and encourage sensible and flexible use of this type of dialysis.

NON-COMPLIANCE

Few patients take all the advice that is given by medical and nursing staff
or follow instructions *all the time*. This probably represents a healthy and
adaptive sign rather than otherwise, unless, of course, patients put themselves at serious risk. Renal patients have little chance of disguising gross
non-compliance, because blood results, blood pressure and weight gain
reveal underdialysis and diet and fluid abuses, as well as failure to take
medication.

Within reason, such non-compliance may be a good sign. However, persistent non-compliance to a dangerous level, often for no discernible reason,
is cause for serious investigation. The commonest causes appear to be:

- Depression – apathy about treatment and life in general.
- A reckless sense of defiance which seems to indicate that since life is
  barely tolerable it really does not matter greatly if one takes risks with
  it.
- Denial. Underlying denial there is often desperation. The patient is
  aware of the reality of the situation but cannot bear to face it squarely.
  Acting as if the painful situation does not exist enables the patient to
  maintain a fantasy that is bearable. Denial is not always dysfunctional.
  It can be a useful coping mechanism. Dying patients, for example, who
  maintain hope and act as if life is going to carry on, may make things
  easier for themselves (and those around them) but denial becomes a
  threat if it leads to dangerous non-compliance.

The depressive reaction is most commonly seen in older patients and
defiance and denial are usually seen in younger patients. All these reactions
seem to be indirect appeals for help and need to be treated as such. Anger
from staff, threats of dire consequences, or lectures on the behaviour
expected of a dialysis patient are unlikely to be helpful. Naturally, patients
need to be given a clear explanation of the reasons for the rules that are
set, and the possible results and risks that they run in choosing to break
those rules, but they also need to have their underlying motives and feelings
explored and respected. Some of the causes for distress may be alleviated
by counselling, changes in medication, adjustment of dialysis regime or
other measures.

SPECIAL PROBLEMS OF PATIENTS FROM ETHNIC MINORITIES

In order to allow patients from cultural backgrounds other than the UK to obtain equal benefits from the health-care system, it is important to be aware of factors which could affect the situation. These include:

- language and understanding
- dietary differences
- attitudes to illness
- family relationships.

It is difficult enough for members of the multidisciplinary team to communicate fully and effectively with those of the same cultural background and language, let alone those who have language problems and different cultural concepts. It is necessary to remain sensitive to the effects of ethnicity, both on understanding and attitudes to illness and treatment (Allison *et al.*, 1983).

Language

The most obvious of these is language. Elderly Indian, Pakistani and Chinese patients, for example, often rely on younger family members for the translation of interviews with medical and nursing staff, and to relay information on symptoms and feelings. Medical advice and information are also given via a third party and may suffer in translation. It is advisable to have a qualified interpreter for any sensitive and important communication, since family members may be too involved to give an impartial and accurate interpretation, relaying nuances of meaning.

All patient information material needs to be available in translation, but it is necessary to check reading ability rather than assuming that by giving a leaflet one has imparted the information.

Diet

Diet, which plays a major role in the management of renal disease, can be a source of considerable problems. Most renal diets are based on native UK eating habits, and are hard to adjust to the religious and cultural requirements of other countries. Many Asian patients prefer to have food brought in by the family during hospital admissions. Vegetarian CAPD patients, who have a greater need to maintain adequate protein intake, sometimes find it hard to do so when pulses are their major source of dietary protein. Specialist dietetic advice is necessary to achieve good serum albumin levels in such diets (see Chapter 9).

Attitudes to Illness

It is usual for Asian families to take a major part in the everyday care of a sick family member (whether at home or in hospital), and for a number of relatives, both young and old, to spend a lot of time at the bedside. Staff used to the less involved attitude of many native UK families may find this unusual or inconvenient, especially if there is a lack of space and facilities on the ward.

Attitudes to illness, and even the conceptual understanding of disease and treatment, may differ from culture to culture, needing the sensitive understanding of the nurse. Cause and effect may be differently perceived. Religious acceptance of illness as a predestined fate to be accepted without attempts to change matters, is a further concept that may cause misunderstandings. Culturally acceptable responses to illness may also differ from country to country. An Asian patient will often cover the whole body including the head, with a blanket, making some staff and other patients uneasy and puzzled. Accepted responses to pain may also differ from one ethnic group to another, leading to an over or under estimation of the subjective suffering involved.

Transplantation will be covered in another chapter, but it should be mentioned here that some ethnic groups may have religious or cultural problems in the concept of either a cadaver or living related graft. Even if these problems do not apply, the likelihood of a well-matched graft is reduced for patients from an ethnic minority, whose tissue type may be uncommon in the UK. It is important that all members of the team remain sensitive to both the needs of the patient and to their own attitudes.

Family Relationships

The family structure and hierarchy should also be taken into account, since some cultures regard any major decision as traditionally the preserve of the senior male member of the family present, leading to an unwillingness on the part of a female patient to determine her own preference or accept responsibility without consultation with a husband, father, uncle or son.

It can be difficult to understand Asian family structure and relationships, since in many families, anyone with a family connection tends to be designated 'a cousin', even, in some cases, where there is no relationship. (In native UK culture the same pattern leads us to call close family friends 'uncles' and 'aunties', without explaining that the title is 'honorary'.) Many patients have relatives, including spouses, in their country of origin and like to visit them every few years. It can therefore be very traumatic to have an illness which precludes travel due to lack of medical facilities at home. If elderly parents die, and the patient is unable to return for the funeral, there can be great distress, not only because of the natural pain of bereavement, but religious implications of duty and respect which carry greater significance than in Western culture.

TRANSPLANTATION

From what has already been said about the stresses of life on dialysis, it is obvious that, for many patients, dialysis is a period of 'marking time' while awaiting transplantation. Almost every study of quality of life so far has shown that successful transplantation offers the best chance of leading a near normal life, and is associated with the highest perceived life satisfaction. Objectively, the quality (although, contrary to the belief of some patients, not the quantity) of life, is greatly increased. Successful transplantation is associated with a number of benefits including:

- highcr chance of employment
- greater energy
- improved mental alertness and concentration
- freedom from a restrictive diet
- the return, in most cases, of sexual capacity
- the possibility of child-bearing.

It would, however, be misleading to regard even successful transplantation as a panacea. Following transplantation, the patient with ESRF *needs* to feel that life is wonderful. A successful transplant is, after all, the nearest to normality that the patient will ever achieve, and has often been the long-awaited 'answer' to the patient's problems, so from a psychological point of view the patient has a need to feel that life has been transformed. The reality is sometimes rather different. Those who want to return to employment find that although declared fit by the doctor, the view of prospective employers is less enthusiastic. Many find it hard to get a job in competition with others. Financially, the position is therefore worse than on dialysis, because, in the UK, DSS disability benefits are often withdrawn, and the patient can only claim basic unemployment benefit. Relationships sometimes become strained, because less tolerance is now shown by spouses and families. The dialysis patient has every right to claim that life is a burden, but gradually and subtly, sympathy is withdrawn from the transplant patient, who should after all be 'grateful for the gift of life' which, whether this is actually stated or not, is seen to have been won at the cost of the death of a cadaveric donor, or through the sacrifice of a living relative. This can be a hard gift to accept, carrying with it a burden of responsibility to make the suffering of others worthwhile. Patients who lose their grafts quite often feel that they have let down not only the team caring for them, but also the donor and donor family.

Immediately post-transplant, provided all goes well, there is usually a euphoric phase, possibly accentuated by steroid immunosuppression, and the sudden 'clearing of the mind' reported by many patients, which has never been fully explained. This is mixed with anxiety that rejection will occur and the graft will be lost. One of the hardest aspects of this stage is the sudden removal of conscious control. The dialysis patient has been conditioned to be very much in control of his or her health through adherence to diet and fluid restrictions, a regular treatment regime, scrupulous care of access and weight and blood pressure measurement. After a transplant, the situation changes dramatically. Apart from regularly taking immunosuppressive medication and attending for follow-up, patients' contribution to the survival of the graft is minimal. They are, as it were, at the mercy of factors beyond conscious control – their own immune response and the effects of the foreign body which now needs to become accepted as part of the self. It is no wonder that many patients become acutely superstitious (the natural human response to forces that cannot be influenced by reason or action). Anxiety can reach almost obsessional levels, and may become displaced from the transplant itself to attach to other health concerns.

The side-effects of immunosuppression may cause little distress, but in some patients have a considerable psychological effect, and, in a very few, produce a psychotic response. The commonest effects are upon body image. Cushingoid changes in the appearance are distressing to both sexes. Facial hair and changes in hair texture are more distressing to women, although the lower levels of drugs now prescribed since the use of Cyclosporin A have made this less evident. Many men choose to grow a beard following transplant, chiefly to disguise the 'moon face'. Weight gain as a result of appetite increase on steroids compounds the body-image problem. Cyclosporin has many advantages as an immunosuppressive agent, but patients can be very distressed by the tremor sometimes associated with this drug.

A good counselling programme should be provided, including access to advice on facial hair removal, treatment for changes in skin texture and advice on skin care to help avoid malignant changes stimulated by exposure to sun. The creation of a positive body image after transplantation is every bit as important as on dialysis.

Counselling may also be needed to help with emotional oversensitivity at this time. Both male and female patients who regarded themselves as previously emotionally controlled are sometimes surprised to find themselves liable to tearful episodes and mood swings, partly due to the drugs and partly due to the very considerable inner turmoil created by the experience of transplantation. The need for sympathetic reassurance and support from the transplant team in the early stages cannot be overestimated.

It is comparatively common for young women who are keen to have children to become pregnant soon after having a transplant. Often they are unmarried and unsupported. It seems that the desire to have a baby over-rides all other considerations for these women and that rational arguments and advice are unlikely to have any part to play against such an imperative. Fear of losing the graft, damaging their own health, risking stillbirth or a seriously premature child, let alone the problems of trying to care for a baby without the security of a permanent relationship, seem completely unimportant. Grafts can be lost due to the strain of pregnancy, especially when undertaken less than a year after transplantation. While it is essential to counsel young women on the risks, advise on birth control and advocate a reasonable delay before becoming pregnant, it seems unlikely that this will prevent some of them from seizing what they see as their only chance of having a child, regardless of the consequences. It is a further way of ratifying their 'normality' following the very artificial and restricted life on dialysis. In the few cases where termination is performed, the feelings of ambivalence are likely to be severe, and may even be directed against the graft itself, whose survival has been protected at the expense of the child.

Graft Loss

The patient whose graft is rapidly rejected experiences an acute disappointment, but is in many ways better able to recover and come to terms than the patient who has several months of unsatisfactory graft function before finally returning to dialysis. In such cases there may have been heavy courses of methyl prednisolone or monoclonal antibodies, numerous biopsies and possibly further surgery to no avail, resulting in a state of physical debility and mental anguish far worse than before the operation. Such patients often say at the time that they regret ever having tried transplantation, yet the great majority return to the transplant list within a few months.

PATIENTS WITH MULTIPLE PATHOLOGY

There are increasing numbers of patients now receiving dialysis for whom renal failure is the most treatable aspect of a serious systemic illness, such as diabetes, scleroderma, primary amyloid or myeloma. A further large patient group consists of those with generalised vascular disease. The complications of these underlying conditions are responsible for many long hospital admissions and a great deal of the morbidity and mortality of patients on dialysis programmes.

The patient with diabetes can be particularly hard to counsel and distressing to nurse. As the disease reaches its late phases, one has no sooner supported a patient through the loss of one limb, when the next becomes problematic. Eyesight may already have been poor, only to be followed by total blindness. Autonomic neuropathy may then lead to diar-rhoea and incontinence, and inability to maintain blood pressure when changing position.

As with all patients on renal replacement therapy, there are two impor-tant aspects for nursing and other staff to consider: the psychological impact of the illness and the practical arrangements that may be necessary to enable the patient to spend time at home. Patients who are aware that their underlying condition is fatal, and that dialysis is a means of prolonging life in the short term, need every help to spend as little time in hospital as possible. This entails involving community nursing, occupational ther-apists, physiotherapists and care managers from Social Services to provide a 'package' of care. This may involve visits from home care staff several times a day, the provision of meals, day centre attendance, respite care in nursing homes and the provision of equipment such as stair lifts, rails and ramps for wheelchair access.

There is occasionally some conflict with community nurses and carers, who express the opinion that the patient is not well enough to be out of hospital, and that it is 'too risky' for the patient to be at home. In their opinion the patient might fall, sustain fractures, succumb to a massive haemorrhage, or a cardiovascular crisis or have some other medical emer-gency. This is, of course, true, but the philosophy of renal units can be at odds with the 'normal' world. Our patients would all have perished without renal replacement. They are alive against the odds, and for them, a degree of risk is an acceptable price to pay for seizing the chance to experience life outside the hospital. A more lengthy admission is unlikely to reduce the chance of sudden and maybe fatal complications. If a patient is happy to take that risk, he or she needs our support.

The strain on spouses and family members is considerable. Many will have jobs and family responsibilities, and may feel guilty if they do not put the patient's needs above their own. Support needs to be given to relatives in this situation, to reduce guilt wherever possible. This entails allowing opportunities for the expression of feelings and encouraging rela-tives to set aside time for themselves. Some will, for example, visit daily from long distances during the patient's admissions to hospital – a time when there is the chance for carers to recharge their own batteries, take much-needed relaxation or catch up with other tasks. This is also a time when unfinished business may need to be resolved. This may be in the form of reconciling old family differences and feuds to secure the future for those who will be left when the patient has died. Another aspect of this may be the desire of common-law partners to marry.

Staff need to be aware of the patient's state of mind, and ready to hear the message that the patient has had enough. It is not unreasonable to choose death from uraemia in preference to a short period of further suffering before succumbing to a more distressing end to life. Some, it is true, are never able to let go, but others may wish to do so while they are still capable of determining their own destiny through rational decision. It may, however, be hard to express this to staff who are unwilling to hear.

Acute Renal Failure and Acute Presentation in ERSF

Providing support

Patients with acute renal failure often come to the renal ward via intensive therapy units, following overwhelming illnesses. Illness severe enough to cause acute renal failure requiring dialysis or haemofiltration is always a crisis for patient and relatives, attended by high levels of anxiety. This is justified, since the mortality in such patients is very high. Once the precipitating illness is controlled and the patient's condition is stable, concern is transferred to the renal failure, and whether the kidneys will recover. During this period, patient and relatives often need emotional support from staff, and reassurance that renal function is expected to return in spite of the need for dialysis over several weeks. From the psychological point of view, it is important to help the spouse to visit as often as possible, both for the sake of the patient and the partner. It is always recognised that children need a parent to be with them, and that recovery is helped by the security this offers. It is seldom realised how lonely and frightened an adult, especially if elderly, can become when seriously ill and separated from their partner and environment.

The patient is often admitted to a unit many miles from home, making visiting expensive. Help with transport costs should be sought from the DSS or charitable funding if hardship is suspected. It is not uncommon for the family of a critically ill patient, admitted for 3–4 weeks, to incur £300–400 in visiting. Staff need to explore the possibilities for inexpensive accommodation in or near the hospital for relatives of such patients. When the patient is finally ready to leave hospital, it is important for a care manager to assess the home circumstances, since the illness may have had permanent debilitating effects. Preparation for this may help to mitigate the emotional blow of returning home, and finding that while home is the same as ever, the person who left it a few weeks ago has changed. Following leg amputations, patients may show a reluctance to go on a visit home to assess future ability to cope. The 'safe and familiar place' has lost its ability to reassure, because it now contains challenges and hazards. Sensitivity, honesty and understanding are needed to build the confidence of someone who feels, rightly, that they will 'never be the same again'.

SUMMARY

The care of renal patients is a highly specialised area of nursing, with unique satisfactions and unique stresses. There is no other field of hospital nursing that involves such intensive involvement with patients over such long periods. High technology may appear to predominate but in spite of, or because of, the dependence of the patient on complicated artificial life-support systems, it is the quality of the human relationships created between the patient and the professional team that determines the success of the whole undertaking. Clinical skills are not enough to give the patient on dialysis the chance to live to the best potential. The commitment of both patient and team is, quite simply, lifelong. As a result, it is an unusually close relationship with all the benefits and disadvantages that this implies. Those who work in renal units have in common a sense of belonging to an extended family group. This is not to say that they are free of conflict, stresses and frustration – rather the reverse. Staff as well as patients need support, and many units recognise this and have good support systems, some formal, some informal.

It is not possible for the renal nurse to avoid a degree of personal involvement. Total detachment from a patient with whom the fight for survival is shared over months, years or even decades is scarcely a realistic proposition. Hospital staff cannot help but admire the tenacity and courage of patients and their spouses, feel frustrated by them and for them, experience anger, exhausted patience, great sadness at battles lost and great happiness at battles won.

REFERENCES

ABRAM, H.S. (1969) The psychiatrist, the treatment of chronic renal failure and the prolongation of life. *Am. J. Psychiat.*, **126**: 57.

ABRAM, H.S. (1970) Survival by machine: the psychological stress of chronic haemodialysis. *Psychiat. Med.*, **1**: 37.

ABRAM, H.S., MOORE, G.L. AND WESTEVELT, F.B. (1971) Suicidal behaviour in chronic dialysis patients. *Am. J. Psychiat.*, **127**: 1199–204.

ALLISON, M., GREGG, D., RANDELL, E., STOUT, J.P. AND WILCOCK D. (1983) *Social work with patients suffering from kidney disease and with their families.* British Association of Social Workers, Birmingham.

AUER, J. (1986) Psychological aspects of elderly renal patients. In *Aspects of Renal Care*, Vol. 1 (eds E. Stevens and P. Monkhouse). Baillière Tindall, Eastbourne.

AUER, J. (1990a) The Oxford–Manchester study of dialysis patients: age, risk factors and treatment method in relation to quality of life. *Scand. J. Urol. Nephrol.*, **131**(Suppl.): 31–7.

AUER, J. (1990b) Psychological problems in chronic illness. In *Social Work*

Practice in Health Care (eds M. Badawi and B. Biamonti). Woodhead Faulkner, Cambridge.

BINIK, Y.M., DEVINS, G.M., BARRE, P.E. *et al.* (1993) Live and learn: patient education delays the need to initiate renal replacement therapy in end stage renal disease. *J. Nerv. Ment. Dis.*, **181**: 371–6.

BRADLEY, C. AND MCGEE, H. (eds) (1994) Improving quality of life in renal failure: ways forward. In *Quality of Life Following Renal Failure* (eds H. McGee and C. Bradley). Chur: Harwood Academic Publishers.

GUDEX, C. (1986) *QALYs and their use by the Health Services.* Discussion Paper 20, University of York Centre for Health Economics, York.

KAPLAN DE NOUR, A. (1983) Staff–patient interactions. In *Psychonephrology,* Vol. 2 (ed. N.B. Levy). Plenum, New York.

KAPLAN DE NOUR, A. (1995) Psychological social and vocational impact of renal failure. In *Quality of Life Following Renal Failure* (eds H. McGee and C. Bradley). Chur: Harwood Academic Publications.

KAPLAN DE NOUR, A. AND CZACKES, J.W. (1968) Emotional problems and reactions of the medical team in a chronic hemodialysis unit. *Lancet,* **ii**: 987.

KLINE, S.A., BURTON, H.J. AND AKHTAR, M. (1986) The elderly patient on dialysis – psychosocial considerations. In *Geriatric Nephrology* (ed. D.G. Oreopoulos). Nijhoff, Boston.

KUBLER ROSS, E. (1970) *On Death and Dying.* Tavistock, London.

LOOMES, G. AND MCKENZIE, L. (1989) The use of QALYs in health care decision making. *Social Science and Medicine,* **28**: 299–308.

NEU, S. AND KJELLSTRAND, C.M. (1986) Stopping long-term dialysis. *N. Engl. J. Med.,* **314**: 14–20.

QUARELLO, F., PICCOLI, G.B., BONELLO, F. *et al.* (1992) Dialysis in the elderly: ten year experience in a large population. *Geriatric Nephrology and Urology,* **2**: 190–1.

SHAMBAUGH, P. AND KANTER, S. (1969) Spouses under stress: group meetings with spouses of patients on haemodialysis. *Am. J. Psychiatry,* **125**: 7.

STOUT, J.P., AUER, J. AND KINCEY, J. (1985) Sexual and marital relationships and dialysis patients. *Perit. Dial. Bulletin,* **7**: 97–9.

WESTLIE, L., UMEN, A., NESTRUD, S. AND KJELLSTRAND, C.M. (1984) Mortality, morbidity and life satisfaction in the very old dialysis patient. *Trans. Am. Soc. Art. Int. Organs,* **30**: 21–31.

WILLIAMS, A. (1985) Economics of coronary artery bypass grafting. *Br. Med. J.,* **291**: 326–9.

CHAPTER 4

ACUTE RENAL FAILURE

INTRODUCTION

The delivery of care for the patient in acute renal failure (ARF) presents a diversity of problems for the nurse responsible for the care. Despite the availiability of various dialysis treatments and different drug therapy, these patients face a mortality rate of anything up to 50%. For those patients who are critically ill, the mortality rate is even greater.

ARF has often been defined as a sudden deterioration in renal function that results in the inability to excrete the products of metabolism that produces a rise in blood urea and other nitrogen waste products (Toto, 1992). Depending on its severity and duration, ARF is often transient in its nature and with careful nursing care the patient can regain normal renal function. However, without the appropriate specialised treatment the patient may be denied the opportunity to make a full recovery and a precipitation of further impairment may lead to chronic or end-stage renal failure (ESRF).

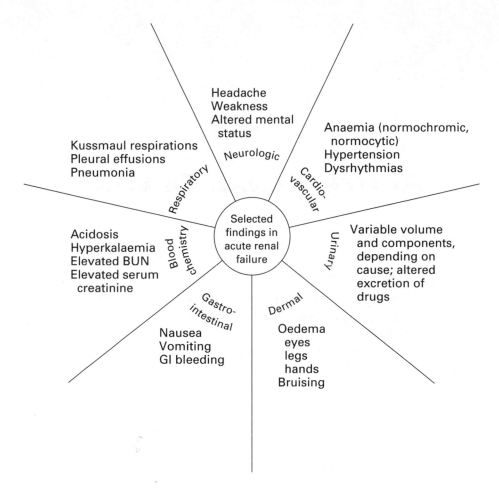

Fig. 4.1 *Signs and symptoms of acute renal failure. BUN, blood urea nitrogen; GI, gastrointestinal. From Brundage D, Renal Disorders. (1992) Mosby Clinical Nurse Series, with permission.*

The aim of this chapter is to emphasise the vital role the nurse plays in the delivery of care for the patient in ARF. The importance of the nurse/patient relationship is vital to the well-being of the patient whereby the nurse can monitor the patient for complications, participate in emergency treatment of fluid and electrolyte balance, assess the patient's progress and response to treatment, and provide physical and emotional support. In this central role the nurse can maintain close links with the patient's family which can be instrumental to a family-centred approach to the patient's treatment. The alliance between the patient, the family and the nurse is paramount in keeping the family informed of the patient's condition, assisting them to understand treatments and to provide psychological support (Fig. 4.1).

MORTALITY

It is essential for nurses to appreciate that ARF is a serious condition, that its mortality rate is still unacceptably high and that the prognosis may vary with the cause and extent of renal failure. Deaths are much more common in patients whose age exceeds 60 years. The lowest rates (10–20% mortality) are reported in renal failure complicating pregnancy or abortion. Results in surgical renal failure, including transfusion reactions, are appreciably worse (50–60% mortality). Death, when tubular necrosis is caused by burns or extensive trauma, is expected in 70% of patients (Ledingham, 1987). The outcome for each individual patient is often unpredictable and, despite new drugs and the availability of dialysis, around 5% of hospitalised patients will face a mortality rate of around 50% (Spiegel, 1991). Stott *et al.* (1972) suggest that the continuing high mortality from ARF is due to changes in both causes and patient mix which may have masked significant improvements in the management of severely ill patients. However, this may be complicated by variations in treatment strategies, case mix and the inclusion of intensive care patients with multi-organ failure (Plate 6). The need for rapid identification of high-risk patients and clinical features is essential so that treatment, which may be vital for survival, can be commenced early. The emphasis here for nursing care is careful attention to the early signs of ARF and the immediate intervention that may avoid further damage.

CLASSIFICATION

ARF may be divided into three major categories in which each category has a physiological location of the insult:

- *Prerenal* – relates to ineffective perfusion of the kidneys which are structurally normal;
- *Renal* – damage to the renal parenchyma, sometimes secondary to prerenal problems;
- *Postrenal* – disordered urinary drainage of both kidneys or of a single functioning kidney.

In addition, an acute impairment may present in the patient with existing chronic renal failure which may lead to further structural damage.

Prerenal Acute Renal Failure

Prerenal causes of ARF are directly related to hypoperfusion states or a decline in the blood supply to the kidneys. The structure of the kidneys is normal (Table 4.1). However, when the renal blood supply is restricted,

Table 4.1 *Acute renal failure: major causes and onset features*

Stage	Causes	Onset features
Prerenal	*Hypovolaemia* Loss of whole blood, or plasma following haemorrhage, trauma, burns, surgery Extracellular fluid loss in dehydration due to bowel obstruction, fistulae, gastroenteritis	Oliguria; anuria; thirst; dry mouth; hypotension, tachycardia; low CVP; tachypnoea; peripheral vasoconstriction,* pallor and coolness; altered level of consciousness
	Septicaemic shock Bacteraemia following surgery, wound infections, peritonitis, cholangitis	*In some patients with septicaemic shock vasodilation is present at the onset and the veins appear full, the skin warm
	Cardiogenic shock Myocardial infarction, arrhythmias, pulmonary embolism, tamponade	
Renal	*Acute ischaemic tubular necrosis* Prolonged 'prerenal' causes Myoglobinaemia (crush injury) Incompatible blood transfusion	Prerenal causes as above, followed by established features oliguria, anuria, dyspnoea due to pulmonary oedema
	Acute nephrotoxic tubular necrosis Poisoning with heavy metals (e.g. mercuric chloride, solvents, paracetamol overdose, ethylene glycol, adverse effects of drugs such as gentamicin, amphotericin) Bacterial toxins *(Clostridium welchi)*	Elevated CVP and JVP Cardiac arrhythmias due to hyperkalaemia Acute uraemic syndrome with bleeding, drowsiness, coma, infection Metabolic acidosis
	Initial damage to glomeruli and small blood vessels Malignant hypertension; acute glomerulonephritis; acute pyelonephritis; polyarteritis	
Postrenal	*Obstruction of lower urinary tract* Benign or malignant prostatic hypertrophy	'Renal' signs above plus those of obstruction Difficulty with micturition
	Obstruction of upper urinary tract Ureteric obstruction due to stricture, calculi, blood clots, extrinsic compression by	Intermittent oliguria – polyuria Complete anuria Back or loin pain Bladder distension if prostatic hypertrophy

Table 4.1 continued

Stage	Causes	Onset features
	pelvic tumours, retroperitoneal fibrosis Intrarenal obstruction of collecting ducts by uric acid crystals, cysteine microcalculi, myeloma protein, sulphonamide crystals	
Acute on chronic impairment	*Underlying chronic renal disease* e.g. Chronic glomerulonephritis, pyelonephritis, diabetic nephropathy, hypertensive nephrosclerosis, chronic analgesic abuse	Established features of chronic failure present at onset (e.g. skin pigmentation, anaemia, wasting, fatigue) Superimposed on these are the classic features of acute impairment
	Acute precipitating event Commonly a recent intercurrent illness (e.g. infection, surgery)	

CVP, central venous pressure; JVP, jugular vein pressure.

glomerular filtration is reduced, causing decreased perfusion of the kidneys. The net effect is a decreased blood flow to the glomeruli which therefore leads to ineffective filtration because of inadequate blood flow. Without an effective renal plasma flow rate the glomeruli are unable to filter waste from the blood but the structure of the renal tubules remains intact (Fig. 4.2).

Urinalysis and urine electrolytes are extremely helpful in distinguishing prerenal from intrarenal causes of ARF. The urinalysis is a mirror of the structural integrity of the renal tubules, and the urine electrolytes reflect the functional ability of the renal tubules (Toto, 1992).

In this prerenal state urine osmolality is high and urinary sodium concentrations are low, which is consistent with renal hypoperfusion and well preserved renal function. If at this stage renal blood flow can be restored then normal renal function will return. However, if the prerenal state is prolonged then this may lead to ischaemic damage due to poor perfusion, which in turn can lead to acute tubular necrosis.

The importance of early recognition and treatment of prerenal failure is vital in preventing the condition progressing to renal failure and a degree of parenchymal damage (Table 4.2).

Renal Failure

This cause is sometimes referred to as parenchymal/intrinsic or intrarenal failure and is associated with structural damage to the glomeruli/vessels

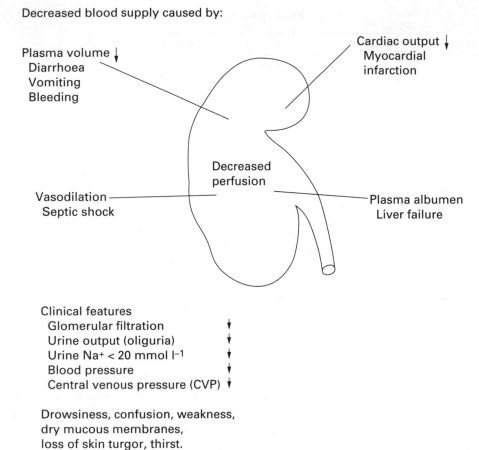

Decreased blood supply caused by:

Plasma volume ↓
  Diarrhoea
  Vomiting
  Bleeding

Cardiac output ↓
  Myocardial
  infarction

Decreased
perfusion

Vasodilation
Septic shock

Plasma albumen
Liver failure

Clinical features
  Glomerular filtration   ↓
  Urine output (oliguria)   ↓
  Urine Na$^+$ < 20 mmol l^{-1} ↓
  Blood pressure   ↓
  Central venous pressure (CVP) ↓

Drowsiness, confusion, weakness,
dry mucous membranes,
loss of skin turgor, thirst.

Fig. 4.2 *Prerenal failure.*

and renal tubules. The difference between pre- and postrenal failure and renal failure is that in renal failure the correction of the aetiology will not guarantee complete recovery of renal function because of damage to the nephron itself. Here the episode of ARF may run a lengthy duration and can often lead to chronic renal failure.

The clinical course of intrinsic renal failure is often complex and, depending upon underlying disorders, the recovery may be prolonged for up to 6 weeks. Table 4.3 highlights the wide variety of causes of intrinsic renal failure which may involve multisystem disease or orginate from a primary renal disorder, but often involve complicating severe illness that causes vasomotor nephropathy.

Some of the specific causes are now discussed (for glomerulonephritis, see Chapter 5).

Table 4.2 Prerenal aetiology

Cardiovascular
- Congestive cardiac failure, myocardial infarction, cardiogenic shock, cardiac tamponade, pulmonary embolism

Vasodilation
- Sepsis, anaphylaxis, ACE inhibitors

Intravascular volume depletion
- Haemorrhage from any cause: i.e. complications of pregnancy, trauma, gastrointestinal bleeding
- Burns: i.e. loss of plasma
- Gastrointestinal losses causing severe vomiting, diarrhoea, acute intestinal obstuction, paralytic ileus, pancreatitis
- Renal losses due to diuretic drugs

Episodes of hypotension following:
- Open heart surgery
- Aortic aneurysm repair

ACE, angiotensin converting enzyme.

Table 4.3 Intrinsic renal failure aetiology

Glomerulonephritis:
- acute poststreptococcal
- systemic lupus erythematosus
- haemolytic uraemic syndrome
- Wegener's granulomatosis
- Goodpasture's syndrome

Vascular:
- vasculitis
- malignant hypertension
- Microangiopathy
- non-steroidal anti-inflammatory drugs
- eclampsia
- renal artery stenosis
- renal vein thrombosis

Tubular ischaemia:
- profound hypotension

Intratubular pigments:
- myoglobin

Intratubular proteins:
- myeloma

Intratubular crystals:
- nephrotoxins

Acute interstitial nephritis

This condition often follows exposure to drugs in the form of antibiotics, analgesics and non-steroidal anti-inflammatory agents. Infections can cause a very similar clinical and pathological picture and these include *Salmonella*, *Streptococcus*, *Meningococcus*, leptospirosis and many viral disorders.

Other categories of interstitial nephritis are caused by systemic disease such as systemic lupus erythematosus and sarcoidosis or present as the primary disease.

Clinical features   Fever, rash, arthralgia, back pain, eosinophilia.

Urinalysis   Blood and protein.

Urine Microscopy   Microhaematuria, white blood cells (WBC) and red blood cells (RBC) casts.

ARF may not develop for some weeks but in some cases renal dysfunction may occur within a few hours after exposure to a causative drug.

Rhabdomyolysis

A major cause of ARF of a toxic nature, rhabdomyolysis is a result of the release of skeletal muscle contents that include myoglobin into the plasma.

Rhabdomyolysis is often caused by trauma, for example crush injury or pressure-induced muscle necrosis. This causes damage to skeletal muscle that allows the pigment myoglobin to be released into the plasma. Myoglobin is a red respiratory pigment and in high plasma levels may become nephrotoxic.

Clinical features   The urine is often brown in colour due to the presence of myoglobin.

Urinalysis   Blood and protein.

Urine microscopy   Pigmented granular casts.

Patients often present with acute illness with fever, weakness, malaise and pain, nausea and vomiting.

Renal failure and liver disease

Acute renal failure is often associated with acute liver injury which may result from:

● paracetamol overdose

- circulatory shock
- severe sepsis leptospirosis.

It may also be seen following surgery on the biliary tract.

For the patient with advanced liver disease the onset of renal failure is often referred to as the hepatorenal syndrome. Septicaemia, fluid and electrolyte imbalance or hypovolaemia from gastrointestinal haemorrhage are common causes of the syndrome.

These patients are often critically ill and require intensive care nursing whereby they may fall into the multi-organ failure category. Renal function may be reversed only by improvement of liver function resulting from partial resolution of the primary disease.

Cortical necrosis

Cortical necrosis may follow any course of intense or prolonged ischaemia, which is a rare condition that is often associated with complication of pregnancy, i.e. placenta abruption, eclampsia or septic abortion. The condition is also associated with sepsis, shock, transfusion reactions and burns.

Renal biopsy reveals a pathology of patchy necrosis of the glomeruli, tubules and small vessels of the renal cortex. The renal medulla remains intact but the renal cortex becomes infarcted and calcifies which may be seen on plain abdominal X-ray.

The return of renal function is often slow but if the cortical necrosis is extensive, recovery is unlikely and the patient will be dependent on dialysis.

Haemolytic uraemic syndrome

This vascular disease refers to a cluster of overlapping conditions which are characterised clinically by renal failure. Haemolytic anaemia and thrombocytopenia occur in haemolytic uraemic syndrome (HUS) and cause thrombosis in the afferent arterioles and glomeruli, together with thickening of the vessel walls. The disease is found in children and in this group the renal prognosis is usually good. In adults with early dialysis the prognosis is good; however, irreversible renal failure is common.

Clinical features   Fever, diarrhoea, vomiting.

Disseminated intravascular coagulation is common along with an extensive consumption of clotting factors and marked prolongation of clotting time. Renal histology may show glomerular ischaemia, thombosis and arteriole narrowing. HUS is discussed fully in the Chapter 5 and Chapter 10.

Acute tubular necrosis

The condition acute tubular necrosis (ATN) accounts for 75% of all intrarenal causes and as its name implies this condition affects the tubules of the kidney. ATN is often caused by prolonged events of prerenal and postrenal conditions, ischaemic or nephrotoxic episodes which damage the tubular portion of the nephron which in itself is the most common cause of ARF (Stark, 1982).

Although the aetiology of ATN varies, the common factor is a reduction in the supply of oxygen and nutrients to the metabolically active tubular cells. This results in the eventual cessation of cell function and patchy necrosis. Fortunately, tubular cells can regenerate and reform the basement membrane. Thus, providing the patient can be kept alive during the regeneration phase, kidney function usually returns to near normal values. Most intrinsic renal disease is caused by acute ischaemia or toxic agents such as drugs or bacterial endotoxins that cause injury to the renal tubules and results in ATN (Table 4.4).

Nephrotoxicity   Toxic insult to the renal tubules can cause direct ATN. Toxic agents in the form of drug therapy are a major cause of ATN and in particular the aminoglycoside and cephalosporin antibiotics. Gentamicin is a common nephrotoxic agent, particularly when used in combination with frusemide. Despite its nephrotoxicity, gentamicin is commonly used in patients with dangerous Gram-negative infections. These agents are primarily excreted by the kidneys and careful monitoring of gentamicin levels before and after each dose is essential so that drug dosage can be adjusted to the correct therapeutic range.

Routine monitoring of blood urea nitrogen and creatinine are therefore necessary when these agents are administered (Table 4.5).

Table 4.4 *Urinary findings in acute tubular necrosis (ATN) and prerenal failure*

Test	ATN	Prerenal failure
Urine microscopy	Brown cellular casts Cellular debris	Normal
Urine sodium (mmol l^{-1})	High (> 40)	Low (< 20)
Urine osmolality	Low (< 400)	High (> 500) Concentrated urine
Urine specific gravity (q.v.)	low (< 1010)	High (> 1020)

Table 4.5 *Nephrotoxins*

- *Heavy metals*: mercury, gold, arsenic, barium, uranium, silver
- *Solvents*: carbon tetrachloride, ethylene glycol
- *Therapeutic agents*: antibiotics (gentami cin, neomycin, amikacin, tobramycin, streptomycin, amphotericin)
- *Iodinated contrast agents*: streptozoticin, cisplatin
- *Chemicals*: hydrogen sulphate, cyanides, copper sulphate, paraquat

Ischaemia   Ischaemic ATN is often associated with inadequate perfusion to the kidney as a result of a fall in mean arterial pressure to below the critical level of 60–70 mmHg. Below this level, the afferent and efferent renal arterioles are unable to maintain their autoregulatory function and this leads to a fall in glomerular filtration rate.

The interruption of blood supply to the kidney often occurs in major vascular surgery whereby the aorta is cross-clamped above the renal arteries. This procedure is likely to cause ischaemia.

Prolonged or severe prerenal failure as mentioned previously are common causes of ATN. If prerenal causes are not corrected the patient may progress to intrarenal damage due to tubular ischaemia.

Postrenal Failure

Postrenal conditions obstruct the flow of urine. Obstruction to a single kidney will not cause renal failure except for those persons with a solitary kidney, therefore obstruction is generally bilateral in order to produce physiological abnormalities. As with prerenal failure, postrenal conditions are reversible when the obstructive lesion is corrected; however, the rapidity of the recovery of renal function depends on the duration and completeness of the obstruction.

Loin pain, alternating oliguria and polyuria, and complete anuria are features sometimes found with the postrenal failure patient.

Like any other hollow viscus the urinary tract may be obstructed by three mechanisms:

- obstruction from within (e.g. a ureteric stone);
- disease of the wall;
- obstruction from outside.

As with prerenal failure it is important to address the obstruction sooner rather than later because in theory postrenal failure is reversible. The longer it persists the less complete is recovery likely to be after the obstruction is relieved (Smith, 1987).

MANAGEMENT OF ACUTE RENAL FAILURE

For the patient who is hypovolaemic or in septic shock, the prime objective is to re-establish normal haemodynamics in an effort to restore renal perfusion.

To prevent ATN in this situation is to prevent shock (Uldall, 1988). Careful fluid replacement in the form of crystalloid (e.g. intravenous saline), colloid (e.g. human albumin) or blood transfusion may be given without delay to not only prevent shock but also maintain and expand plasma volume and improve renal blood flow.

Careful fluid replacement must incorporate close monitoring of the patient. Careful measurement of blood pressure, pulse, respirations and temperature plus accurate fluid balance is important in monitoring fluid status.

Direct measurement of central venous pressure (CVP) if a central line is present will help manage fluid replacement safely and give a good indication for fluid replacement. The CVP will be low in volume depletion, therefore with careful fluid replacement the aim would be to elevate this to 5–8 cm of water.

Inotropic agents such as dopamine and dobutamine to increase renal blood flow are sometimes prescribed as a 'renal dose' at 3–5 mcg kg^{-1} min^{-1} to increase renal perfusion and in turn increase the urine output. Again, it is important to monitor the patient including vital signs within the appropriate range for the individual: normal skin colour, turgor and temperature; a relaxed, sedate body posture and behaviour; and a cardiac rhythm and rate that is consistent with the patient's fluid and electrolyte status.

The ARF patient may develop several dangerous conditions:

- hyperkalaemia
- volume overload
- metabolic acidosis
- uraemia
- infection.

Hyperkalaemia

Hyperkalaemia and hypokalaemia can occur in ARF, but more often than not hyperkalaemia is a lethal complication in ARF. The normal range of serum potassium is between 3.5 and 5.0 mmol l^{-1}. The kidney is primarily the major organ that maintains potassium levels via selective tubular reabsorption. The failing kidney cannot excrete potassium effectively, particularly if the patient is oliguric or, even worse, anuric. Extremes in the potassium level are often seen in the critically ill patient and are further complicated by metabolic acidosis, tissue hypoxia, infection, blood transfusions and potassium-containing drugs.

Watch out for changes on the patient's electrocardiogram (ECG) monitor (Fig. 4.3):

- hyperkalaemia
- widened QRS complex
- tall dented T wave
- flattened or loss of P wave.

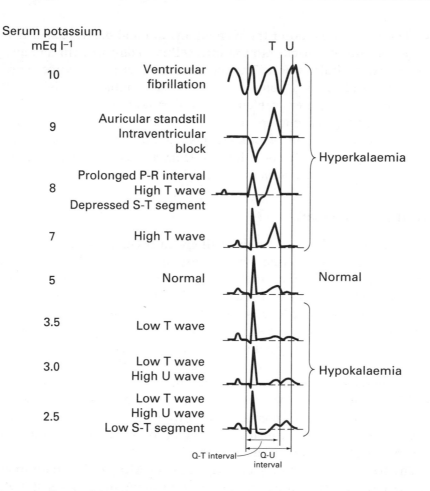

Fig. 4.3 *Effects of hyper- and hypokalaemia on the electrocardiogram. Reproduced from Birch and Winsor, 1996, with permission.*

Myocardial hyperexcitability may cause arrhythmias initially, but later bradycardia and conduction defects can precede cardiac arrest if the serum potassium rises to 7 mmol l[-1].

Haemodialysis is often preferred in the treatment of hyperkalaemia, which may take time if the patient does not have vascular access for dialysis or needs to be transferred to a renal speciality. Therefore, the following patient-care management may be prescribed in an effort to reduce the patient's serum potassium:

● Oral or rectal potassium exchange agents in the form of calcium resonium may be administered. The mode of action of calcium resonium is to exchange potassium ions with calcium ions in the gut. Potassium exchange resin can have a constipating effect so it is essential to avoid faecal impaction or bowel obstruction by promoting adequate bowel elimination.

- The administration of intravenous insulin and dextrose will help move potassium ions back into the intracellular compartment and away from the extracellular spaces. The infusion of hypertonic dextrose and insulin may be given as a bolus dose or by slow infusion; it is important to monitor the patient's blood sugar during and after the treatment as hyper/hypoglycaemic episodes often occur.
- The administration of intravenous calcium may also be prescribed to help reverse the effects of hyperkalaemia as calcium has a direct antagonist effect on the action of potassium.

Volume Overload

Volume overload in ARF is most likely to occur in patients who are oliguric and is characterised by the expansion of the extracellular fluid compartments. The increased accumulation of water and electrolytes in the extracellular fluid is associated with the inability to excrete sodium; therefore, volume overload is where there is a failure to excrete water and sodium which leads to the expansion of the extracellular compartment. The increase in total sodium concentration will cause more water to be drawn into the extracellular fluid to re-establish the proper sodium to water ratio. Increases in sodium and water manifest in the extracellular space and in particular the intravascular space. The expansion of blood volume will result in the transference of fluid from the intravascular to the interstitial compartments causing peripheral oedema due to the abnormal expansion of the interstitial fluid space.

The patient who is in the oliguric phase of ARF needs careful monitoring of their intake and output in an effort to maintain or re-establish a fluid and electrolyte balance. The nurse assessment of the patient's fluid status will help determine the management of the patient's fluid balance. For the patient with fluid overload, accurate measurements of blood pressure are recorded and increases in systolic blood pressure reported. CVP will be raised, indicating an increase in fluid volume.

Shortness of breath and in particular orthopnoea are indicative of pulmonary oedema. The presence of oedema may be seen in the feet, legs and sacral pad. When there is generalised oedema the term 'anasarca' is sometimes used to indicate the magnitude of oedema in all parts of the body. It is vital to protect the skin and maintain its integrity as oedematous tissue receives less oxygen and is more susceptible to breakdown and infection. It is essential to carry out risk assessment and implement early application of pressure area care. For high-risk patients the use of sophisticated beds will not only protect the skin integrity but add additional comfort for the patient who needs careful handling. Some also provide a patient weight facility that proves invaluable for monitoring fluid balance in the critically ill patient.

Name (label)

DEPARTMENT OF NEPHROLOGY
FLUID CHART

Nursing instructions
500 ml + previous
days output
Date

Time	INTAKE Oral	I.V.I			Running total	OUTPUT Urine	Bowels	Vomit		Running total	Balance
01.00											
02.00	50										+50
03.00											
04.00						100				100	
05.00											
06.00	100	100 ml antibiotic			250						+150
07.00		infusion									
08.00											
09.00								+			
10.00	100	500 ml human			350	50	Diarrhoea ++			150	+200
11.00		albumen									
12.00		over						200		350	
13.00	1	4 h									
14.00					850						0
15.00	50				900						
16.00						100	Diarrhoea ++			450	
17.00											
18.00		100 ml antibiotic			1000			100		550	+450
19.00		infusion									
20.00	50				1050						
21.00											
22.00					1050	100				650	+400
23.00											
24.00											
Total	350				1050	350		300		650	+400

Fig. 4.4 *Department of Nephrology fluid chart.*

The assessment of fluid requirements should be based not only on accurate fluid charts but also on the daily weight of the patient and clinical signs of over- or underhydration. Rapid daily gains and losses in weight are usually related to changes in fluid volume. Because of the difficulties of obtaining accurate figures for intake and output, serial weights are often more reliable. It is useful to try and weigh the patient at the same time each day and make sure the patient is wearing the same amount of clothing.

Fluid intake is usually regulated to the volume of the previous day's output of urine plus 500 ml for insensible loss. This is a good working rule, but it must be used with flexibility to allow for the patient who may be febrile, has diarrhoea, has a draining wound or is being nursed in a hot environment. It is an advantage to calculate total intake and output throughout the 24 h period so as to maintain hydration without producing volume overload. To help maintain accuracy all nursing staff, the patient and visitors can be involved and instructed in the importance of accurate recording of intake and output (Fig. 4.4).

Metabolic Acidosis

The patient in ARF often presents with a metabolic acidosis, which depending on its severity may require intervention.

Acidosis in renal failure occurs when the renal tubules fail to regenerate bicarbonate and to secrete hydrogen ions into the urine. This causes an acid–base imbalance that occurs when acids increase and the normal acid–base ratio changes. A low arterial blood pH and bicarbonate is the combination of the increase of metabolic acids and their reaction with sodium bicarbonate that forms carbonic acid. This reaction generates water and carbon dioxide which is excreted in the lungs. However, in renal failure there is a loss of bicarbonate ions causing a diminished bicarbonate–carbon dioxide ratio that results in a lowered arterial blood pH. This metabolic imbalance leads to respiratory compensation whereby there is an increase in the rate and depth of respiration in an effort to excrete carbon dioxide; this is often referred to as 'Kussmaul' respirations.

In some instances correction of metabolic acidosis can be treated with an infusion of sodium bicarbonate, but the benefits of producing a rise in serum pH and buffering capacity are counterbalanced by the addition of sodium and the increased risk of fluid overload. Therefore, acidosis is most effectively treated with haemodialysis using bicarbonate as the buffer.

Uraemia

The retention of nitrogenous waste products from protein metabolism will produce acute uraemia in the ARF patient and is often referred to as azotemia. Associated with the rise of blood urea nitrogen (BUN) are a multitude of problems that are often referred to as the 'acute uraemic syndrome'. These often include:

- gastrointestinal problems: nausea, vomiting, hiccoughs;
- bleeding: reduction in clotting factors and platelet synthesis which may cause haematemisis, malaena, skin purpura, pericardia bleeding;
- risk of infection: pneumonia, urinary tract infections, wound infection;
- neurological problems: confusion, decreased responsiveness, twitching and irritability.

BUN along with creatinine are commonly measured to indicate a level of renal function. To control and minimise the complications of a rising BUN and creatinine in ARF dialysis is indicated to maintain patient BUN level below 25 mmol l^{-1} and a creatinine level of below 500 mmol l^{-1}.

The need to institute dialysis early will help stabilise the patient and allow for the re-establishment of adequate nutrition. The therapeutic emphasis towards increased feeding of such patients has led to the need for more frequent dialysis to manage fluid status and rising BUN (Whitworth and Lawrence, 1987). The majority of patients are extremely catabolic. Many will be suffering the symptoms of nausea and vomiting caused by uraemia and whilst these can be controlled to some extent using drug therapy, anorexia will still be present. It is therefore important to commence feeding as soon as possible to avoid further breakdown of muscle mass and consequent wasting (De Burgh, 1992).

Dietary restrictions will help control uraemia but it is vital to provide adequate calories to maintain nutrition in an effort to prevent the patient being catabolic. Whilst it is necessary to restrict potassium, sodium and fluid intake, it is rarely necessary to restrict protein and the use of oral supplements is encouraged. For the patient who is unable to eat then total parenteral nutrition (TPN) or when possible enteral nutrition using a fine-bore nasogastric feeding tube will be an essential part of the management (see p. 120).

Dialysis

For patients in ARF the decision to initiate dialysis is usually made on clinical grounds; however, it is usually essential in the presence of a rapid rise in blood urea, uncontrolled acidosis, fluid overload and hyperkalaemia.

Indications for dialysis

- fluid overload – pulmonary oedema, peripheral oedema, anasarca;
- uraemic symptoms – nausea, vomiting, drowsiness, twitching;
- hyperkalaemia – serum potassium level above 6 mmol l^{-1};
- acidosis – arterial pH less than 7.1 and serum bicarbonate level less than 12 mmol l^{-1}.
- 'space making' for transfusions, nutrition, infusions.

Haemodialysis plays a pivotal role in the management of those patients who require dialysis. Patients often receive bicarbonate dialysis via a double-lumen haemodialysis catheter that has been inserted into the internal jugular, subclavian or femoral vein.

Careful assessment and planning of acute dialysis is essential to minimise related complications such as hypotension, nausea, vomiting, headaches, bleeding, disequilibrium, seizures or cardiac arrest.

For those patients who are haemodynamically unstable the use of continuous veno venous haemofiltration (CVVH) provides a continuous rather than an intermittent treatment that will allow for the removal of fluid and maintain control of urea, creatinine and electrolytes. The use of CVVH can be effective in the treatment of ARF, particularly in the intensive care situation whereby the critically ill patient can be complicated by multi-organ failure that may involve the kidneys, liver, lungs, heart and pancreas. The prognosis of these patients depends on several factors that may enhance their chances of survival:

- anticipation and early prevention of electolyte imbalance;
- recognition of pre-existing renal disease;
- avoidance of nephrotoxic agents – aminoglycosides, angiotensin converting enzyme (ACE) inhibitors;

- early restoration of circulating volume and cardiac output;
- early diagnosis and vigorous treatment of sepsis.

Infection

Careful attention to the prevention of infection is essential in the care for the patient in ARF because sepsis is the single most contributive cause of death for this immunocompromised patient. Twenty per cent of all deaths in ARF are directly attributable to infection (Goodinson, 1985).

Invasive lines in the form of CVP, Swan–Ganz or feeding lines are often difficult to avoid in the critically ill patient and are often essential if haemodialysis is being carried out. Therefore, it is important to assess the need for removal of lines/catheter if at all possible; for example, is there an essential need for an indwelling urinary catheter, or is the patient oliguric/anuric, and can the urine output be monitored without an indwelling catheter?

Careful management of vascular access for dialysis is essential as these offer direct access to the patient's blood. These temporary venous catheters are inserted in the subclavian or internal jugular veins and are a potential source for infection. The femoral veins are often used as an alternative site for vascular access, but their position in the groin should only be short term as they are more prone to infection and restrict the patient's mobility. Care of vascular access is resticted to specialist nursing staff who are familiar with the care of these catheters and their importance when used for dialysis therapies.

Central lines/feeding lines have the same problems as the temporary dialysis catheter and are again a potential source of infection. The insertion of nasogastric fine-bore feeding tube (when possible) for enteral feeding is an ideal alternative to TPN.

Good meticulous nursing skills can help monitor the patient for early signs of infection. Intravenous catheters and wound sites require careful attention using aseptic techniques when using or redressing wound sites. Accurate measurement of vital signs is important and any rise in the patient's temperature must be taken seriously and reported to medical staff.

The early ambulation of patients is essential to avoid the complications of bed rest and in particular chest infection and maintaining skin integrity. This is often easier said than done for the critical patient but must be given a high priority despite the difficulties.

THE CLINICAL COURSE OF ACUTE RENAL FAILURE

The clinical course of ARF has traditionally been separated into several distinct phases (Finn, 1990):

(1) the onset phase
(2) the oliguric/non-oliguric phase
(3) the diuretic phase
(4) the recovery phase.

The Onset Phase

The onset or initial phase of ARF is the period of time from the precipitating event to the onset of oliguria. The duration of this phase is variable and depends upon the cause of renal failure. For example, in the case of an ischaemic event the onset phase may last up to 2 days, whereas in the case of a nephrotoxic insult it may last for several days. The urine output at this stage is not necessarily decreased; however, the collection and examination of urine at this stage may reveal the presence of renal disease, give clues to the nature of disease if one is present, provide a valuable tool in following the progress of disease, and give an immediate assessment of renal function (Schoengrund and Balzer, 1985).

The Oliguric Phase (Fig. 4.5)

During this second stage the patient's urinary volume is less than 400 ml per day but this may vary and in some cases the patient may be anuric. It is useful to consider the parameter used for determining oliguria and the significance of a urine volume of 400 ml per day (Table 4.6). This indicates that the necessary amount of solute cannot be excreted in relation to the insufficient urine volume and therefore will not maintain homeostasis in a normal adult. The total amount of solute produced per day by a normal adult on a normal diet is about 600–650 mOsmol. If the adult has normal renal function, then the kidneys can maximally concentrate urine at a level of about 1200–1300 mOsmol l^{-1}. Thus, the normal adult's kidneys could excrete the total solute load in about 500 ml of water. For the patient in ARF, the kidneys cannot excrete the total solute load because of the inability to maximally concentrate the urine.

The duration of the oliguric phase may be variable and may last anything up to 6–8 weeks. However, the longer this phase continues then the prognosis for renal recovery is poor (King, 1994).

Table 4.6 Types of urine output

Anuria	No urine output
Oliguria	Less than 400 ml per day
Non oliguria	Greater than 400 ml per day
Polyuria	Normal or high urine output

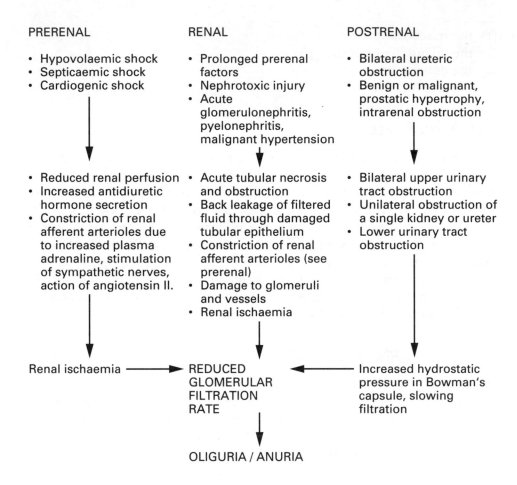

Fig. 4.5 *Acute renal failure: mechanisms involved in the genesis of oliguria.*

The non-oliguric phase can usually be associated with nephrotoxic agents and often present with an adequate urine output. The advantage for this patient is that the kidneys are more capable of managing fluid and electrolytes and may not require frequent episodes of dialysis. Although the urine volume is not reduced, the ability to produce a concentrated urine is severely impaired and total solute excretion is reduced.

For the patient in the oliguric and non-oliguric phase it is essential to emphasise the importance of strict fluid and electrolyte balance and that careful monitoring of intake and output, changes in body weight, presence of oedema, respiration rate and breathlessness will help fluid balance.

The Diuretic Phase

The diuretic phase is marked by the increase of urine output over 24 h with subsequent increases in urine flow rates over a period of hours or days (Finn,

1990). At this stage urine volumes will increase and it is not uncommon to have a daily volume of 3 l in total and again it is essential to maintain adequate hydration at this point until the kidneys return to normal function. As with the oliguric/non-oliguric phase the monitoring of fluid balance should follow the rule of 500 ml plus previous day's urine output in 24 h. Urine specimens for creatinine clearance collected over a 24 h period calculated alongside serum clearance will measure renal function and monitor selective reabsorption (see Chapter 6). It may be also necessary to lift dietary restrictions and reintroduce sodium and potassium into the diet.

The Recovery Phase

Once the patient's blood urea nitrogen and serum creatinine have subsided after several days of diuresis, this indicates the end of the oliguric phase and the beginning of the recovery phase. The rapidity of the changes in blood urea nitrogen and serum creatinine ratios can be related to the time and magnitude of the preceding diuresis and the metabolic state of the individual. Those patients who are markedly catabolic and whose endogenous nitrogen loads are high will take a longer period of time to clear these substances from the blood.

Of the patients who recover from ARF, up to 50% are left with some degree of permanent kidney damage, and a number of these patients will develop chronic renal failure in the future (Baer and Lancaster, 1992).

NUTRITIONAL MANAGEMENT OF ACUTE RENAL FAILURE

Protein calorie malnutrition has been implicated as one of the contributing factors to the high mortality rate seen in ARF (Mault et al., 1983). Generalised nutritional deficiencies, which can occur rapidly in the setting of higher metabolic demands, are associated with increased infections (Chandra, 1983), reduced or delayed wound healing (Windsor, 1988b) and loss of muscle strength (Windsor, 1988a)

New modalities of dialysis are now available that facilitate the delivery of full calorie and protein support, allowing the abandonment of previous dietary restrictions which were based on the principles of treating patients with chronic renal failure.

Metabolic Consequences

Critically ill patients with ARF have increased demands for both calories and protein. These result from the underlying disease processes and derangement in macronutrient metabolism that leads to an inadequate use of available nutrients.

Hyperglycaemia is common due to a combination of insulin resistance and accelerated hepatic gluconeogenesis, resulting from the conversion of amino acids released during protein catabolism into glucose (Wilmore, 1976). In addition, lipid metabolism is altered with an impaired ability to use free fatty acids and triglycerides probably due to decreased activity of lipoprotein and hepatic triglyceride lipases (Druml et al., 1992). Insulin resistance, secondary hyperparathyroidism (Pietiak et al., 1978), increased levels of catecholamines, glucagon and corticosteroids (Schaefer et al., 1989) and possibly the presence of metabolic acidosis (Mitch, 1989) may all be important in accelerating protein degradation. Loss of kidney function also renders some amino acids, normally synthesised by the kidney, to become conditionally indispensable.

Nutritional Assessment

In the critically ill patient with ARF, the following assessment tools can be useful but they need to be interpreted with caution and not considered in isolation:

1. Anthropometric measurements usually involve monitoring weight, tricep skinfolds, mid-arm circumference and mid-arm muscle circumference. The presence of fluid overload and fluid shifts in patients with anuric or oliguric ARF may compromise these measurements.
2. Visceral proteins – albumin, transferrin and prealbumin – have been used to assess protein status but levels of serum proteins invariably decrease with stress, injury, infection or inflammation (Ricketts and Bull, 1962) and therefore in the critical care setting changes in these hepatic transport proteins may result from the therapeutic effect of nutritional support or from the underlying disease process.
3. Depressed total lymphocyte count and delayed cutaneous sensitivity to skin test antigens are also thought to be indicators of protein malnutrition (Twomey et al., 1982). However, uraemic toxicity may impair the immune response making conclusions difficult to draw.

Calculation of Requirements

Energy

Requirements, determined by the underlying disease, are calculated by working out the patient's basic metabolic rate (BMR) from standard equations (Schofield, 1985). Modifications to cover stress, activity, the energy requirements of feeding and temperature can be added to the BMR (Elia, 1990). To avoid overfeeding, the provision of carbohydrate energy during the dialysis therapy also needs to be taken into account. Dextrose absorption during renal replacement therapy (RRT) varies with the type of dialysis therapy from zero or very little in conventional intermittent haemodialysis to 45% net dextrose absorption during continuous arteriovenous haemodialysis (CAVHD) with 1.5 and 2.5% dialysate solutions (Sigler and Teehan, 1987). In peritoneal dialysis dextrose absorption varies with the volume and dextrose concentration of dialysate. An average of 182 ± 61 g dextrose is absorbed per day during continuous ambulatory peritoneal dialysis (Grodstein et al., 1981).

If total parenteral nutrition (TPN) has been instigated then the changes in lipid metabolism associated with renal failure should not prevent the use of lipid emulsions. Usually 1 g fat kg^{-1} body weight (BW) day^{-1} does not increase the plasma triglyceride levels substantially (Druml, 1987). Sponsel and Conger (1995) state that up to 30–40% of total calories can be supplied by lipids but no more than 60% (Sponsel and Conger, 1995).

Protein

It is important to emphasise that there is no role, in catabolic ARF, for the restriction of protein intake in order to avoid or reduce the frequency of renal support.

The optimal requirement for protein is influenced by the illness causing the ARF, the extent of protein catabolism and the type and frequency of dialysis. In 1980, Elwyn produced estimations of protein requirements according to the degree of catabolism (Table 4.7).

Table 4.7 Estimation of the protein/nitrogen requirements in acute renal failure.

Change in BMR	Protein (g kg^{-1} BW)	Nitrogen (g kg^{-1} BW)
Normal (up to 25%)	1.0	0.16
Intermediate (25–55%)	1.3–1.9	0.2–0.3
Hypermetabolic (45–100%)	2.0–3.0	0.3–0.5

Druml (1993) states that the maximal protein intake should be 1.5 g kg^{-1} BW day^{-1} but for patients requiring regular haemodialysis or continuous therapy, protein intake should be increased by 0.2 g kg^{-1} BW day^{-1} to compensate for substrate losses during therapy.

Electrolytes

The electrolyte content of the nutritional prescription should be adjusted based on each individual patient and whether the patient is on RRT. Sodium should not be greatly restricted unless oedema is present. If the patient is being dialysed then sodium will be removed from the patient, enabling a balance to be achieved.

Serum levels of potassium, magnesium and phosphorus generally are elevated in patients with ARF but can decrease as a result of intracellular shifts associated with carbohydrate delivery and anabolism. Additionally, low levels of phosphorus due to increased clearance with continuous RRT are often seen. Frequent monitoring to assess the need for supplementation is essential.

Vitamins and trace elements

Vitamin A toxicity has been reported in chronic renal failure (Farrington *et al.*, 1981) and because of the unlikely possibility of vitamin A deficiency occurring in the short term it is generally thought prudent to limit the intake in ARF. With regards to the other fat soluble vitamins, vitamin D requirements have not been established and vitamin K has been reported on occasions to be deficient and may therefore need supplementing. There is a potential for deficiency of water soluble vitamins (Bs and Folic Acid) with the exception of vitamin C. Large doses of vitamin C have resulted in oxalate deposition and supplementation of no greater than $100 \, \text{mg day}^{-1}$ is recommended (Friedman *et al.*, 1983). The requirements for trace elements in ARF are not well defined.

Fluid

Patients with ARF are frequently anuric and hence monitoring of fluid balance and restriction of intake is often necessary. The development of continuous RRT has allowed fluid to be more easily managed without the need for the tight restrictions that previously meant having to limit nutritional support.

Route of Feeding

The enteral route should be used whenever possible as enteral feeding helps to maintain the gastrointestinal barrier and prevents translocation of bacteria and systemic infection (Deitch *et al.*, 1987). In addition TPN has been associated with a number of disadvantages including metabolic disturbances, blunting of the immune response, increased sepsis rates and much higher costs.

The development of concentrated, low electrolyte feeds (as detailed in Table 9.8, p. 343), have proven invaluable in allowing delivery of optimal protein and calories with the minimum of fluid and electrolytes. However, these special feeds are not normally needed if the patient is receiving continuous RRT.

SUMMARY

The impact of acute renal failure on the patient and their family is often unexpected and despite the avalanche of technical progress it still remains a serious disease with a high mortality rate. All patients require nutritional support to maintain protein stores. In ARF it is not renal insufficiency per se that determines the need for nutritional support but the type and severity of the underlying disease and the degree of associated hypercatabolism. Understanding the nutritional requirements, careful interpretation of nutritional assessment and familiarity with the various forms of RRT will greatly improve the success of nutritional therapy although the optimal nutritional regimen has not yet been defined. The key element for the nurse is to balance the humanistic caring skills with the technological and clinical expertise required to optimise the patient's survival during this stressful time. This responsibility often falls upon senior nurses whose role is not only concurrent with a multidisciplinary team but acts as a supervisory role for junior nurses who will benefit from the learning experience. The emphasis here is to ensure safety and the well-being for the patient not only by careful nursing, nutritional and medical care, but also incorporating experience and education that will promote nursing values.

REFERENCES

BAER, C.L. AND LANCASTER, L.E. (1992) Acute renal failure. *Critical Care Quarterly*, **14**(4): 1.

BIRCH AND WINSOR, T. (1996) *A Primer of Electrocardiography*. Lea & Febiger, Philadelphia.

DE BURGH, (1992) The nursing management of acute renal failure. *Care of the Critically Ill*, **8**(1): 15–17.

CHANDRA, R.K. (1983) Nutrition, immunity and infection: present knowledge and future direction. *Lancet*, **1**: 688–91.

DEITCH, E.A., WINTERTON, J. AND BERG, R. (1987) The gut as a portal of entry for bacteremia. Role of protein malnutrition. *Ann. Surg.*, **205**: 681–92.

DRUML, W. (1987) Lipid metabolism and amino acid metabolism in acute renal failure. *Klin Ernahr*, **28**: 1.

DRUML, W. (1993) Nutritional support in acute renal failure. In *Nutrition & the Kidney*, 2nd edn. Little, Brown.

DRUML, W., FISCHER, M., SERTL, S. *et al.* (1992) Fat elimination in acute renal failure: long-chain vs short-chain triglycerides. *Am. J. Clin. Nutr.*, **55**: 468–72.

ELIA, M. (1990) Artificial Nutrition al Support. *Med. Int.*, **82**: 3392–6.

FARRINGTON, K., MILLER, P., VARQHESEZ. *et al.* (1981) Vitamin A toxicity and hypercalcemia in chronic renal failure. *Br. Med. J.*, **282**: 1999–2002.

FINN, W.F. (1990) Diagnosis and management of acute tubular necrosis. *Medical Clinics of North America*, **74**(4).

FRIEDMAN, A.L., CHESNEY, R.W., GILBERT, E.F. *et al.* (1983) Secondary oxalosis as a complication of parenteral alimentation in acute renal failure. *Am. J. Nephrol.*, **3**: 248–53.

GOODINSON, S. (1985) Emergency dialysis in acute renal failure. Nursing (London). *J. Clin. Prac. Ed. Man.*, 3(32): 8.

GRODSTEIN, G.P., BLUMENKRANTZ, M.J., KOPPLE, J.D. *et al.* (1981) Glucose absorption during continuous ambulatory peritoneal dialysis. *Kidney Int.*, **19**: 564–7.

KING, B. (1994) Acute renal failure. *Registered Nurse*, **March 1995**: 35–9.

LEDINGHAM, J.J.G. (1987) Acute renal failure. In *Oxford Textbook of Medicine* 2nd edn (eds D.J. Wetherall and J.G.G. Ledingham). Oxford University Press, Oxford.

MAULT, J.R., DECHERT, R.E., CLARK, S.F. *et al.* (1983) Starvation: a major contribution to mortality in acute renal failure. *Trans. Am. Soc. Artif. Intern. Organs*, **29**: 390–5.

MITCH, W.E. (1989) Protein and amino acid metabolism in uremia: influence of metabolic acidosis. *Kid. Int. suppl.* **27**: 205–7.

PIETIAK, J., KOKOT, F. AND KUSKA, J. (1978) Serum 25-hydroxyvitamin D and parathyroid hormone in patients with acute renal failure. *Horm. Metab. Res.*, **13**: 178.

RICKETTS, C.R. AND BULL, S.P. (1962) Studies of plasma protein metabolism. *Clin. Sci.*, **23**: 411–23.

SCHAEFER, R.M. *et al.* (1989) Reduced protein catabolism by the antigluco-corticoid RU 38 486 in acutely uremic rats. *Kid. Int. suppl.*, **27**: S208–11.

SCHOENGRUND, L. AND BALZER, P. (1985) *Renal problems in Critical Care*. John Wiley, New York.

SCHOFIELD, W.N. (1985) Predicting basal metabolic rate. New standards and review of previous work. *Hum. Nutr. Clin. Nutr.*, **44**: 1–19.

SIGLER, M.H. AND TEEHAN, B.P. (1987) Solute transport in continuous hemodialysis. A new treatment for acute renal failure. *Kid. Int.*, **32**: 562–71.

SMITH, K. (1987) *Renal Disease. A Conceptual Approach*. Churchill Livingstone, New York.

SPIEGEL, D.M. (1991) Determinants of survival and recovery in acute renal failure patients dialysed in intensive care units. *American Journal of Nephrology*, **11**(1): 44–7.

SPONSEL, H. AND CONGER, J.D. (1995) (Jan). Is parenteral nutrition therapy of value in acute renal failure? (review). *Am. J. of Kid. Dis.*, **25**(1): 96–102.

STARK, J.L. (1982) How to succeed against acute renal failure. *Nursing*, **82**: 26–55.

STOTT, R.B., OGGS, C.S., CAMERON, J.S. AND BEWICK, M. (1972) Why the persistently high mortality rate in acute renal failure? *Lancet*, **2**: 75–7.

TOTO, K.H. (1992) Acute renal failure. A question of location. *American Journal of Nursing*, **November**: 44–53.

TWOMEY, P., ZIEGLER, D. AND ROMBEAU, J. (1982) Utility of skin testing in nutritional assessment: a critical review. *J. Parenter. Enter. Nutr.*, **6**: 50–8.

ULDALL, R. (1988) *Renal Nursing*, 3rd edn. Blackwell Scientific Publications, London.

WHITWORTH, J. AND LAWRENCE, J. (1987) *Textbook of Renal Disease.* Churchill Livingstone, London.

WILMORE, D.W. (1976) Carbohydrate metabolism in trauma. *Clin. Endocrinol. Metab.*, **5**: 731–45.

WINDSOR, J.A. AND HILL, G.L. (1988a) Grip strength: a measure of the proportion of protein loss in surgical patients *Br. J. Surg.*, **75**: 880–2.

WINDSOR, J.A., KNIGHT, G.S. AND HILL, G.L. (1988b) Wound healing response in surgical patients: recent food intake is more important than nutritional status. *Br. J. Surg.*, **75**: 135–7.

CHAPTER 5

CHRONIC RENAL FAILURE

INTRODUCTION

This chapter aims to define the term 'chronic renal failure' and the classification and causes of the main renal diseases. The complications and management of patients with chronic renal failure are also reviewed. The nursing care in relation to the dialysis needs of the patient is discussed in Chapters 7 and 8.

DEFINITION OF CHRONIC RENAL FAILURE

Chronic renal failure is a result of a number of pathological processes causing irreversible damage to kidney tissue. There is mass destruction of nephrons, so that the kidneys are unable to maintain fluid and electrolyte balance and excrete waste products from the body.

Chronic renal failure is caused by a slow progressive kidney disease over a course of many years (perhaps 10–20). There may be an insidious onset of renal failure with the minimum of symptoms developing in the patient on the approach to end-stage renal failure. The main renal diseases are now discussed in more detail.

DISEASES AND PROCESSES CAUSING KIDNEY FAILURE

URINARY TRACT INFECTIONS

Urinary tract infections are the most common of all bacterial infections and the main cause of end-stage renal failure. A urinary tract infection is the invasion of the urinary tract and renal interstitium by pathogenic Gram-negative organisms. Common bacteria that cause the infections are *Escherichia coli*, *Klebsiella proteus*, *Enterobacter* and *Pseudomonas*. Predisposing factors attributed to the development of a urinary tract infection can include:

- *Structure of urinary tract.* The incidence of urinary tract infections is higher in females than in males. Females have shorter urethras that are close to the rectum and there is no production of the protective prostatic fluid that is found in males.
- *Obstruction.* Any obstruction to the outflow of urine and impaired bladder emptying increase the risk of infection in the urinary tract as a result of urinary stasis producing a culture medium for bacteria.

- *Chronic illness/disease*. Chronic illness or disease alters the metabolism of tissues, assists in the development of urinary tract obstructions and damages the structure and impairs the function of the kidney.
- *Instrumentation*. Urinary catheterisation and invasive procedures for diagnostic investigations such as cystoscopies can predispose to infection by introducing bacteria to the urinary tract.

Cystitis and Urethritis

Cystitis is the inflammation of the urinary bladder and occurs more frequently in females.

Clinical features and management of care for the patient

The patient passes small amounts of urine frequently accompanied with dysuria. There will be a sensation in the bladder, postmicturition, of not feeling completely empty and suprapubic pain will be experienced. The urine has a strong odour and is cloudy with the presence of blood and leukocytes.

A mid-stream specimen of urine should be taken, which may reveal pus cells and bacteria on microscopy and culture. Appropriate antibiotic therapy should be commenced according to sensitivity of organism. In conjunction with antibiotics, patients should be advised to increase their daily intake of fluids to a least 3 l and females should receive appropriate health education on perineal hygiene and the importance of early recognition and reporting of the symptoms of a urinary tract infection.

After two episodes of cystitis, further investigations and examination of the patient's urinary tract would be advisable to detect for structural or functional defect that could predispose to urinary tract infections occurring.

Clinical symptoms in the patient that resemble cystitis, but where there is no bacterial growth cultured from the urine, may indicate that the patient has urethritis, caused by sensitivity to perfumed soaps, bath preparations or possibly infection from a sexually transmitted disease.

Acute Pyelonephritis

This is a bacterial infection of kidney tissue with the infection beginning in the lower urinary tract and ascending to the kidney(s). Acute pyelonephritis is commonly associated with pregnancy, obstruction, instrumentation or trauma to the urinary tract and in patients with a chronic illness.

Clinical features and management of care for the patient

The patient often complains of similar symptoms to cystitis but with accompanying rigors, fever (temperature 39–40°C, malaise, elevated white cell count and loin pain over the affected kidney(s)).

A mid-stream specimen of urine for culture and antibiotic sensitivity should be collected from the patient before antibiotics are given either orally or intravenously. The infection may also cause the patient considerable discomfort and appropriate analgesia may be required.

To maintain a daily fluid intake of 3 l (preventing urinary stasis), the patient may require an intravenous infusion to supplement the oral intake. Appropriate health education should be discussed with female patients regarding perineal hygiene.

On completion of antibiotics, urine should be recultured at regular intervals to ensure that the infection has been eradicated, particularly if the patient is recognised to be at risk of developing further episodes of pyelonephritis.

Disease progression and prognosis

Acute pyelonephritis may temporarily affect renal function. The process of the patient developing chronic renal failure from repeated attacks of acute pyelonephritis occurs over many years or after several extensive and severe infections. Any underlying systemic disease or urinary tract abnormality should be investigated and treated appropriately, so that infections do not reoccur.

Chronic Pyelonephritis

Chronic pyelonephritis is the result of repeated infections of the urinary tract. There is widespread destruction of nephrons and replacement with scar tissue eventually causing end-stage renal failure. For the majority of patients, the disease starts in early childhood and is due to uteric reflux and infection, but symptoms of the disease may not present clinically until adulthood. In adults, chronic pyelonephritis is a complication of obstruction in the renal tract, because of stone formation or structural abnormalities, both causing stasis of urine.

Clinical features and management of care for the patients

The patient will present with pyrexia and rigors and loin pain over the affected kidney(s). Symptoms of a lower urinary tract infection may also be present.

Antibiotics can be given to treat the acute phase of the infection, but there is little evidence to prove that prophylactic antibiotics slow down the onset of chronic renal failure.

Diagnostic investigations

Straight abdominal X-rays will show the irregular outline of the kidneys, clubbed calyces and unequal size, all occurring as a result of chronic infection and scar tissue (Fig. 5.1).

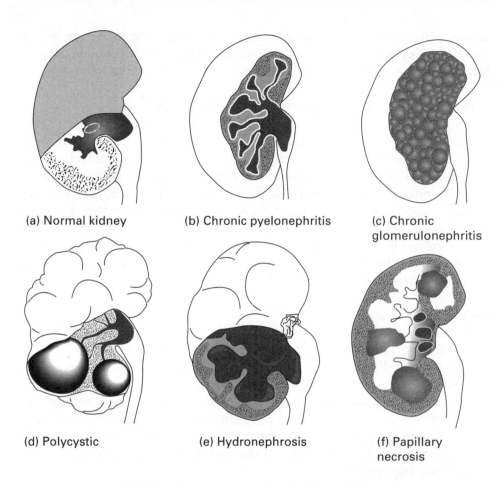

(a) Normal kidney   (b) Chronic pyelonephritis   (c) Chronic glomerulonephritis

(d) Polycystic   (e) Hydronephrosis   (f) Papillary necrosis

Fig 5.1 *Kidney appearance in health and disease.*

An intravenous pyelogram and a cystoscopy (see Chapter 6), will be of assistance in determining whether there is any structural abnormality present which would require surgical correction.

Disease progression and prognosis

If the chronic infections are only affecting one kidney, the disease is usually prolonged but benign. Bilateral chronic infection will ensure that chronic renal failure is of a rapid onset.

Reflux Nephropathy

Chronic renal failure can be caused by reflux nephropathy, a congenital anatomical abnormality where there is incompetence of the sphincter at the junction of the ureter with the bladder, allowing the reflux of urine (vesico ureteric reflux) back up the ureter and in to the renal pelvis of the kidney (intrarenal reflux). Infection may develop and the formation of scar tissue will eventually cause chronic renal failure. Reflux can be uni- or bilateral and is present at birth, rarely developing in adults.

Clinical features and management of care for the patient

In children whose reflux is minimal and does not cause infections, the reflux may disappear as they get older and may never be detected. In children with severe and bilateral reflux, repeated urinary tract infections are common and the resulting scar tissue formation in the kidneys leads to chronic renal failure as adulthood is reached. A child who has repeated urinary tract infections should have the cause investigated and a micturating cystogram will demonstrate the reflux of urine up the ureter(s). Infections can be treated with antibiotics but if the reflux is severe, surgical correction will be needed to halt the progress of scar tissue formation and progressive renal impairment.

Classification

- Grade 1 – reflux partly up ureter;
- Grade 2 – reflux up to pelvis and calyces without dilation;
- Grade 3 – reflux up to pelvis and calyces with mild to moderate dilation of ureters;
- Grade 4 – moderate dilation and tortuosity of ureter, pelvis and calyces;
- Grade 5 – gross dilation and tortuosity of ureter, pelvis and calyces. Papillae in renal medulla no longer visible in calyces. At this stage the glomeruli are also sclerosed and the patient will start to develop signs of renal impairment.

ANALGESIC NEPHROPATHY

Chronic renal failure can be caused by an excessive and long-term intake of aspirin and/or analgesics containing phenacetin. The nephropathy is characterised by renal papillary necrosis (Fig. 5.1) and chronic interstitial nephritis.

Clinical features and management of care for the patient

The first signs of renal impairment are haematuria, sterile pyuria and polyuria. Repeated urinary tract infections can also occur which need to be treated to slow down the progression of scar tissue formation.

Other clinical manifestations that require treatment include hypertension, which is caused by renal artery stenosis or thrombosis. Patients also present with severe premature atherosclerosis with associated ischaemic heart, cerebrovascular and peripheral vascular disease, all as a result of the analgesic abuse.

The first line of treatment for analgesic nephropathy would require the patient to stop taking the analgesic medication. Non-steroidal anti-inflammatory drugs (NSAIDS), should also be avoided, due to their nephrotoxic effects. To ensure that the analgesic abuse has ceased, the patient's urine can be tested for the presence of salicyates.

Renal replacement therapy may be the eventual outcome for patients who have analgesic nephropathy but many patients will only need long-term outpatient follow-ups to monitor renal function.

RENAL TUBULAR DISORDERS

Renal Tubular Acidosis

This disease is caused by a specific tubular abnormality which prevents the excretion of acid, ultimately resulting in a systemic metabolic acidosis. Two types of tubular acidosis are discussed.

Type One – Distal Tubular Acidosis

Clinical features and management of care for the patient
This disease is inherited as an autosomal dominant trait. A chronic hyper-chloraemic systemic acidosis exists in the patient, with the distal tubules failing to reduce the urinary pH. There is also reduced urinary concentration ability with increased potassium and calcium excretion leading to hypokalaemia, urolithiasis and osteomalacia. Renal function will appear normal but if the condition is left untreated the patient may develop chronic renal failure.

The aim of treatment is to correct the systemic acidosis and maintain a normal acid–base balance. Hypokalaemia and hypocalcaemia can be corrected with supplements and the acidosis can be corrected with oral sodium bicarbonate, which will be required indefinitely.

Type Two – Proximal Tubular Acidosis

Clinical features and management of care for the patient
This is usually a hereditary disorder where there is widespread proximal tubule dysfunction. There is a systemic, metabolic hyperchloraemic acidosis and an alkaline urine, but there is also a deficient bicarbonate reabsorption mechanism in the proximal tubule, resulting in bicarbonaturia. There is also some increase in the urinary excretion of potassium and calcium, again resulting in hypokalaemia and urolithiasis.

Alkali and potassium supplementation is required to correct the acidosis and hypokalaemia and will be given on a long-term basis.

GLOMERULAR DISEASES

Glomerulonephritis

In the past 20 years, there have been many advances made in the ability to differentiate between the various types of glomerulonephritis. This may suggest that the classification of glomerular disease is in a constant state of evolution and change. This section aims to clarify any confusion that may exist.

Glomerulonephritis may be defined as a bilateral, diffuse disease of the kidneys. It predominately affects the glomeruli, where there is a non-bacterial, inflammatory response, which is not due to an infection but occurs as a result of antigen/antibody reactions. The cause of the various glomerulonephritides can be classified into two types: primary glomerular disease or secondary glomerular disease.

Primary glomerular disease occurs when the structure or function of the glomerular capillary network has been damaged. It is also a collection of disorders where the glomeruli is the only, or the majority of tissue, that is involved. Examples of primary glomerular diseases are:

- acute glomerulonephritis – poststreptococcal/non-poststreptococcal
- rapidly progressive (crescenteric) glomeruonephritis
- minimal change disease*
- mesangial proliferative glomerulonephritis*
- membranous glomerulonephritis*
- focal glomerulosclerosis*
- chronic glomerulonephritis.

(*histological lesions seen in the nephrotic syndrome.)

Secondary glomerular disease is where the glomerular involvement is secondary to a systemic disease or hereditary disorder. Examples of secondary glomerular disease are:

- systemic lupus erythematosus
- Goodpasture's syndrome
- polyarteritis nodosa
- Wegner's granulomatosis
- amyloidosis
- Henoch–Schonlein purpura
- sickle cell disease*
- Alport's syndrome*

(*hereditary disorders.)

Disease process in glomerulonephritis

The various glomerular diseases are characterised by one or more of four basic tissue reactions:

- *Cellular proliferation.* There is an increase in the number of cells in the glomerular tuft and is a common response in glomerular diseases. The cells that are involved are endothelial, mesangial and epithelial.
- *Thickening of the basement membrane.* 'Thickening' is the general term that is given to the alterations that are seen in the basement membrane caused by glomerulonephritis and occur as a result of diabetic nephropathy or the deposition of circulating immune responses (seen in systemic lupus erythematosus).
- *Leukocytic exudation.* There is infiltration of the glomerulus by leukocytes, neutrophils and monocytes.
- *Sclerosis.* There is deposition of eosinphilic acelluar material in the glomerulus causing irreversible damage to the glomerular tuft.

Because many of the glomerulonephritides are of unknown aetiology, they will be classified by the histological characteristics given above. The areas of these changes in the kidney that are found on biopsy are described as:

- diffuse – changes that affect the entire glomerulus and all of the glomeruli;
- focal – changes affecting some, but not all of the glomeruli;
- global – all glomeruli are affected;
- mesangial – changes affecting the mesangial region only;
- segmental – changes affecting a portion of the glomerulus.

Acute Glomerulonephritis

In most types of glomerulonephritis, the major immunoglobulin (or antibody) IgG, found in the serum, can be detected in the glomerular capillary walls, occurring as a result of an antigen/antibody reaction, where aggregates (or groups of complexes) are formed, then circulate throughout the body, with some complexes eventually lodging themselves in the glomerulus, inducing an inflammatory response.

In acute glomerulonephritis, the stimulus of this reaction is a 'group A' streptococcal infection of the throat or skin. It is classified as a poststreptococcal glomerulonephritis and it is this type of acute glomerulonephritis that is now examined in more detail.

Poststreptococcal Glomerulonephritis (see Plate 1)

There is an abrupt onset of the disease, but the patient is usually able to give a recent history of 10–14 days of a throat or skin infection. The disease may also occur after numerous bacterial, viral and parasitic infections.

Children over the age of 2 years are more likely to be affected but the disease does occur in adults.

Disease process

The streptococci act as an antigen and generate circulating antibodies, which are deposited in the glomeruli, causing damage to the kidney. There is an increase in the production of endothelial cells lining the glomerulus, with infiltration by leukocytes and thickening of the glomerular basement membrane. This results in scarring and a reduction in the filtering surface of the kidney. On visual examination, the kidneys appear large and swollen with an irregular outer surface.

There is a latent period of around 10–14 days between the onset of the streptococcal throat or skin infection and the development of the glomerulonephritis and this is due to the primary immune response to bacterial antigens entering the body.

Clinical features and management of care for the patient

The patient will pass gross haematuria in the form of smoky or red urine. This will occur during the initial streptococcal infection and again, 10–14 days afterwards. Proteinuria may also be present, but is usually less than 3.5 g day^{-1}. The formation of oedema and oliguria accompanied by hypertension is a result of sodium and water retention. The oedema is usually facial, giving a 'puffy' appearance especially on rising in the morning. Patients may also have circulatory congestion causing dyspnoea, cardiomyeagealy and pulmonary oedema.

To control oedema the patient will need to have fluids and sodium intake restricted. Loop diuretics such as frusemide may be prescribed to encourage a diuresis, which in turn reduces circulatory congestion and oedema.

Hypertension may be present in a patient with acute glomerulonephritis but it is usually mild and presents at the beginning of the disease process and reduces when the patient shows signs of recovery by passing urine again. This is usually within days or weeks, but antihypertensive medication may sometimes be required.

Any deterioration in renal function is due to the obstruction of the glomerular capillary lumina by endothelial proliferation and swelling. Renal blood flow may be slightly reduced or even normal in some patients.

Diagnostic investigations

The patient may be able to give a recent history of a throat or skin infection and swabs of these areas may confirm the presence of a 'group A' streptococci infection in the patient. Macroscopic or microscopic haematuria will be confirmed, but urine is usually sterile in acute glomerulonephritis, so a mid-stream specimen of urine may not be required.

Serum urea, electrolytes and creatinine will assess renal function and determine the extent of any renal damage.

A renal biopsy may be required if the symptoms continue 2–3 weeks after the initial onset, to ensure that chronic glomerulonephritis or rapidly progressive glomerulonephritis has not developed.

Disease progression and prognosis

Without complications, most patients who have acute glomerulonephritis can expect to have a diuresis within a week after the onset of the symptoms; however, some patients will have persistent proteinuria for up to a year after the onset of the disease and may also develop nephrotic syndrome or chronic renal impairment because of the progression into rapidly progressive glomerulonephritis, which is now discussed.

Rapidly Progressive Glomerulonephritis

Rapidly progressive glomerulonephritis (RPGN) is a clinical, pathological syndrome where the glomerular damage is associated with a rapid but progressive deterioration in a patient's renal function and the presence of oliguria or anuria. Without effective treatment, end-stage renal failure will develop in weeks and months, rather than years. The syndrome of RPGN may also occur in association with systemic diseases that affect glomerular function, for example Goodpasture's syndrome, Wegner's granulomatosis; systemic lupus erythematosus; polyarteritis nodosa.

Disease process

In RPGN, there is extensive involvement of the glomeruli which are surrounded and compressed by large crescenteric growths. The crescents are formed by the overproduction of epithelial cells of the Bowman's capsule and also by the infiltration of monocytes.

Clinical features and management of care for the patient

The patient with RPGN will usually present with acute renal failure and symptoms that are associated with the systemic diseases already listed. Haematuria is common, with the presence of proteinuria variable. Oedema and associated hypertension may be present in the patient.

The main objective in treating patients who have the disease is to remove the antiglomerular basement membrane antibodies, which can be achieved by the initiation of plasma exchanges (see Chapter 7).

Administration of oral cytotoxic drugs and corticosteriods can be of benefit in the treatment of this condition, but dialysis may also be needed if renal impairment is present.

Disease progression and prognosis

On examination of kidney tissue from a renal biopsy, the presence of crescents in large numbers is usually a sign of a poor prognosis from the recovery of the disease and chronic dialysis will be necessary.

Minimal Change Glomerulonephritis

This glomerular disease occurs commonly in children between the ages of 2 and 6 years and is the principal cause of childhood nephrotic syndrome, although minimal change glomerulonephritis can also develop in adults.

The cause of minimal change glomerulonephritis is not clear, but it is thought that it could be due to the patient suffering an allergic reaction to a substance or an immunological deficiency.

Clinical features and management of care for the patient

There is a rapid onset of the nephrotic syndrome in the patient. There is severe oedema (but without associated hypertension), which can be removed by the administration of diuretics, but intermittent ultrafiltration may also be required.

Corticosteroids will suppress the minimal change glomerulonephritis and achieve a remission. However, if the patient's condition is unresponsive to treatment or if severe side-effects develop from the steroids, oral cyclophosphamide could be considered.

A renal biopsy confirms the diagnosis of minimal change glomerulonephritis and should be performed when the patient's generalised oedema has reduced.

Disease progression and prognosis

After the first remission of the disease has been achieved with drug therapy, the patient may develop a relapse, but this possibility will diminish with the progression of time and relapses can be effectively treated with similar treatment protocols.

The glomerular disease is called 'minimal change' because little or no abnormalities can be detected in the glomeruli on biopsy examination and patients do not usually develop chronic renal failure.

Membranous Glomerulonephritis

In many cases of this glomerular disease no cause can be found, but some aetiological factors can include drugs and heavy metal poisoning (e.g. mercury), malignancies and infections (e.g. hepatitis B virus).

Patients are usually adults, with the disease not normally being found in children. Membranous glomerulonephritis has an insidious onset without any systemic disease being present and develops slowly – over a course of up to 20 years in some cases.

Disease process

Membranous glomerulonephritis is characterised by widespread thickening of the capillary walls of the glomeruli, caused by the deposition of complexes of antigen/antibody complements.

Clinical features and management of care for the patient

There are no specific clinical signs in patients, but often haematuria and proteinuria will be present. The clinical signs of the nephrotic syndrome may present if proteinuria increases as the disease progresses, but then only to reduce as renal function deteriorates. Levels of antinuclear and anti-glomerular basement membrane antibodies can assist in the diagnosis. A renal biopsy will confirm the presence of membranous glomerulonephritis.

The overall aim in the management of care for the patient is to remove the causative factor of the disease, but corticosteroids may also have some beneficial effect on its progression.

Disease progression and prognosis

Glomerular filtration rates in patients with membranous glomerular nephritis may be normal for the first few years, but then may slowly deteriorate as the sclerosis of the glomerolus increases. Spontaneous remissions will occur in rare cases and this may be permanent if the original causative factor is removed; however, in many patients dialysis is inevitable.

Focal Glomerulosclerosis

This can be a cause of the nephrotic syndrome and is associated with a slow but progressive deterioration in renal function with the origin often unknown. Secondary causes may include analgesic or heroin abuse, sickle cell disease, Alport's syndrome and sarcoidosis.

Clinical features and management of care for the patient

The patient usually presents with the nephrotic syndrome, but with no other specific features. Hypertension is common, as is haematuria and proteinuria.

The prognosis of this disease is influenced by the severity of proteinuria and development of the nephrotic syndrome. There is no response to steroids or immunosuppression therapy.

Chronic Glomerulonephritis

Chronic glomerulonephritis is the clinical term given for wide range of glomerular diseases that have a protracted course with the on-going destruction of nephrons. Chronic glomerulonephritis may develop following an episode of acute glomerulonephritis, or the nephrotic syndrome. It may also occur without any history of renal disease.

Disease process

Chronic glomerulonephritis is characterised by slow progressive destruction or sclerosis of the glomeruli and a gradual loss of renal function. The kidneys gradually reduce in size, with tubular atrophy, chronic interstitial inflammation and arteriosclerosis (Fig. 5.1). The cause is often unknown, as renal biopsies are rarely performed on 'small kidneys'.

Clinical features and management of care for the patient

As some patients progress through the latent stage of chronic glomerulo-nephritis, they may only experience a slow onset of dependent oedema, dyspnoea on exertion and headaches due to hypertension. Once a definite deterioration in renal function is noted and a diagnosis made, the onset of end-stage renal failure can be rapid.

Disease progression and prognosis   The progression of chronic glomerulonephritis may vary considerably in patients. Some present with few symptoms such as proteinuria or haematuria and develop deteriorating renal function over a course of up to 15–20 years (called the latent stage) until dialysis is required.

THE NEPHROTIC SYNDROME

The nephrotic syndrome is not a disease, but a collection of symptoms. It is characterised by:

- heavy proteinuria (greater than 3.5 g in 24 h)
- a reduction in plasma proteins
- severe and generalised oedema.

The nephrotic syndrome may develop in a patient with a primary renal disease of unknown cause (idiopathic nephrotic syndrome) or it may be associated with other conditions in which kidney involvement is secondary, such as amyloidosis or diabetes mellitus (Fig. 5.2).

Pathology of the disease process

The nephrotic syndrome is the result of glomerular damage increasing the glomerular basement membrane permeability, allowing large amounts of small albumin molecules to pass through into the urine. As the disease progresses, larger molecular weight proteins leak through the glomerular basement membrane and glomerular filtration rates may also reduce as the glomerular damage increases.

   As the protein continues to be excreted, the serum albumin decreases (hypoalbuminaemia). This in turn leads to a low plasma osmotic pressure and diffusion of fluid into the tissue spaces causing generalised oedema.

   A reduction in the circulating blood volume stimulates the release of aldosterone from the adrenal cortex, which is responsible for the retention of sodium and water. Retained fluid also passes out of the capillaries into the tissues, causing more oedema (Fig. 5.3).

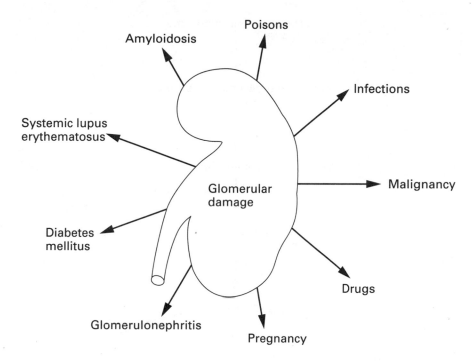

Fig 5.2 *Causes of the nephrotic syndrome.*

In the early stages of the nephrotic syndrome, the protein leak may be the only disorder of renal function, but with some glomerular lesions, the disease progresses and nephrons are destroyed, eventually leading to end-stage renal failure and the patient requiring chronic dialysis.

Clinical features and management of care for the patient

Oedema   In the early stages of the nephrotic syndrome, the patient may complain of swollen eyes first thing in the morning and swollen feet and ankles at the end of the day. As the disease progresses, or as a result of poor symptom control, the oedema becomes more generalised, causing pleural and peritoneal effusions and sacral oedema, and lower limbs may leak serous fluid through the skin's surface.

Fluid removal will be the treatment of priority for patients, but diuretic therapy needs to be administered carefully with the patient being closely monitored, as profound hypoalbuminaemia may cause a reduced circulating blood volume, triggering a hypotensive response in some patients, following the administration of large doses of intravenous diuretics (e.g. frusemide). Infusions of small volumes of intravenous salt-poor albumin prior to the administration of diuretics will increase plasma volume and restore a diuretic response in the patient. This regime gives an overall increase in

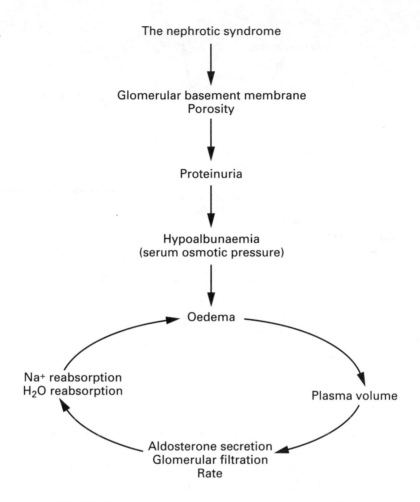

The nephrotic syndrome

Glomerular basement membrane
Porosity

Proteinuria

Hypoalbunaemia
(serum osmotic pressure)

Oedema

Na+ reabsorption
H₂O reabsorption

Plasma volume

Aldosterone secretion
Glomerular filtration
Rate

Fig 5.3 *Oedema formation in the nephrotic syndrome.*

the efficiency of the diuretics, but in the majority of the patients the albumin that is given is excreted after 24–48 h.

All patients with severe oedema, and receiving aggressive diuretics, should be weighed daily and have 4 hourly, lying and standing blood pressure recordings to observe for deficits caused by a reduced plasma volume.

Muscle wasting   The loss of skeletal muscles becomes apparent when the generalised oedema has subsided. Muscle wasting is a result of protein mobilisation into the circulating blood volume to counteract the effects of proteinuria.

Breathlessness   Patients with the nephrotic syndrome may be breathless at rest and on exertion, due to the development of pleural effusions, caused by the increasing oedema. The excessive weight gain caused by fluid retention may also give difficulty with breathing.

Pleural effusions can be tapped and the patient's breathing pattern should improve as the oedema reduces.

Proteinuria   Urine has a frothy appearance, due to the high protein content (usually greater than 3.5 g in 24 h) and as a consequence hypoalbuminaemia develops. Hyperlipidaemia is also a clinical sign of the nephrotic syndrome, as body fat stores are mobilised to assist with the synthesis of protein whilst there is a negative nitrogen balance caused by proteinuria.

Weight loss and malnutrition   The gastrointestinal tract becomes congested because of the oedema and the patient may complain of chronic nausea, vomiting and poor appetite. This will eventually result in weight loss and malnutrition and is exacerbated by the heavy proteinuria.

A dietetic referral should be made and the patient encouraged to take a high calorie diet with a protein allowance compensating for the protein loss. Meals should be small and taken at frequent intervals to aid digestion.

Tiredness and lethargy   These symptoms may be attributed to a combination of a reduced calorie intake due to anorexia, muscle wasting and weakness. Generalised oedema may result in the patient carrying up to 10 kg of extra body weight, using up more energy. Patients should be allowed plenty of rest and be encouraged to follow the dietary advice given to them to maintain maximum energy and optimum health.

Intravascular clotting   There is a risk of spontaneous intravascular clotting in a patient with the nephrotic syndrome due to the increase in circulating lipoproteins and cholesterol. Platelet counts are also slightly elevated and they become sticky so that 'clumping' occurs. There is also a higher concentration of fibrinogen.

During episodes of hospitalisation and immobility because of enforced bedrest, prophylactic anticoagulation of patients (usually with subcutaneous heparin) is a protocol that can be performed to reduce the risk of clot formation. This treatment can be given in conjunction with the patient wearing antiembolic stockings which increases the venous return in the lower limbs, again reducing the risk of clot formation.

Diagnostic investigations
A full history from the patient and a clinical examination may discover whether there was any preceding illness or allergies to drug therapies that may have caused the nephrotic syndrome.

Urinalysis will confirm the presence of proteinuria and a 24 h urine collection for protein selectivity and creatinine clearance will determine the severity of the syndrome in the patient. Serum urea, electrolytes and creatinine will assess renal function and a reduced serum albumin and elevated cholesterol levels in the patient will assist in the diagnosis. A renal biopsy should only be performed when the patient's sacral oedema has reduced.

The glomerular lesion that has caused the nephrotic syndrome can be treated by removing or suppressing the antibody/antigen reaction. This can be achieved by the administration of steroids or immunosuppressive agents or by plasma exchange.

SECONDARY GLOMERULAR DISEASES

Systemic Lupus Erythematosus (SLE)

Lupus is an autoimmune, multisystem disorder of the connective tissue, affecting the heart, kidneys, joints, central nervous system and the blood. It occurs predominately in women, particularly adolescents and young adults, and it has a familial tendency. The characteristic pattern of the disease is one of exacerbation and remission.

Disease process
Renal involvement develops in over half of the patients with lupus and occurs because of the antinuclear antibodies formation of autoimmune complexes, which are deposited in the glomerular capillaries. Immune complexes are also found on the walls of small arterioles and capillaries in connective tissue and serous membranes, eventually leading to necrosis.

Clinical features and management of care for the patient

Renal involvement   The clinical symptoms of renal impairment in lupus are variable and include gross/microscopic haematuria, acute nephritis, nephrotic syndrome or chronic renal impairment.

Central nervous system   The patient may present with neuropsychiatric disorders or convulsions. Cerebrovascular accidents may occur, resulting in hemiplegia.

Blood   Anaemia may be a clinical symptom in the patient, as well as other blood disorders such as thrombocytopenia, neutropenia, leukocytosis and leucopenia.

Joints   The patient may have restricted and painful movement due to polyarthralgia and polyarthritis, affecting the small finger joints.

Skin   Erythema over the bridge of the patient's nose/cheeks and continuing over the ears and neck or other parts of the body exposed to ultraviolet light is a classic sign of lupus and the rash is often referred to as the 'butterfly rash'.

The patient may also experience itching, skin lesions and alopecia during the acute episodes of the disease.

Heart and circulation   Raynaud's disease may be present in the patient who has lupus. If the heart is also involved in the disease process, pericarditis, myocarditis and endocarditis can be serious complications.

General symptoms   The patient may complain of moderate to severe fever, generalised weakness, weight loss and fatigue.

The extrarenal manifestations of lupus are effectively treated with corticosteroids. High doses are initially required and then slowly reduced to a maintenance dose. Immunosuppressive drugs and plasmapheresis can also be beneficial in the treatment of lupus.

Diagnostic investigations

These should include the following:

- the patient should be asked to recall any recent history of drug allergies;
- serum DNA and anti-DNA binding tests and antinuclear factor;
- blood for presence of rheumatoid factor and white cell count;
- urinalysis to detect for haematuria/proteinuria.

Disease progression and prognosis

The overall prognosis for patients with lupus is improving. Those patients who have the disease diagnosed early usually have only minimal changes seen on renal biopsy tissue. In these cases, it is uncommon for the renal involvement to progress further. If the disease develops in the patient and end-stage renal failure occurs, peritoneal dialysis or haemodialysis can be selected. In patients who have a renal transplant, lupus does not reoccur in the graft.

Goodpasture's Syndrome

This is a rare disease that is characterised by a rapid onset of deteriorating renal function in association with haemoptysis and severe dyspnoea.

Disease process

It is thought that there is a development of an antibody which attacks the glomerular basement membrane and alveolar capillary membrane. In the early stages or in a mild form of the disease, the deterioration in renal function is caused by focal and segmental necrotising glomerulonephritis, causing haematuria and a reduced glomerular filtration rate.

In severe forms of the disease there is extensive necrosis, fibrin deposition and the formation of epithelial crescents similar to those found in rapidly progressive glomerulonephritis.

Disease progression and prognosis

If left undiagnosed or untreated, the crescenteric glomerulonephritis will progress, eventually causing end-stage renal failure, with the other symptom of Goodpasture's syndrome – haemoptysis – still occurring intermittently.

Cytotoxic drugs and corticosteroids may be administered to initiate a remission, but plasma exchanges are also effective in removing the antibody that causes Goodpasture's syndrome.

Necrotising Vasculitis

Necrotising vasculitis represents a group of disorders that cause inflammation and necrosis to vessel walls of arteries, veins and capillaries.

There are many types of vasculitis, but the main types that involve the kidneys are polyarteritis nodosa (or classic) and Wegner's granulomatosis.

Polyarteritis Nodosa

This type of vasculitis has a multisystem involvement and is characterised by the small- and medium-sized vessels developing arteritic lesions that are widely disseminated throughout the body and which eventually cause aneurysm formation, rupture, haemorrhage, thrombosis and recanalisation and infarction of renal tissue.

Clinical features and management of care for the patient

General clinical features of the disease will include fever and weight loss, hypertension and tachycardia. The patient may have severe abdominal pain due to mesenteric arteritis and develop gangrene on their extremities as the vessels in their limbs become diseased. Proteinuria associated with deteriorating renal function indicates renal involvement.

The treatment will require the patient to have high dose corticosteroids and immunosuppressive drugs such as cyclophosphamide.

Diagnostic investigations

Diagnosis of the disease is usually by muscle, skin, nerve or renal biopsy. Renal arteriography may also reveal small aneurysms which are diagnostic characteristics of polyarteritis nodosa.

Wegner's Granulomatosis

This is a severe disease that can occur at any age, but appears to be more prevalent in older males, the onset being in middle age.

Disease process

Wegner's granulomatosis is a rare necrotising vasculitis with necrotising granulomatous arteritis of the upper and lower respiratory tract and deteriorating renal function that is due to focal and diffuse necrotising glomerulonephritis with crescent formation.

The process occurs because of immune complexes being deposited in the artery walls, damaging the endothelium and occluding the vessels. Necrotising granulomas in the lungs develop in association with necrotising glomerulonephritis.

Clinical features and management of care for the patient

The patient will experience severe ear, upper and lower respiratory tract symptoms of:

- epistaxis/otitis media
- haemoptysis and pleurisy and dyspnoea
- chest pain/pericarditis
- arthralgia.

Symptoms indicating renal involvement will include haematuria or proteinuria and hypertension. The patient can be treated with corticosteroids and cytotoxic drugs and initiation of plasma exchange can slow down the progression of the disease.

RENAL AMYLOIDOSIS

Amyloidosis is the term given to a group of chronic infiltrative disorders characterised by the presence of deposits of an abnormal protein called amyloid, which is the result of chronic infections or inflammation. Amyloid is deposited in tissues and infiltrates all organs of the body including the kidney and is possibly related to an immunological disturbance, as the amyloid material contains a fragment of a light chain of immunoglobulin molecules. Renal involvement in amyloidosis occurs when there is an accumulation of amyloid which progressively replaces the glomerulus.

Disease classification
Amyloidosis can be classified as a primary disease or as a secondary disease where it complicates various systemic disorders.

Primary Amyloidosis

In primary amyloidosis there is no underlying cause of the disease and the deposition of amyloid will involve multiple organs such as the gastrointestinal tract, heart, liver, kidneys, spleen and peripheral nerves. Primary amyloidosis affects men and women equally, between the ages of 20 and 40 years, and is occasionally familial. Patients will present with various symptoms depending on which organ has been infiltrated with the amyloid.

Secondary Amyloidosis

Infiltration of amyloid occurs in the liver, spleen, kidneys, adrenals, small intestine, arteries and skin. The disease will have an underlying cause and is associated with:

- chronic infective conditions such as osteomyelitis and tuberculosis;
- chronic non-infective inflammatory conditions such as rheumatoid arthritis, ulcerative colitis and ankylosing spondylitis;
- neoplastic conditions – Hodgkin's disease, myeloma;
- familial amyloid disease (complication of the familial Mediterranean fever).

Clinical features and management of care for the patient
The patient may present with hypoalbuminaemia which can be due to several causes:

- heavy proteinuria from the nephrotic syndrome;
- reduced protein synthesis by the liver as a consequence of hepatic amyloidosis;
- impaired absorption of amino acids because of amyloid deposits in the mucous membrane of the small intestine; hypotension may be present in the patient and is due to amyloid deposition in the sympathetic chains. A sudden deterioration in renal function may be indicative of a renal thrombosis formation which develops in the intrarenal veins.

Diagnostic investigations
A clinical examination will find the possible cause of amyloidosis such as septic lesions or chronic inflammatory conditions.

Urinalysis will determine the presence of proteinuria and a 24-h urine collection for protein selectivity and creatinine clearance will assist in confirming if the patient has the nephrotic syndrome. Serum urea, electrolytes and creatinine will also assess present renal function.

Characteristic deposits of amyloid will be found in kidney tissue from a renal biopsy but if this investigation is inappropriate, a rectal biopsy can be performed which will detect amyloid material in the rectal tissue.

Disease progression and prognosis

There is no satisfactory form of treatment for amyloidosis. Steroids have been found to be ineffective but the appropriate treatment should be given for the nephrotic syndrome and chronic renal failure. Spontaneous remissions are rare but they can occur, especially if the underlying cause of chronic infection is treated effectively. Amyloidosis also reoccurs in the grafts of renal transplant patients.

Distribution of amyloid in the kidney found on renal biopsy determines the severity of the disease. On microscopy, if amyloid is widespread interstitially and in the vessels, the prognosis is poor. If the amyloid is predominately in the glomeruli the prognosis improves.

MULTIPLE MYELOMA AND RENAL INVOLVEMENT

In multiple myeloma there is a malignant proliferation of plasma cells producing large quantities of monoclonal immunoglobulins which are then deposited in the glomerular capillaries. Monoclonal light chains are also excessively produced and are filtered and precipitated in the renal tubules, forming casts causing a cellular reaction because of their toxicity. The mononclonal light chains are also known as Bence–Jones protein.

Clinical features and management of care for the patient

Acute or chronic renal failure will affect over half of the patients with multiple myeloma and is exacerbated by hypercalcaemia (due to bone reabsorption), hyperuricaemia and the development of amyloidosis. Renal involvement can be confirmed by the presence of Bence–Jones proteinuria.

Immunosuppression in the form of cytotoxic drugs and steroids can be used to treat the patient.

SICKLE CELL DISEASE

Sickle cell disease is a severe inherited disorder of haemoglobin synthesis and is associated with a variety of symptoms, such as anaemia, pain in the abdomen, joints, muscles and bones. Patients with sickle cell disease or sickle cell trait (the carrier state) also have functional changes present in the kidney that can progress to chronic renal impairment, although glomerular lesions are unusual in patients with the sickle cell trait.

Disease process (sickle cell trait)

Haematuria is caused by medullary ischaemia resulting from intravascular sickling of erythrocytes in the medulla of the kidney. There is also a urinary concentration deficit where urine is unable to be concentrated and is passed in large dilute quantities.

Disease process (sickle cell disease)

Enlarged and congested glomeruli with sickled erythrocytes within the capillary lumen prevents urinary concentration. The sickling of erythrocytes in the renal capillary bed causes ischaemia and infarction of renal tissue. Papillary necrosis develops slowly and the sickled cells cause decreased perfusion leading to the eventual necrosis of the papilla.

Clinical features and management of care for the patient

Clinical features of glomerular involvement in patients with sickle cell disease will include proteinuria and haematuria with the nephrotic syndrome developing in some patients. The course of the renal disease usually takes the form of slow but progressive glomerulosclerosis.

Disease progression and prognosis

There is, as yet, no specific or effective form of treatment available for those patients with sickle cell glomerular disease. Sickle cell crisis still occurs in those patients who have undergone renal transplantation.

VASCULAR DISEASES OF THE KIDNEY AND HYPERTENSION

Abnormal processes or diseases that cause narrowing to the lumen of renal blood vessels and a reduction in blood flow to the renal cortex will ultimately reduce the glomerular filtration rate and cause deterioration in renal function. The causative factors can include renal artery stenosis or nephrosclerosis (sclerosis of the renal arterioles).

Renal Artery Stenosis

This can be a cause of hypertension and occurs when there is narrowing of the lumen of arteries that supply the kidneys by a process called arteriosclerosis. The changes that take place include:

- *Atherosclerosis*. Lipids and fibrous tissue lining the main renal artery and its larger branches.
- *Hyaline arteriolar sclerosis*. Thickening vessel walls due to the deposition of hyaline material, narrowing the lumen. Occurs naturally after 50 years of age, but is also seen earlier in diabetics.

- *Thickening of small arteries*. Increase of fibrous tissue in the media of arteries, narrowing the lumen. Obstruction to the renal blood flow can also be caused by:
- *Vasculitis*. Necrosis and inflammation of the vessel walls because of immunological changes.
- *Embolism*. The kidney is a common site of embolism from circulating cardiac thrombi.
- *Thrombosis*. Intravascular coagulation in the arterioles and glomerular capillaries of the kidney, which will result in renal tissue infarction.

Disease progression and prognosis

In renal artery stenosis there is a major reduction in renal perfusion. This alteration results in increased renin secretion and activation of the renin/angiotensin/aldosterone system (see Chapter 2). If left untreated, accelerated hypertension will develop, resulting in further pathological changes and damage to the kidneys.

Renal artery stenosis can be treated by angioplasty of the renal artery with intra-arterial balloon catheters. If this is unsuccessful, removal of the small and diseased kidney can be performed.

Nephrosclerosis

Hypertension can cause nephrosclerosis and is a major precipitating factor of renal disease. Hypertension that is not treated leads to sclerosis of the renal arterioles and the blood supply to glomeruli, tubules and interstitium gradually decreases. Scar tissue develops in the kidney, resulting in loss of renal function and eventually chronic renal failure.

Scleroderma

Scleroderma, or systemic sclerosis, is an uncommon disease affecting the vascular system. Its characteristics include the excessive deposition of collagen in the dermis and viscera mainly in the gastrointestinal tract. There is also small vessel arteritis particularly involving the kidneys which takes the form of glomerulonephritis.

The cause is unknown, but it is thought that there are immunological pathogenic mechanisms involved.

Clinical features and management of care for the patient

In the initial stage of the disease, oedema develops in the fingers of patients and is followed by stiffness of the joints. The skin then becomes waxy in appearance, but remains rigid. The sclerosis eventually spreads to the forearms, face, upper trunk, and to the feet and legs. Visceral involvement can lead to dysphasia, pulmonary fibrosis and possibly cardiac complications.

Renal involvement in scleroderma is common and is dominated by hypertension, with a small number of patients developing malignant hypertension and rapidly progressive renal failure.

Steroids are of no benefit in patients with this unpleasant disease, but the hypertension can be treated with the usual regimes of antihypertensive drugs and as a consequence effective blood pressure control will reduce the complications of the disease, but chronic dialysis is usually an inevitable outcome.

ADULT POLYCYSTIC DISEASE

Adult polycystic disease is a congenital, progressive condition where both kidneys enlarge with the development of multiple cysts that cause a slow deterioration in renal function and eventually end-stage renal failure.

Adult polycystic disease is an autosomal dominant trait, occurring equally in men and women and transmitted by both sexes. If one parent is affected, 50% of the offspring will develop the disease in later life.

Adults with the disorder develop symptoms by the time they are 30 or 40 years and the progression into end-stage renal failure will be 10–15 years after the symptoms first arise.

Familial screening can result in the early detection of the disease, enabling medical care which prevents and slows down the progression towards the patient requiring chronic dialysis.

Disease process
Both kidneys are considerably enlarged and consist of a compact mass of cysts which are scattered equally throughout the cortex and medulla (Fig. 5.1). The cysts increase in size and eventually rupture, allowing infections and scar tissue formation and reducing the number of functioning nephrons.

The enlarged cysts compress the normal renal tissue and hypertensive changes and glomerulosclerosis occur. Cysts are filled with watery fluid which may be clear, bloodstained from a recent haemorrhage, brown from an old haemorrhage or filled with pus.

Liver cysts may be found in patients with polycystic kidneys and there is also a significant association with aneurysms of the cerebral arteries.

Clinical features and management of care for the patient

Pain   The patient with polycystic kidneys may complain of abdominal distension or discomfort following minor physical trauma that can cause frank or microscopic haematuria. Flank pain is associated with the large cysts rupturing and any blood clots that are passed will cause the patient to experience 'colic'-type pain.

Mild analgesia may be sufficient to relieve the discomfort, but pain caused by the cysts rupturing or clot retention from frank haematuria may require the patient to have opiate medication.

Haematuria   Mild to frank haematuria with clot formation will occur if the blood-filled cysts rupture, in the presence of renal stones or infection of the renal tract. Mild proteinuria is always present in the mid to late stages of the disease and may be the first abnormality that draws attention to the polycystic disease in the patient when undergoing a routine medical examination. A short period of bed rest and assistance with the patient's activities of daily living are advised if the patient experiences light haematuria and is otherwise asymptomatic.

Patients with adult polycystic disease who suffer with chronic blood loss do not usually have profound anaemia as there is an increase in erythropoietin production by the cysts. Patients who are susceptible to physical trauma to their abdomen are advised to modify their lifestyle and physical activity to reduce the risk of haemorrhage.

Urinary tract infections   Repeated urinary tract infections are common complications, and occur as a result of ruptured cysts becoming infected. Septicaemia is a rare complication of infected cysts and could occur following delayed antibiotic treatment. To prevent urinary tract infections, female patients should receive health education with perineal hygiene and all patients should be advised on the importance of a high fluid intake to prevent urinary stasis and how to recognise the signs of a urinary tract infection.

Hypertension   Secondary hypertension is common in patients with polycystic disease and may deteriorate as end-stage renal failure approaches. Hypertension can also accelerate renal damage.

Diagnostic investigations

- There may be a familial history of the disease and on physical examination, bilateral enlarged polycystic kidneys will be abdominally palpated with ease and have a characteristic knobbly feel. Many patients will also have an increase in their abdominal girth size.
- Urinalysis confirms the presence of haematuria and proteinuria.
- Serum urea, electrolytes and creatinine assess renal function.
- A straight X-ray of the kidneys, ureters and bladder and a retrograde pyelogram confirms the size and irregular outline of the kidneys. An intravenous pyelogram will illustrate the distortion of the renal pelvis and calyces by the cysts.
- Abdominal ultrasounds or a computed axial tomography scan (CAT scan) will detail the cyst development by distinguishing between solid and

liquid renal masses and show the distribution of large and small cysts. A CAT scan will also confirm liver or cerebral involvement.

Management of renal replacement therapy

When a patient with polycystic kidney disease reaches end-stage renal failure, haemodialysis is usually the preferred treatment option, although when heparin is given to maintain patency of the extracorporeal circuit, it may aggravate further haemorrhage from the cysts.

Continuous ambulatory peritoneal dialysis (CAPD) is not usually a suitable treatment option, as the enlarged polycystic kidneys reduce the amount of intra-abdominal space for dialysis fluid and repeated peritonitis may occur as a result of the pus-filled cysts rupturing.

Uni/bilateral nephrectomies are usually only performed if the cystic kidneys cause persistent infections, haemorrhage or chronic pain – especially if the patient wishes to be considered for a renal transplant.

The familial tendency of polycystic kidney disease may mean that the patient will have an insight into the disease process and dialysis treatments and as a result may be very anxious. Family members may have died as a result of complications of the disease.

Prevention is the only way of reducing the incidence of adult polycystic disease and some families may be offered genetic counselling or familial screening. However, information gained may be of minimal comfort to a patient facing the possibility of dialysis within the next 20–30 years.

DIABETIC NEPHROPATHY

Diabetic nephropathy is the term used to describe damage to the kidney structure and function that occurs as a result of the long-term complications of diabetes mellitus.

Pathology of disease process

The appearance of proteinuria in a diabetic patient will indicate that renal impairment is present. The progression towards end-stage renal failure is inevitable and may be rapid. Proteinuria usually develops 10–20 years after the initial onset of diabetes. If proteinuria does not appear after 30 years, the patient is no longer considered to be at risk of developing diabetic nephropathy.

The kidneys may be of normal size or slightly larger than normal and the glomerular lesions that occur are:

● Pyelonephritis, the most common lesion found in diabetic patients, causing chronic renal failure and a result of autonomic neuropathy in the bladder.

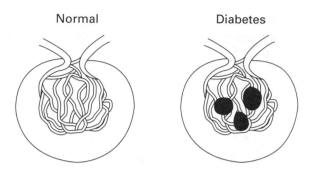

Fig 5.4 *Histological changes in the glomerulus of the kidney in diabetic nephropathy.*

- Diffuse intercapillary glomerulosclerosis, causing thickening and sclerosis of the basement membrane of the glomerular capillary and proliferation of the mesangial cells.
- The glomerulus becoming increasingly replaced and destroyed by the deposition of nodules of a glycoprotein material – 'nodular glomerulosclerosis' (or Kimmeisteil Wilson nodules) (Fig. 5.4).
- Arteriosclerosis develops in the arteries supplying the glomerulus due to hyaline deposits in the afferent and efferent arterioles causing ischaemia and accelerating the disease process.
- Papillary necrosis (Fig. 5.1).

Clinical features and management of care for the patient

Urinary tract infections   Patients with diabetic nephropathy may be more susceptible to developing urinary tract infections, causing further renal damage. The repeated infections may be a result of incomplete emptying of the patient's bladder following micturition because of autonomic neuropathy (i.e. neurogenic bladder). This in turn allows urine to become stagnant, encouraging bacterial growth and infection.

Renal failure and glucose control   The kidneys have an important role in the metabolism of insulin and as the glomerular filtration rate decreases in renal failure, so does the delivery of insulin to the proximal tubule cells where it is metabolised. Consequently, the circulating half-life of insulin increases with higher levels in the body after any given dose. Insulin requirements or oral hypoglycaemic agents should therefore be decreased so that hypoglycaemia does not occur.

Progressive uraemia and its unpleasant side-effects of nausea and vomiting may mean that the patient can only tolerate a reduced calorie intake and will need less insulin to prevent hypoglycaemia.

With altered insulin and glucose metabolism, many diabetic patients with deteriorating renal function may appear to have an improved glucose control (i.e. stable diabetes). Good blood glucose control in patients with glomerulosclerosis has been proven to prevent or to slow down the progression towards end-stage renal failure.

MANAGEMENT OF RENAL REPLACEMENT THERAPY

HAEMODIALYSIS

Haemodialysis is not often a treatment option in patients with diabetic nephropathy as peripheral vascular disease and neuropathy, both long-term complications of diabetes, may make the creation and maintenance of vascular access very difficult. For diabetic patients for whom haemodialysis is the only treatment option available, permanent forms of access such as grafts or Tenckhoff subclavian catheters may be necessary to ensure adequate and long-term dialysis access.

Cardiac disease, another complication of diabetes, may also be a contraindication to the patient receiving haemodialysis. Intermittent dialysis and fluid removal puts the patient at risk of cardiovascular instability and haemodialysis intolerance.

CONTINUOUS AMBULATORY PERITONEAL DIALYSIS (CAPD)

CAPD is usually the treatment of choice for patients with diabetic nephropathy. The treatment, being continuous, is ideal for those patients who are haemodynamically unstable or have few sites suitable for vascular access.

Retinal disease may cause the patient to become visually impaired or blind. At one time this would have been indicative that the treatment option would be haemodialysis, because of the difficulties of training and coping independently with CAPD. Many mechanical devices are now available to assist the patient in performing CAPD exchanges independently and safely.

Pathology of Chronic Renal Failure

When the glomerular filtration rate falls below 5% of normal in adults with chronic renal failure, chronic health problems will be experienced which can be treated conservatively until dialysis is required.

The management of chronic renal failure and its complications is now discussed.

MANAGEMENT OF CHRONIC RENAL FAILURE

The aim of management of chronic renal failure is to delay the progression towards end-stage renal failure and dialysis. This can be attained by:

- treatment of lesion causing renal failure (see previous notes);
- blood pressure control;
- avoidance of nephrotoxic agents;
- dietary restriction of protein (see Chapter 9);
- nursing and medical management of extrarenal manifestations of chronic renal failure.

The management of these treatments is now discussed in turn.

BLOOD PRESSURE CONTROL

The control of hypertension is the treatment of priority in patients with chronic renal failure in preventing the progression of renal failure and cardiovascular complications. Health education pertaining to cessation of smoking and alcohol, healthy eating and regular exercise for weight control is just as important in patients with chronic renal failure as in other patients with hypertension.

AVOIDANCE OF NEPHROTOXIC AGENTS

The avoidance of nephrotoxic drugs in patients with chronic renal failure is very important in the prevention of accelerated renal failure. If patients have to take drugs that are known to be nephrotoxic, drug levels and renal function should be closely monitored, and if renal function deteriorates suddenly, the drug should be discontinued (for mechanisms of drug-induced toxicity refer to Appendix One).

NURSING AND MEDICAL MANAGEMENT OF EXTRARENAL MANIFESTATIONS

Haemotologic Abnormalities (Anaemia)

Chronic renal failure will affect three types of cells in the blood:

- erythrocytes – causing anaemia;
- leukocytes – causing immunosuppression;
- platelets – causing bleeding tendencies.

Anaemia in advanced chronic renal failure is usually normocytic and normochronic and due to primary causes such as reduced erythropoietin production, uraemic toxins inhibiting erythropoiesis and haemolysis due to uraemic changes to the red cell membrane.

Treatment

- Correct contributing factors to anaemia, e.g. gastrointestinal bleeding or iron, folate or vitamin B12 deficiency.
- Maintain adequate nutrition.
- Administer blood transfusions when haemoglobulin falls to a predetermined level set by clinicians, or administer recombinant erythropoietin as prescribed until desired haemocrit is achieved and then continue with a maintenance dose.
- A persistent anaemia may be indicative of the patient commencing chronic dialysis.

Gastrointestinal Disorders

Gastrointestinal disorders in patients with chronic renal failure are common, especially as the patient approaches end stage. A wide range of symptoms are experienced due to uraemia and include anorexia, nausea and vomiting, a metallic taste in the mouth and hiccoughs.

Heartburn may be caused by the side-effects of oral iron supplements and phosphate binders but could also be due to peptic ulcer formation.

Constipation is common, because of a combination of a low residue diet (necessary for a reduced potassium intake), decreased fluid allowance and reduced physical activity due to chronic tiredness and lethargy.

Bleeding from the gastrointestinal tract can occur in advanced chronic renal failure causing haematemesis or malaena. Urea is excreted in the gut and is broken down, releasing ammonia which acts as an irritant.

Treatment

Patient education is required on the importance of medications to relieve the symptoms which are safe to take in chronic renal failure, as many preparations can be bought without a prescription but can cause complications in renal patients.

If nausea, vomiting and weight loss are persistent because of uraemia, dialysis may be the only effective treatment available.

Dermatological Disorders

Generalised uraemic pruritus is a distressing symptom in patients with chronic renal failure, with often little relief gained from drugs. Deposition of calcium and phosphorus in the skin and sweat glands excreting urea are thought to be causative factors of pruritus, but dry skin and drug allergies must not be overlooked as causes.

Platelet defects and capillary permeability, both complications of renal failure, can cause bleeding and bruising of the skin, especially if there is continued scratching. Many patients with advanced chronic renal failure also have a yellow tinge to their skin which is a combined result of hypermelanosis and the deposition of pigments in the skin (urochrome and carotene) that are usually excreted by the kidneys.

Treatment

Although the medications included in Appendix One may give some relief from pruritus, commencement of dialysis may be the only long-term relief.

Renal Osteodystrophy (Renal Bone Disease)

In patients with chronic renal failure there is an abnormality of vitamin D metabolism, causing deficient calcium levels, skeletal damage and bone pain.

In normal health, vitamin D (cholecalciferol) is metabolised in the liver to 25-hydroxycholecalciferol which is then activated to 1.25 dihydroxycholecalciferol (1.25-(OH) D3) in the kidney, allowing calcium and phosphates to be absorbed from the gut. In renal failure this process is impaired and therefore calcium is unable to be absorbed, resulting in a low serum calcium (hypocalcaemia).

Again in normal health, a low serum calcium triggers a response in the parathyroid glands and parathormone is released, inducing renal retention of calcium. In renal failure this response does not occur and an excess of parathormone is released, eventually leaching calcium from the bones.

Phosphate retention (hyperphosphataemia) in chronic renal failure provides further stimulus for hyperparathyroidism and exacerbating hypocalcaemia by allowing the precipitation into soft tissue. Persistent metabolic acidosis in advanced renal failure reduces bone carbonate buffers and causes a loss of calcium from the bone, as calcium is more soluble in acid conditions (see Chapter 2).

Treatment

The aim of treatment is to maintain calcium and phosphate levels within normal ranges, thus preventing hyperparathyroidism.

After correcting the metabolic acidosis, plasma phosphate and calcium levels can be controlled by oral phosphate binders, calcium supplements and the introduction of dietary restrictions (see Chapter 9). However, some patients remain hypocalcaemic and require oral vitamin D preparations to aid calcium absorption from the gut, but care must be taken not to induce hypercalcaemia.

Volume Disorders

During the progression of chronic renal failure, some nephrons remain intact while others continue to be destroyed. The remaining undamaged nephrons hypertrophy and produce an increased volume of filtrate with increased tubular reabsorption even though there is a reduction in the glomerular filtration rate. This process allows the kidney to continue to function until three-quarters of the nephrons are destroyed.

In patients with advanced chronic renal failure with blood urea maintained above $40 \, \text{mmol} \, 1^{-1}$, the solute load becomes greater than can be reabsorbed, producing an osmotic diuresis accompanied by polyuria of up to $3 \, 1$ in a 24-h period. The urine is dilute as the kidney's concentration ability is lost and the patient will have nocturia.

As more nephrons are destroyed, oliguria occurs with the retention of waste products. The patient develops a wide variety of biochemical, haematological and endocrinal disorders and clinical features of fluid overload.

Treatment

Fluid retention/oedema   Fluid restrictions may be required in association with diuretics. Loop diuretics such as frusemide or bumetanide will increase sodium excretion from the kidneys and prevent sodium retention.

Polyuria   During episodes of polyuria or fluid loss from diarrhoea or persistent vomiting, volume replacement should be administered to prevent a further reduction in renal perfusion and worsening of kidney function.

Dialysis   When volume overload is unresponsive to treatment, the commencement of dialysis is usually indicated.

Potassium Disorders

Excess potassium is normally removed by renal excretion, but as chronic renal failure progresses, excretion of urinary potassium decreases because of a reduced glomerular filtration rate or a distal tubular defect in diseases such as diabetes mellitus or tubulointerstitial abnormalities, ultimately resulting in hyperkalaemia.

Hyperkalaemia (serum potassium above $6.0 \, mmol \, l^{-1}$) can occur in advanced chronic renal failure following episodes of acute illness or infection, or dietary indiscretions if a potassium restriction has been enforced.

Chronic metabolic acidosis also causes potassium to shift out of cells and into the extracellular fluid, causing hyperkalaemia.

Treatment

- If metabolic acidosis is present, this should be corrected first, which will then assist in reducing the serum potassium to safe limits.
- If chronic hyperkalaemia is present, dietary advice may be indicated so that high potassium foods are avoided (see Chapter 9).
- Potassium-sparing diuretics should be discontinued immediately in patients with hyperkalaemia. These drugs block the distal potassium transfer so that potassium is retained.
- The patient with advanced renal failure should be monitored by the physicians very closely. If hyperkalaemia develops, drugs can be given which may negate the need for immediate dialysis.

Treatment of chronic hyperkalaemia

- *Exchange resins* – calcium polystyrene sulphonate/sodium polystyrene sulphonate (calcium resonium or resonium A). Oral exchange resins are not absorbed, but exchange potassium for calcium or sodium from the gastrointestinal tract. The choice of calcium or sodium depends on the level of hypercalcaemia or sodium/fluid overload in the patient. Serum calcium should be monitored in patients with chronic renal failure and either type of exchange resin should be discontinued when the patient's serum potassium falls to $5 \, mmol \, l^{-1}$.

Treatment of acute hyperkalaemia

- *Glucose and insulin infusion.* Insulin shifts potassium back into the cells and glucose prevents hypoglycaemia. The effect of reducing potassium can last up to 2 h.
- *Intravenous calcium gluconate 10%/calcium chloride 10 ml.* Calcium reduces the cardiotoxic effects of potassium, protecting cardiac muscle and preventing arrythmias.
- *Intravenous infusion of sodium bicarbonate.* This treatment will temporarily reduce serum potassium, especially in patients with acidosis, but it should only be given where there is no fluid overload present.

For drug doses please refer to Appendix One.

Metabolic Acidosis

In normal health, acid–base balance is maintained mainly by the excretion into the renal tubules of excess acid (hydrogen or H^+ ions) where the following processes then take place:

- reabsorption of filtered bicarbonate;
- increased production of ammonia that combines with H^+ ions and is then excreted in the form of ammonium salts;
- formation of a titratable acid;
- reduction of tubular fluid pH.

In chronic renal failure, a mild metabolic acidosis may be present, as the normal renal tissue that exists is not sufficient to perform the above functions efficiently. Metabolic acidosis may also be worse in patients who have renal tubular diseases such as renal tubular acidosis.

Signs and symptoms

- Blood pH – less than 7.35.
- Hyperkalaemia may be present as metabolic acidosis shifts potassium from the cells into the extracellular fluid.
- Signs of renal bone disease may exist as metabolic acidosis reduces the bone carbonate buffers, allowing calcium to be lost from the bones which is more soluble in an acid environment.
- Acidosis causes a gasping form of breathing in the patient known as 'Kussmaul's respirations' in an attempt to breathe off the excess acid through expired carbon dioxide.

Treatment

- In the acute situation, intravenous sodium bicarbonate can correct the acidosis but the sodium can cause hypernatraemia leading to fluid retention and hypertension.
- Persistent metabolic acidosis can indicate terminal chronic renal failure and the need to commence dialysis.

Cardiovascular Complications

Hypertension

Hypertension in chronic renal failure can be the result of an increased cardiac output because of sodium retention and fluid overload or as a complication of severe anaemia. Vasopressor functions of the kidney and the production of renin can also have a major role in the development of hypertension.

Pericarditis

Chronic uraemia can predispose to pericarditis. The patient will initially present with a pericardial friction rub and if not treated by reducing the urea by dialysis, a cardiac tamponade can develop which is life threatening.

Heart Failure

Heart failure may be due to prolonged and severe hypertension and volume overload, coronary artery disease, severe electrolyte disorders or cardiomyopathy.

Disorders of the Central Nervous System

Nervous system dysfunction in chronic renal failure can cause numerous mental disabilities such as a poor memory function, loss of concentration, and slower mental ability.

Physical disabilities result in peripheral neuropathies affecting the feet and legs of a patient with chronic renal failure because of longstanding uraemia and develop in the form of 'restless legs' and parathesia.

More serious neurological problems can arise in the presence of fluid overload and hypertension in advanced renal failure, often in the form of convulsions and cerebral oedema.

Treatment

All the above complications can be reduced or prevented by the introduction of early dialysis in the uraemic patient.

Loss of Sexual Function

In women with chronic renal failure, loss of sexual function may take the form of infertility due to amenorrhoea and other menstrual abnormalities. They may also suffer loss of libido; however, if pregnancy occurs, there is a high risk of early miscarriage because of the effects of uraemia. There is also a risk to the mother's health as it is possible that the progression of the renal failure will accelerate because of extra workload on the damaged kidneys.

In males, the incidence of infertility and impotence increases with age and the advancement of chronic renal failure. There are multiple causes of impotence which can include poor nutrition, anxiety, side-effects of antihypertensive drugs and reduced plasma testosterone.

INDICATIONS FOR DIALYSIS

Patients who have advanced uraemia will require dialysis when conservative management of the symptoms of chronic renal failure no longer maintains quality of life in the patient.

To enable medical staff to decide when chronic dialysis should be initiated, the following guidelines may be used:

- *Uraemic pericarditis.* Patients with uraemic pericarditis and a pericardial friction rub need to commence dialysis as soon as possible as any delay may cause the patient to develop a cardiac tamponade.
- *Malnutrition.* The presence of persistent nausea, vomiting and lack of appetite may cause chronic weight loss and malnutrition in the patient with advanced chronic renal failure. The prescription of antiemetic drugs does not usually prevent these symptoms.
- *Fluid overload* – fluid overload that is unresponsive to diuretic therapy.
- *Disorders of the central nervous system* – if the patient is showing signs of deteriorating mental ability and peripheral neuropathy.
- *Hyperkalaemia* – persistent hyperkalaemia that is not controlled with medication.
- *Metabolic acidosis* – acidosis that is not reduced with the maximum dose of oral bicarbonate.
- *Other indications.* Many centres have guidelines to commence dialysis when the glomerular filtration rate and creatinine clearance falls to a predetermined level.

Patients requiring chronic dialysis need education and information on dietary restrictions, dialysis access, medications and the proposed dialysis treatment of either CAPD or haemodialysis. Suggested methods for the delivery of information is given in Chapters 7 and 8.

CARE OF THE PATIENT WITH END-STAGE RENAL FAILURE WITHOUT DIALYSIS

In end-stage renal failure the maintenance of life can only be ensured by dialysis or renal transplantation. However, the initiation of such treatments may not always be feasible or indeed acceptable to the patient. Nursing care must be provided for the patient who is dying from renal failure. The major objectives in caring for the terminally ill should be to maintain the comfort and safety of the patient and provide support for the family. In the early stages of terminal care the patient can be free of dietary and fluid restrictions although the accumulation of fluid may cause some discomfort.

The patient may also wish to continue with the medications that reduce the unpleasant effects of uraemia or other systemic disorders.

Extra care must be taken to prevent skin excoriation and breakdown, as healing is unlikely to take place in the presence of chronic uraemia. As death approaches, the patient may become confused and drowsy, with a comatose state occurring before the patient dies.

Strategies to provide psychological support to patients with terminal renal failure are discussed in Chapter 3.

SUMMARY

Once chronic renal failure has been diagnosed, progression of the disease is inevitable. Dialysis or transplantation is the only choice if life is to be sustained. It is imperative that doctors and nurses involve both the patient and the carers in the decision and that all the information necessary to enable the patient to make an informed choice is freely available.

If treatment is accepted, the patient will be continually monitored throughout their life, through changes in the modes of treatment, whatever the outcome, to ensure complications are kept to a minimum and quality of life is maximised.

CHAPTER 6

INVESTIGATIONS IN RENAL FAILURE

INTRODUCTION

Patients referred to a nephrologist are subjected to a bewildering array of diagnostic tests and procedures. Nurses working in this area should familiarise themselves with a knowledge of these investigations in order to be able adequately to explain these procedures to the patient; consent then will be truly 'informed consent'. The knowledgeable patient is likely to be more compliant and relaxed than the uninformed patient.

Many patients who have progressive renal disease show no outward signs or symptoms and do not feel unwell until the disease is well advanced. Unusual results of blood and urine tests carried out at routine medical examinations may warrant referral, whether they be pre-employment, pre-life insurance or preoperative or during visits to a general practitioner for other reasons. Diabetics are referred by the diabetologists when signs of renal involvement become evident, and patients being treated for hypertension are referred when blood sampling reveals early signs of renal disease. Numerous other disorders cause renal impairment as a secondary feature.

Patients in acute renal failure (see Chapter 4) for whatever cause, also come under the remit of a nephrologist; urgent diagnosis and treatment in potentially life-threatening situations are vital. Sometimes only a battery of investigations will help in the diagnosis.

The tests explained in this chapter include those involving blood and urine, invasive diagnostic investigations, X-rays, scans, isotope studies and methods of evaluating glomerular filtration rate. Investigations which are carried out prior to erythropoietin (EPO) therapy are also discussed as well as those which should be used in cases of diminished or non-response to EPO therapy.

Nurses are responsible for the correct procedure of many investigations, so an understanding of the nature of these tests is vital, as is the ability to recognise abnormal results.

Patients are monitored according to their individual needs, ranging from an annual outpatient visit to a weekly visit if dialysis is imminent. Ideally, a diagnosis should be made early in the patient's care and may be obvious to the nephrologist, whilst other diagnoses may only become apparent in the light of the results of many investigations.

The end-stage renal failure patient is subjected to constant investigation to monitor the effectiveness of dialysis treatment, with the objective of giving the patient maximum benefit from treatment with the minimum of side-effects, in order to maintain a reasonable quality of life.

VENESECTION

Traditionally, venesection has not been regarded as a procedure routinely performed by nurses in the UK, the exception being those nurses carrying out what was known as an 'extended role'. The collecting of blood samples was considered to be within the role of the medical staff and phlebotomists. However, in 1994 the UK Department of Health recommended that amongst the redefining of the nurse's activities, venesection should now be considered a routine nursing procedure, to be shared with the medical staff in the absence of a phlebotomist (Greenhalgh Report, 1994). In the renal field, as urgent blood test results can be vital to the successful treatment of the patient, nurses who can demonstrate competency have extended their scope of practice to include venesection (UKCC, 1992).

Before embarking on the collection of blood samples there are several factors which should be considered:

- the safety of health care personnel;
- the safety and comfort of the patient;
- the correct collection system.

Safety of Health Care Personnel

In order that the danger of blood-borne infection is kept to a minimum, universal precautions should be observed at all times; that is, all patients' body fluids should be assumed to be carriers of infective organisms (Department of Health, 1990). Disposable gloves (also aprons and eye shields in some situations) should be worn as appropriate and attention paid to proper handwashing before and after each procedure.

Safety closed blood collection systems are now available, for example the Sarstedt 'Monovette'® and Becton Dickinson 'Vacutainer'®. Closed systems avoid the need to transfer blood from syringe to laboratory sample tube, the blood collection device fulfilling both functions. The use of syringes and needles with the decanting of blood from syringe to blood tube should only be used when absolutely necessary. Local protocol may demand that samples from patients known to be infected with HIV, or hepatitis B or C and other contagious organisms, be identified by use of internationally recognised yellow 'biohazard labels' and be processed at the end of a laboratory run. On completion of the procedure, no attempt should be made to reshield the needle; it should be immediately discarded into a suitable sharps box. Needle-stick injury is still an unnecessary form of accident (BMA, 1990).

Choice of Vein

When carrying out venesection on a patient with renal disease, great care must be taken of veins as they may be needed in the future for fistula formation for haemodialysis. For this reason the cephalic vein in the forearm must be avoided for both venesection and intravenous infusion. The veins of the antecubital fossa should be used for venesection whenever possible, with the veins of the upper aspect of the hand as second choice, although this can be a painful site for the patient (Fig. 6.1). Arteriovenous fistula sites should not be needled except for dialysis purposes, to exclude the slight danger of infection or haematoma which may render the fistula unsuitable for dialysis in either the short or long term.

The Correct Collection Procedure

Prior to attempting venesection, the correct method of collection should be ascertained and all necessary equipment assembled. There are many designated tubes available; blood sent to the laboratory in the wrong tube

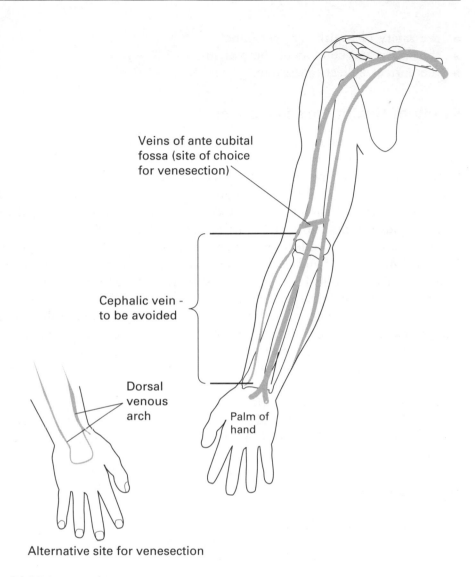

Veins of ante cubital fossa (site of choice for venesection)

Cephalic vein - to be avoided

Dorsal venous arch

Palm of hand

Alternative site for venesection

Fig 6.1 *Veins of the arm.*

cannot be processed, time and money is wasted and unnecessary discomfort caused to the patient in repeating the procedure. Check unfamiliar tests with the laboratory before commencing.

If difficulties arise in collecting a blood sample from a patient it is advisable that only two attempts should be made before calling for assistance from a more experienced member of staff.

Equipment required for venesection

- tourniquet
- (local anaesthetic cream, e.g. EMLA® (Astra) for paediatric use)

- preinjection swabs
- cotton wool balls
- plaster dressing
- Monovette® or Vacutainer® type blood taking system with needle (or 21G needle, syringe and sample container)
- sharps box
- disposable gloves
- request form.

Procedure

1. Inform patient of blood sampling requirement and gain verbal consent.
2. Wash hands and put on gloves.
3. Support chosen arm. Palpate vein in antecubital fossa – 'the vein you feel is more reliable than the vein you see' is a good maxim!
4. Apply tourniquet (only as tight as is necessary to cause venous congestion; if applied too tightly blood cells may be damaged causing false results, and unnecessary bruising and pain to the patient may occur).
5. Clean area with preinjection swab, then dry with cotton wool ball (alcohol in swab may alter blood result).
6. Insert needle into vein with 'eye' of needle uppermost.
7. Withdraw blood with as little pressure as possible (if using a vacuumed system the tubes will fill automatically).
8. Release tourniquet before withdrawing needle (otherwise a haematoma may form). If using vacuum system, detach tube from needle before withdrawing needle from skin.
9. Immediately apply pressure to the puncture site with a cotton wool ball. Do not let patient bend elbow to stop blood flow, as this often causes formation of a haematoma.
10. Dispose of needle into sharps box.
11. Label blood tubes, making sure that those containing anticoagulant are gently inverted a few times to ensure adequate mixing.
12. Apply plaster dressing to puncture site (or use other suitable dressing if the patient is allergic to plaster).

Points for consideration

If difficulty is encountered in locating a suitable vein

- Apply gentle slapping to chosen site.
- Ask patient to open and close fist several times.
- Hang arm down towards floor for a few minutes.
- In cold weather keep clothing intact until last moment, or immerse the chosen arm in warm water to encourage peripheral circulation.

Blood sampling pre-, during and posthaemodialysis using arteriovenous fistula or graft

Predialysis.   The blood sample should be collected using the dialysis needle immediately after insertion, before flushing with normal saline.

Mid-dialysis.   Mid-dialysis sampling can be done by stopping the blood pump, and taking the blood sample from the arterial port in the blood line (in the section of line prior to any addition of heparin). Some centres prefer to take the blood sample from the arterial needle after stopping the blood pump, clamping both lines and disconnecting the arterial blood line for the connection of the sampling syringe.

Postdialysis.   Blood samples are taken from the arterial needle on disconnection before the washback procedure is carried out.

Blood sampling pre-, during and posthaemodialysis using temporary vascular access dialysis catheters, or semipermanent vascular catheters

Predialysis.   Blood samples should be taken after all heparin and clotted material has been discarded, just prior to commencing dialysis (see Chapter 7).

Mid-dialysis samples.   Stop blood pump and then clamp the lines, disconnect the line flowing from the patient to the machine and unclamp in order to take blood sample. Reconnect blood lines, open clamps and resume dialysis.

Postdialysis sampling.   As mid-dialysis sampling, but after sampling the blood lines should be flushed and a heparin lock inserted as local protocol.

Blood samples from dialysis access lines must be free of anticoagulants (e.g. heparin), free of clotted material, be blood directly from the patient and not the machine and must not be recirculated blood. Blood for any clotting tests should be taken predialysis from another site such as the back of the hand or antecubital fossa, as any heparin contamination will falsify the result.
   Haemodialysis samples should all have 'pre-, mid- or postdialysis sample' clearly marked on the request form to avoid confusion.

Important

- Always check the correct collection tube and request form is to hand.
- Know whether the sample has to be delivered immediately to the laboratory, or can be stored – at room temperature, in a fridge or on ice.

- Should the patient be fasting?
- Use minimum pressure with a tourniquet to avoid haemolysis and other cell damage, and also to minimise bruising of the patient.
- Ensure the sample is correctly labelled. Do not add extra adhesive labels to the sample tube as they may become jammed in laboratory equipment causing breakage and spillage. Added labels also make serum separation difficult.
- Use 'biohazard labels' for known contaminated samples. However, all samples should be treated as potentially hazardous.

BIOCHEMICAL BLOOD TESTS

Normal Values

These are listed in Table 6.1. *These may vary locally and be expressed in alternative units of measurement. Paediatric normal values should be checked as these vary with age.*

The biochemical study of blood samples from patients with renal disease can be very informative as the products of metabolism, which in health are excreted by the kidney, may be retained or altered. Blood analyses may provide a diagnosis; therefore, all patients with renal disease will be subjected to blood sampling. Serum or heparinised plasma samples are suitable for the majority of biochemistry investigations.

Blood to be separated for *serum* samples is collected in a plain clotting tube (no additives) or in a tube containing beads treated with a clotting activator, serum being the extracellular fluid of clotted blood.

Table 6.1 *Analysis of normal blood sample*

Urea (blood urea nitrogen)	2.5–6.4 mmol l^{-1}
children	1.1–6.4 mmol l^{-1}
Creatinine	70–120 µmol l^{-1}
children (increasing with age)	27–88 µmol l^{-1}
Sodium	135–147 mmol l^{-1}
Potassium	3.5–5 mmol l^{-1}
Calcium	2.1–2.6 mmol l^{-1}
Phosphate	0.8–1.4 mmol l^{-1}
Uric acid	♀ 200–350 µmol l^{-1}
Uric acid	♂ 260–500 µmol l^{-1}
Bicarbonate	22–30 mmol l^{-1}
Cholesterol	3.5–5.7 mmol l^{-1}
Triglycerides	0.45–2.0 mmol l^{-1}
Total protein	60–80 g l^{-1}
Albumin	35–55 g l^{-1}

Blood to be separated for *plasma* samples is collected in a tube containing lithium heparin or beads treated with lithium heparin, plasma being the extracellular fluid of anticoagulated blood. The beads form a layer between the blood clot and serum\plasma after centrifugation, which allows the withdrawal of the serum by pipette (by mechanised or manual methods) for the appropriate analysis. Some tubes contain a gel for the same purpose to act as a barrier between cells and plasma or serum.

Many of the following analyses can be taken from *one 5 ml blood sample* as modern laboratory equipment only requires minute samples for each test. In children, many tests can be carried out on 0.5–1 ml of blood.

Tests frequently used in the renal field with normal values (*these may be subject to local variation and expressed in different units*) are described below.

Renal Failure Profile

The following tests (urea, creatinine, sodium, potassium, calcium, phosphate, bicarbonate and albumin) are often requested together, the result being generated from one 5 ml blood sample in a plain or lithium heparin tube. Some centres may include other tests under this heading.

Urea

Urea (normal range 2.5–6.4 mmol l^{-1}) is one of the principal end-products of protein metabolism. Urea is formed in the liver, carried by the blood and excreted by the kidneys in the urine. Raised blood urea indicates failure of the kidneys and usually increases in tandem with creatinine levels in chronic renal failure, but not inevitably, as urea levels may remain within normal limits whilst creatinine levels increase.

Urea can rise dramatically in previously healthy individuals who experience overwhelming infection or major crush injuries and are admitted to hospital in acute renal failure.

A slight rise in urea may be seen if a very high protein diet is consumed, and in low protein diets a lower level of blood urea may be observed. Certain drugs, such as corticosteroids and tetracycline, can cause a sudden rise in blood urea, especially if the patient is already in chronic renal failure.

Creatinine

Creatinine (normal range 70–120 µmol l^{-1}) is produced by the breakdown of creatine phosphate in muscle by catabolism and is excreted by the kidney. Raised creatinine can reliably be used as a specific indicator of kidney malfunction as it is fairly constant from day to day, with a slow, steady rise in the progressive renal failure patient. With advancing age, however, a higher level of serum creatinine may be expected.

Creatinine levels in the progressive renal failure patient may eventually rise to a level where it is considered expedient to commence dialysis. This may be in the region of 800–1000 µmol l⁻¹ but varies with each patient and the policy of the attending medical staff. Creatinine levels can be plotted on a log graph at regular intervals over a period of time, as a predictor of the time scale for renal support treatment to commence.

Large quantities of meat products consumed in the diet can produce a rise in creatinine.

Sodium

Sodium (normal range 135–147 mmol l⁻¹) is the principal electrolyte (Na⁺) of the extracellular fluid of the blood, maintaining osmotic pressure, acid–base balance and it aids the transmission of nerve impulses. Sodium is taken into the body with the diet and is regulated and conserved or excreted by the kidneys. *Hyponatremia* (< 135 mmol l⁻¹) can be an indication of excess body fluid, and is also often present in burns, diarrhoea, vomiting, nephritis and diabetic acidosis.

Hypernatremia (> 148 mmol l⁻¹) can be an indication of dehydration and insufficient water intake, diabetes insipidus or excessive intravenous isotonic fluids in renal failure. Patients may be proportionally hypernatraemic or hyponatraemic without an altered fluid state.

Potassium

Potassium (normal range 3.5–5 mmol l⁻¹) is the principal electrolyte (K⁺) of the intracellular fluid, with only low concentrations (2%) circulating in the extracellular fluid. Potassium is provided by the diet and excreted mainly by the kidneys, where an automatic adjustment of the body potassium content is maintained – a small amount is also lost in the faeces. Potassium is necessary to maintain nerve conduction and plays a major role in control of cardiac output. Potassium levels usually remain normal if a urine output in excess of 1500 ml day⁻¹ can be maintained. *Hypokalemia* (< 3.5 mmol l⁻¹) may be found in cases of diarrhoea, vomiting, renal tubular acidosis, in diuretic usage, intravenous fluid administration without added potassium, and when excess insulin causes an increase in cellular uptake of potassium. Hypokalaemia can cause cardiac arrhythmias.

Hyperkalaemia (> 5.5 mmol l⁻¹) may be seen in renal failure, burns, insulin deficiency, post-traumatic conditions – surgical and accidental, disseminated intravascular coagulation and any condition where cell damage has occurred to leak intracellular potassium into the serum. In the renal failure patient a potassium level > 6.5 mmol l⁻¹ is cause for clinical alert and the swift instigation of dialysis or other treatments to reduce this level. If left unattended the patient may suffer cardiac arrest caused by the arrhythmic effect of potassium build-up, due to the inefficiency or lack of kidney function. *Blood samples for accurate potassium analysis should be delivered swiftly to the laboratory or if impossible, separated and stored, to prevent leaching of intracellular potassium into the serum.*

Calcium

Calcium (normal range total Ca^{2+} 2.1–2.6 mmol l^{-1}) is provided by the diet, and is excreted by the kidneys. Most of the body calcium is found in the skeleton but a small proportion is circulated in the blood. About 50% of serum calcium is protein bound and 50% is ionised. Ionised serum calcium is responsible for muscle contraction, cardiac function and blood clotting.

In the healthy subject calcium homeostasis is controlled by the parathyroid hormone and the influence of vitamin D and the hormone calcitonin.

Hypocalcaemia is found in chronic renal failure where phosphate retention is present (calcium carbonate is given to alleviate this) (see Chapter 9). Chronic hypocalcaemia causes an excess of parathyroid hormone to be excreted into the bloodstream which in turn releases calcium from the bone, resulting in renal bone disease often in conjunction with vitamin D deficiency in renal patients. In nephrotic syndrome low levels of calcium will be found due to albumin leaking into the urine taking bound calcium with it. In the nephrotic patient the ratio of protein bound and ionised calcium will remain the same. The acidosis of chronic renal failure is an added cause of loss of bone calcium. *Hypercalcaemia* can be an indication of hyperparathyroidism, sarcoidosis or malignancy. High levels of calcium can cause renal stones and renal tubular disease.

Phosphate

Phosphorus is found in the diet. Phosphate (normal value PO_2 0.8–1.4 mmol l^{-1}) is mainly combined with calcium in the skeletal bone. It is controlled (as is calcium) by the parathyroid hormone and apart from its skeletal function has a part in the metabolism of glucose and lipids. Phosphates are excreted by the kidney. When phosphate is increased, calcium is lowered and vice versa.

Hypophosphataemia may be found in the patient with renal tubular disease who loses phosphate, possibly leading to osteomalacia. *Hyperphosphataemia* will be found in conjunction with hypocalcaemia and thus in many types of renal failure.

Other Biochemical Blood Tests

Uric acid

Uric acid (normal value ♀ 200–350 µmol l^{-1}, ♂ 260–500 µmol l^{-1}) is an end-product of purine metabolism and is excreted mainly by the kidney, but in part by the bowel. In gout, uric acid is produced to excess. Patients in renal failure have an impaired ability to excrete uric acid and a high serum level may be found in association with raised urea and creatinine.

Increased serum uric acid is also found in eclampsia of pregnancy, leukaemia, multiple myeloma, various cancers and in acute shock. Five millilitres of clotted blood are required.

Bicarbonate
The normal value of HCO_3 is 22–30 mmol l^{-1}. Low plasma HCO_3 indicates metabolic acidosis caused by chronic renal failure with an inability to adequately excrete hydrogen ions. Five millilitres of clotted blood are required.

Plasma total proteins
The normal value of plasma total proteins is 60–80 g l^{-1}. Hyperproteinaemia (increase of total plasma protein) with a normal albumin/globulin ratio may occur in dehydration. If total protein increases with albumin/globulin ratio falling (i.e. a raised globulin), it may indicate autoimmune disease such as systemic lupus erythematosus, shock, chronic infection or myeloma. Hypoproteinaemia associated with low *albumin* (normal value 35–55 g l^{-1}) levels may be found in the many conditions associated with nephrotic syndrome where protein leakage occurs from the kidney into the urine. Also decreased total protein in conjunction with low albumin may be found in liver disease, burns and haemorrhage.

Lipids
The normal values are: total cholesterol 3.5–5.7 mmol l^{-1}; triglycerides 0.45–2.0 mmol l^{-1}. Hyperlipidaemia is often found in renal patients, especially those with nephrotic syndrome and in transplanted patients. A major cause of morbidity and mortality in renal patients can be attributed to cardiovascular events, one of the risk factors being hyperlipidaemia. A 5-ml fasting blood sample should be collected in a lithium heparin tube.

Parathyroid hormone
See below in section on EPO investigation.

Other blood tests
These are frequently required as many renal diseases are only one manifestation of a systemic disease. Therefore, tests specific to certain diseases may be required (e.g. conditions involving the immune system, metabolic disorders, malignancies and infections).

HAEMATOLOGY

Haematological tests give information about anaemias, haematological malignancies and clotting disorders. Infections, inflammatory disease and other conditions can be indicated by changes in total and differential white cell counts. Normal values are shown in Table 6.2 (*there may be slight local variations, especially in paediatric normal range*).

Table 6.2 *Normal values – haematological tests*

Haemoglobin	♂ 13.5–18 g dl^{-1}
	♀ 11.5–16.5 g dl^{-1}
Haematocrit	♂ 40–55%
	♀ 35–45%
Platelets	150–350 × 10^9 1^{-1}
Reticulocytes	0.5–2.5% of total erythrocytes
Erythrocytes (RBC)	♂ 4.2–5.4 × 10^{12} 1^{-1}; ♀ 3.6–5.0 × 10^{12} 1^{-1}
Leucocytes (WBC)	5–10^9 1^{-1}
WBC differential	Neutrophil granulocytes 40–75%
	Eosinophil granulocytes 1–6%
	Basophil granulocytes 0–1%
	Lymphocytes 20–45%
	Monocytes 2–10%

RBC, red blood cells; WBC, white blood cells.

Full Blood Count (FBC)

This test provides information regarding the red blood cell size, composition and number, often providing evidence of renal anaemia in the chronic renal failure patient. White cell numbers and differentiation are also calculated. It may be appropriate to investigate further those values falling outside normal parameters. Platelet concentration is also estimated in this test. Two and a half millilitres of blood in a potassium ethylene diamine tetra-acetic acid (EDTA) tube are required, well mixed by inverting several times (further information regarding FBC, reticulocytes, etc. is given in the EPO investigations section below).

Coagulation

In circulating blood a series of mechanisms are constantly in force to achieve the correct balance to maintain fluidity and yet provide the means for clot formation as appropriate when damage to a vessel occurs.

Prior to many procedures carried out on renal patients such as kidney biopsy, it is standard procedure to ascertain normal clotting mechanisms – included in this group will be *platelets* (normal 150–400 × 10^9 1^{-1} are included in the FBC). Platelets adhere to each other and initiate the clotting cascade when damaged endothelium is encountered. Platelet deficiency (thrombocytopenia) is a common cause of prolonged bleeding.

Blood for other coagulation studies likely to be encountered in renal investigations (e.g. bleeding times (normal < 10 min); partial thromboplastin time (PTT); activated partial thromboplastin time (APTT); fibrinogen and international normalised ratio (INR)) should be collected in a tube containing the anticoagulant trisodium citrate. Most methods in current use require a very precise amount of blood in coagulation tests; the blood sample should exactly reach the marked line. Never take blood for coagulation studies during or immediately posthaemodialysis or from heparinised lines (e.g. temporary or permanent dialysis catheters) as the result will be falsified – use a vein instead.

ERYTHROPOIETIN

Tests to be Performed Before Commencing Therapy

Recombinant erythropoietin (EPO) is now recognised as the standard treatment for the patient who is suffering from renal anaemia – anaemia caused by endogenous erythropoietin deficiency. Prior to commencement of EPO therapy, some basic investigations have to be completed in order to correct any deficiencies which may prevent an adequate response to this very expensive therapy.

Full blood count
A 2.5-ml sample of venous blood is taken into a tube containing the anticoagulant potassium EDTA, and well mixed by inverting the tube several times to prevent clotting.

Haemoglobin
Haemoglobin (normal values – ♂ 13.5–18 g dl^{-1}, ♀ 11.5–16.5 g dl^{-1}) should be checked to ensure that anaemia is present. The level at which it is considered that EPO should justifiably be given varies from one centre to another, but a haemoglobin of less than 8 g dl^{-1} or haematocrit below 25% is commonly given as a guideline. The aim is to increase the haemoglobin to 10–11.5 g dl^{-1} or even higher in the continuous ambulatory peritoneal dialysis (CAPD) patient (Sundal and Kaesar, 1989). Hypochromic microcytic erythrocytes are typical in the patient with renal anaemia.

Haematocrit
Haematocrit (normal value – ♂ 40–54%, ♀ 35–47%) is the percentage of red cells in the whole blood volume, which will be low in the patient with renal anaemia, running in parallel with the low level of haemoglobin. When the patient responds to the effect of EPO, a rise in haematocrit will be seen in conjunction with a rise in haemoglobin and red blood cells (RBC).

Other Tests

Having ascertained that the patient has renal anaemia, the next step is to carry out certain investigations to check that there is no condition present which may prevent or reduce the effect of EPO. These tests should be repeated if diminished or non-response to EPO occurs at a later date.

Haematinics

In order to maintain the haem component of the healthy red blood cell, an adequate amount of available and stored iron must be present. There are several tests which can be carried out to determine this very important factor – the main cause of non-response to EPO has been found to be low available iron.

Ferritin   The normal range in health is $15–300\ \mu g\ l^{-1}$, but the renal patient needs a minimum of $100\ \mu g\ l^{-1}$ (Macdougall et al., 1989). A 5-ml sample of blood is sent to the laboratory in a plain tube with no anticoagulant. Ferritin is the main stored iron form found in all tissues, but especially in the liver, spleen and bone marrow. Ferritin found in the serum relates to the amount of stored iron, but is not necessarily an accurate assessment of available iron.

Unless ferritin levels are at least $100\ \mu g\ l^{-1}$ prior to the commencement of EPO therapy, response will be short lived. Ferritin levels should be kept in excess of this figure (using iron supplementation, either oral or intravenous) to allow adequate erythropoiesis.

Transferrin   Iron is transported by the specific plasma protein transferrin (or siderophilin). A useful test of available iron for red cell production is the transferrin saturation rate. To calculate transferrin saturation rate, which should be in excess of 20% (Macdougall et al., 1989) for efficient EPO response the following calculation can be made:

$$\frac{\text{Serum iron } (\mu g\ l^{-1}) \times 395}{\text{Transferrin } (mg\ dl^{-1})}$$

$$= \text{Transferrin saturation rate}$$

for example:
$$\frac{\text{Serum iron } (19.6\ \mu g\ l^{-1}) \times 395}{\text{Transferrin } (180\ mg\ dl^{-1})}$$

$$= \text{Transferrin saturation rate } 43\%$$

Serum iron   Serum iron (normal value $14–28\ \mu mol\ l^{-1}$) in the chronic renal failure patient is of no great significance (except in iron overload) but is necessary for calculating transferrin saturation rate. Five millilitres of venous blood in a lithium heparin tube are required for serum iron and transferrin estimation.

Iron overload   Patients who have been subjected to frequent blood transfusions are often found to be iron overloaded. The administration of EPO is an efficient method of using up the unrequired stored and available iron. The other method of removing this excess iron (or aluminium – see below,) from the system is the use of desferroxamine, which chelates the iron. Desferroxamine is used to good effect to decrease iron overload in patients with conditions demanding constant blood transfusions as in haemoglobinopathies (i.e. sickle cell anaemia).

Reticulocytes

Reticulocytes (normal range ♂ 0.5–1.5%, ♀ 0.5–2.5%) are immature red blood cells newly released from the bone marrow, and can be recognised as such for about 48 h before reaching a mature state. The blood sample must be freshly drawn, using a EDTA tube as in a full blood count. Patients with renal anaemia have a depressed reticulocyte count prior to EPO therapy and a rise should be seen when the stimulation of erythrocyte production occurs as a response to EPO. If no response occurs further investigation should be considered.

Aluminium

The normal range is less than $20 \, \mu g \, l^{-1}$. In dialysis patients who have been prescribed aluminium hydroxide as a phosphate binder, or have used dialysate containing aluminium or water with high aluminium levels, a high serum aluminium level may be exhibited. Aluminium has been implicated in osteomalacic bone disease, dialysis dementia and, importantly in EPO therapy, unresponsiveness due to hypoplasia of the bone marrow (Rao *et al.*, 1993). Owing to the current acceptance that aluminium ingestion should be kept to a minimum, especially for the kidney patient, measures have been taken to provide purer water and dialysate. Aluminium hydroxide has mainly been discontinued as a phosphate binder in favour of calcium carbonate. However, serum aluminium levels should still be checked. Venous samples (10 ml) are collected in a plain plastic tube, as samples can become contaminated by the aluminium content of glass.

Parathyroid hormone

Normal values of parathyroid hormone (parathormone – PTH) vary according to the local assay method being used.

PTH is a hormone produced in the parathyroid gland and is concerned with the regulation of extracellular calcium. This test is useful in establishing whether hypercalcaemia is due to an overactive parathyroid. Increased PTH is found in chronic renal failure, vitamin D deficiency and osteomalacia. Hyperparathyroidism has been implicated in reduced response to EPO therapy due to bone marrow fibrosis (Rao *et al.*, 1993).

Blood (10 ml) should be collected in a plain tube and *delivered immediately to the laboratory* for analysis or, if impossible, kept on ice for a maximum of 30 min.

Other reasons for low or non-response to EPO therapy may be underlying infection or inflammation, immunosuppressive drugs, and chronic blood loss (e.g. haemorrhoids, menorrhagia, gastro-intestinal bleeding.) These possibilities should be investigated.

URINE INVESTIGATIONS

Urine plays an important part as an indicator in the renal disease process and provides much valuable information in renal disorders, as most substances found in the blood are also present in the urine, albeit in different concentrations. Table 6.3 lists the normal volumes of urine passed per day.

Table 6.3 *Normal volumes of urine*

Healthy adult	$1–1.5 \, l \, day^{-1}$
Newborn baby	$50–300 \, ml \, day^{-1}$
Infant	$350–550 \, ml \, day^{-1}$
Child	$500–1000 \, ml \, day^{-1}$
Adolescent	$700–1400 \, ml \, day^{-1}$

Urine is composed of about 95% water and 5% solids, mainly urea and sodium chloride, is slightly acid (pH 6.0) and has a specific gravity (SG) of 1.010–1.030 (SG of water = 1.000).

Urinalysis

Appearance
Urine can vary in colour from pale straw to dark amber:

- *Pale urine* is dilute either

    (a) because of heavy fluid intake;
    (b) polyuria due to renal disease where the tubules fail to reabsorb water;
    (c) diabetes – insipidus or mellitus.

- *Dark urine* may indicate

    (a) concentration due to fluid depletion;
    (b) presence of bile.

- *Haematuria* can vary in appearance from 'smoky' to 'tea' to red, either bright or dark.
- *Coloured urine* can be caused by beetroot in the diet and other vegetable food dyes, porphyria and some drugs, for example orange-coloured urine caused by Rifampicin.
- *Frothy urine* indicates heavy proteinuria.
- *Smoky urine* may indicate the presence of bleeding from the kidney.
- *Deposits* which occur when the urine sample is left to stand may be crystals of phosphate, oxalate or urates, or due to pus in the presence of infection.

Dipstick tests

Dipstick tests can be carried out in the clinic or ward situation as well as in the laboratory. Dipsticks are available which accurately show the presence of a variety of substances which may occur in the urine (e.g. protein, glucose, ketones, blood) as well as giving the pH of the urine sample. The stick should be briefly dipped into a *fresh sample of urine* and read after 1 min or according to the manufacturer's instructions. The results are then compared with those supplied on the instruction sheet.

Caution: These kits are very reliable providing that the container is always kept dry and capped between use, the strips are only briefly dipped into the urine sample and the expiratory date is not exceeded.

The majority of biochemical laboratory tests performed on blood samples can also be carried out on urine – usually taken from a mixed 24-h urine collection (see creatinine clearance below).

Osmolality

Osmolality (normal 500–850 mOsmol kg^{-1}) measurement indicates the kidney's ability in concentration and dilution and is considered more reliable than measuring the specific gravity. Collection methods vary from one centre to another.

Proteinuria

No more than a trace of protein should be found in the normal collection (i.e. less than 25 mg 24 h^{-1}, mainly albumin). However, proteinuria may be present up to 150 mg in 24 h before a dipstick test shows a positive reading. (The procedure for collecting the 24-h sample is the same as detailed for creatinine clearance.) The urine should be kept refrigerated during the collection period to minimise bacterial growth.

Persistent proteinuria is a common sign of many forms of renal disease. In nephrotic syndrome, proteinuria may be as high as 4–30 g 24 h^{-1}.

Microalbuminuria

Microalbuminuria, persistent small amounts of albumin not determined by the usual dip-stick test, is of importance as a predictor of renal involvement in the patient with insulin dependent diabetes mellitus (IDDM). Whereas a *normal* sample of urine may contain albumin 2.5–25 mg 24 h^{-1}, *micro*albuminuria is in the range 26–150 mg 24 h^{-1} and *macro*albuminuria is generally more than 150 mg 24 h^{-1}.

IDDM patients who have an albumin excretion of between 50 and 250 mg 24 h^{-1} have a 20-fold greater risk of developing diabetic nephropathy than do patients with an excretion rate below this figure (Viberti and Walker, 1992). Laboratory testing for microalbuminuria, therefore, is of importance in the care of the diabetic patient.

Urine Microscopy and Culture

Microscopy will reveal information from the sediment found in urine – casts, crystals, blood cells and bacteria. The site of origin of casts can often be determined indicating the type and extent of damage to the kidney. The 10-ml sample is taken from a fresh mid-stream collection of urine and centrifuged, the sediment being examined.

If micro-organisms are found to be present in the urine specimen, usually determined by the Gram's-staining method, the laboratory will provide information as to which antibiotic is most appropriate. It is important that the urine sample is collected before the commencement of a broad-spectrum antibiotic, which may be given in the interim period before a specific sensitivity is ascertained.

A positive microscopy sample shows at least 10 000 organisms ml^{-1}; below this figure is not considered significant. However, with very dilute urine, a false-negative result may occur despite infection being present.

Specimens should be sent to the laboratory in a sterile universal container, preferably containing boric acid. All containers used in the collection must be sterile to avoid contamination which may give a false result. Because urine is an excellent growing medium for bacteria, the sample should be taken to the laboratory as soon after collection as possible, or refrigerated. A boric acid-containing tube should be used if possible, which prevents decay or growth of organisms in the urine sample. A suitably worded explanation and instructions for a mid-stream collection should be given to the patient. The first voided urine of the day is most suitable for culture as this will be the most concentrated.

KIDNEY FUNCTION TESTS

In chronic renal disease a regular assessment of kidney function can be useful in assessing change and in predicting the time scale or likelihood of dialysis. Glomerular filtration rate (GFR) tends to decrease in a linear fashion over time in progressive renal disease and so, by extrapolation, predictions can be made as to when end-stage renal failure may occur.

Knowledge of the amount of nephron damage is useful in guiding the nephrologist's choice of suitable drug regimen. When there is more than 30% of nephron loss, certain drugs should be avoided or used with caution due to slow excretion of the drug or its metabolites.

Many research studies and clinical trials of pharmaceuticals depend on regular GFR calculations to monitor the effect of treatments with regard to renal function.

Kidney function investigations discussed here include creatinine clearance, the [51]chromium ethylene diamine tetra-acetic acid glomerular filtration rate (^{51}Cr EDTA GFR), the inulin clearance test and the 'renalyser' analysis.

Creatinine Clearance

The principle of clearance is that an estimation of a known substance in the plasma is compared with the amount in the urine. This substance must only be excreted in the urine. The calculation by which the clearance of the substance occurs can be measured thus:

$$\frac{\text{Urine concentration of substance } (U) \times \text{Volume of urine in 24 h } (V)}{\text{Plasma concentration of substance } (P)}$$

Because creatinine is believed to be manufactured at a fairly constant rate by the muscle mass, is circulating in the blood stream and is filtered by the glomeruli (although a very small amount excreted is by the tubules), this is the usual substance measured and when used in the above example is known as creatinine clearance.

About 50% of nephrons will have lost their function before an appreciable alteration occurs in the result of the creatinine clearance test. The normal value of creatinine clearance should be between 70 and 125 ml min^{-1}, function lessening with age. A creatinine clearance result of less than 10 ml min^{-1} is an indication for the commencement of renal replacement therapy.

Procedure

A 24-h urine collection is made which will provide the urinary creatinine content (U) and volume (V). A blood sample should be taken to indicate the plasma creatinine (P).

Patient information for 24-h urine collection   The patient should be given an explanation of the reason for the test and what is expected of them. One (or more) 2-l collection bottles containing no additives or preservatives should be given to the patient. Whereas male patients can usually void straight into the bottle, female patients should be provided with a suitable receptacle in which they can catch the urine. The patient must be instructed to discard the first urine of the day (on day 1) into the lavatory and then collect all urine passed for the next 24 h into the bottle provided. The following morning (day 2), the first sample should be collected and then the collection is complete. The completed urine collection should be labelled with the date and time of start and completion of the collection as well as the usual details such as name, identity number and date of birth.

The urine collection and the blood sample should be delivered together to the laboratory with the request form, which should specify creatinine clearance test. The above formula is then applied which will calculate the creatinine clearance.

Precautions necessary to obtain an accurate result   This test is comparatively inexpensive to perform, but unless great care is taken to obtain a total 24-h urine collection the result is useless. If the amount of urine collected appears extremely scanty, it may well be that the patient did not understand that any urine passed during the night should also be collected, or they may have forgotten one sample – such collections are of no value, and if sent for analysis the result will be misleading.

In the elderly, confused, incontinent or handicapped patient it can be difficult to ensure a complete collection. Even a ward-based patient may be prone to provide an incomplete collection due to inadequate communication between staff, or patient incontinence.

Patients with renal disease may pass copious quantities of urine and should be provided with an adequate supply of collection bottles, or a full 24-h collection may not be achieved.

It is useful to provide written instructions in all languages commonly used in the locality in order to ensure full understanding and compliance.

In infants and small children, a urine collection bag may be adhered to the clean, dry cream-free skin. If a child is unable to void, suprapubic aspiration of the full bladder can be carried out. Rarely, catheterisation is used in adults and children if all other methods have failed to produce the required urine specimen.

Creatinine clearance tends to decrease in accuracy as renal failure progresses, usually with an overestimation of GFR.

⁵¹Chromium EDTA GFR

A more accurate method of assessing renal function than the creatinine clearance test is the ⁵¹Cr EDTA GFR. The normal range as with the creatinine clearance test is a clearance of 70–125 ml min⁻¹.

Patient preparation

The patient should be informed of the reason for this test, the fact that a small dose of a radio-isotope will be injected, and the necessity of a series of blood samples over a 4-h period, and consent should be sought.

Procedure

The radio-labelled substance is given by intravenous injection followed by a 10-ml bolus of normal saline into a vein of the antecubital fossa. The time of injection must be carefully noted. The patient's weight and height must also be recorded to enable the result to be normalised for the individual patient's body surface area.

Over the 4 h following the injection the usual procedure is for four blood samples to be drawn from the opposite arm to the injection of the radio-isotope. (This is to avoid contamination from any activity still lingering around the injection site, which will falsify the result.)

A cannula is inserted into the vein chosen for sampling to avoid constant puncturing of the vein. Blood samples (10 ml) are taken at intervals such as 2, 2.5, 3 and 4 h from the isotope injection, into a lithium heparin tube. After each blood collection the vein is kept patent by flushing the cannula with heparinised saline, which also necessitates withdrawing and discarding about 5 ml of blood before the next sample is drawn. After the 4-h period the cannula is removed and the patient can leave the department.

The four blood samples should be sent to the radio-isotope laboratory for analysis together with the syringe used for giving the isotope and any other equipment which may have been contaminated with the isotope. This is necessary for disposal according to safe practice. Request forms should state the exact time that the injection was given, the exact time that all blood samples were drawn together with the patient's weight, height, age and identity details. This test has to be arranged in conjunction with the radio-pharmacy, so that the injection can be specially prepared. Analysis of the blood samples for a result is also carried out within the radio-isotope department.

Whilst the ⁵¹Cr EDTA GFR is considered to be very accurate, only personnel who have completed a radiation protection course in accordance with the Ionising Radiation Regulations 1988 (POPUMET) are permitted to administer radiolabelled substances.

Inulin Clearance Test

The most precise test of renal clearance is considered to be the inulin clearance test. Inulin, an inert sugar harvested from plants, when given by intravenous injection is not metabolised, is not secreted or reabsorbed by the tubules, but is filtered solely by the glomerulus. This test is now reserved as a research technique where total accuracy is required and so will not be detailed here apart from a few important points.

Inulin is usually presented in a 50-ml ampoule and is dose/weight calculated. At room temperature, inulin precipitates out and a white crystalline substance can be seen suspended in clear fluid. To prepare for injection the ampoules must be placed in a water bath and gently heated over about 20 min until the precipitate has disappeared. The inulin is then allowed to cool to blood heat before being injected – to maintain the balance between precipitation and overheating is not easy!

A bolus injection of inulin is given followed by a timed infusion to create a steady state, with blood sampling at certain time points. Owing to this being a complicated, labour-intensive test, with recovered inulin difficult to measure, this method of GFR is reserved for research purposes only. However, renewed attempts are being made to provide simplified tests on the inulin test principle due to increased restrictions in the medical use of radionuclides (^{51}Cr EDTA GFR).

'Renalyser' Method

This is a computerised X-ray spectrophotometric technique which measures iodine content of plasma. A measured iodine-containing contrast medium (e.g. Iohexol®), which is only excreted by glomerular filtration, is injected into a vein. It must be first ascertained that the patient is not allergic to iodine. Blood sampling is carried out at timed intervals over 4 h after injection, as in the ^{51}Cr EDTA GFR. The result is believed to be comparable in accuracy with the ^{51}Cr EDTA GFR without resorting to the use of radioactive isotopes (Brown and O'Reilly, 1991).

RENAL BIOPSY

Patients who are referred to the nephrology outpatient clinic with proteinuria, haematuria or renal impairment with no obvious cause require a renal biopsy in order that the nephrologist can make a diagnosis and commence appropriate treatment (Plate 1). Patients referred in acute renal failure may be subjected to renal biopsy to provide a diagnosis. Whilst in experienced hands renal biopsy is a fairly safe procedure, there are risks which should be taken into consideration. Risks of renal biopsy, greater in the acute renal failure patient, are perirenal haematoma, prolonged and severe bleeding needing blood transfusion and possible surgery, irreparable damage to the kidney requiring its surgical removal (1 in 1000) and, rarely, death can result.

Patients who have only one functioning native kidney are not usually subjected to biopsy, as the risk of damage to that kidney during biopsy may not be justified in order to gain a diagnosis.

Patient Preparation

Information regarding the benefits and risks attached to this procedure should be given to the patient, who should be allowed the opportunity to ask questions and time to consider the implications before consenting to the biopsy. Child patients under 16 years need written parental consent.

Patients are usually admitted to the ward on the day planned for biopsy and a further explanation of the exact procedure and what is expected of the patient should be given prior to signature of a consent form. Children are fasted for 4 h prebiopsy as they will be sedated with a preparation such as Midazolam following a mild premedication. It is helpful that in order to gain full compliance, whilst still in the ward, the patient should be asked to practise deep breathing and breath holding. Unless the patient can co-operate with breath holding on demand, the procedure should not be attempted, as the danger of malplacement of the sharp biopsy needle causing laceration or haemorrhage becomes a possibility.

Blood samples should be taken for bleeding times, full blood count, plasma viscosity (International Normalised Ratio (INR)), and group and save, full biochemical and immunology profile. Biopsies *should not* proceed if any bleeding disorder is present (platelets $< 100 \times 10^9 \, l^{-1}$, INR > 1.2, bleeding time > 10 min, or if the blood pressure exceeds 160/95, as the highly vascular kidney can haemorrhage even when clotting times are within normal limits.

Equipment

Equipment may vary according to local requirements:

- surgeon's sterile gown and gloves;
- basic dressing pack containing cotton wool balls, gauze squares, forceps, gallipot, sterile paper towel. Lithotomy sheet;
- methylated spirit (do not use iodine-containing solutions, as iodine damages the ultrasound probe);
- 2% lignocaine;
- hypodermic needles 21G and 25G. Syringes 10 ml;
- spinal needle 22G;

- Baxter 'Trucut'® type biopsy needle 11.4 cm or automatic system;
- scalpel blade no. 11;
- wide Elastoplast and gauze for dressing;
- sandbags for positioning patient.

For specimens
- microscope slide or Petri dish with normal saline 'puddle' (to keep sample moist);
- specimen pots containing:

    (a) electron microscopy fixative (keep cold in fridge);
    (b) 10% formalin (for histology);
    (c) normal saline (for immunofluorescence).

Procedure

The patient will be asked to empty his/her bladder before the procedure. Percutaneous renal biopsy is usually done in a ward treatment or side room, or X-ray department, under local anaesthetic. The patient lies in a prone position, with a pillow under the upper abdomen to isolate the kidney, perhaps supported with sandbags to prevent movement. The kidney (usually left) is identified by ultrasound as to position and depth and the skin is marked as to where the needle should be inserted. After cleaning the ultrasound gel from the skin, using a full aseptic technique, the area is cleansed with methylated spirit, the area infiltrated with lignocaine as a local anaesthetic and a spinal needle inserted into the lumbar muscle layer until the needle is noted to swing with the patient's respirations. The patient should be asked to hold their breath whilst the needle is advanced 5 mm at a time, leaving the needle to swing free when the patient breathes in and out. When the needle has located the kidney, more local anaesthetic should be injected.

The spinal needle is then withdrawn, a small incision made at the needle exit site and a 'Trucut'® renal biopsy needle is inserted along the pathway made by the spinal needle in the same manner, advances made as the patient holds their breath. When the kidney is again located, the biopsy is taken with the patient holding his/her breath. The biopsy needle is withdrawn and the specimen obtained is immediately placed on a slide and viewed under a dissecting microscope to ascertain that cortex has been obtained, large enough (about 5 mm length) to divide into three samples. If not enough cortex has been obtained, the biopsy needle will have to be inserted again until a suitable strip of cortex containing sufficient glomeruli has been identified. *Samples* are sent to the laboratory for histology (in a 10% formalin pot), for immunofluorescence (in sterile normal saline) and electron microscopy (in specific glutaraldehyde fixative, kept cold). These samples should be delivered immediately (minutes, not hours) to the laboratory, which must have had advance warning of the biopsy.

Finally, after the needle has been withdrawn, a pressure dressing is applied and the patient asked to remain flat in bed. The patient will need much encouragement and reassurance during the renal biopsy procedure as it can be painful, despite local anaesthetic. A friendly hand to hold and quiet encouragement to co-operate with breathing requirements from the attending nurse can be very reassuring.

Occasionally, an open renal biopsy is performed in the operating theatre under general anaesthetic, the biopsy being obtained through a surgical loin incision. This is reserved for the patient who would be unable to co-operate with instructions during the percutaneous method, but the risks of operation are outweighed by the need to establish the histology of the renal disease.

Patient Care Following Renal Biopsy

It is usual practice to keep patients in the ward on bedrest for 24 h following this procedure. Haemorrhage is the main complication following renal biopsy; the wound site should be frequently checked for surface bleeding, the observation of blood pressure and pulse should be carried out until stable, for example on the time scale of every 15 min for 2 h, then every 30 min for 2 h and then hourly for 4 h. The signs and symptoms giving an indication of internal bleeding are a rise or fall in blood pressure and dull aching pain in the abdomen, back or shoulder. The patient should be warned that some degree of haematuria will occur initially, but only persisting or heavy haematuria is of significance. Small urine samples from each void should be retained in transparent specimen containers for observation of diminishing haematuria and dipstick testing. It is becoming common practice for suitable patients to be admitted to day case units for this procedure. These patients must be carefully chosen and must fully understand instructions for aftercare at home. The patient should be advised not to do any strenuous activity for 2 weeks following renal biopsy.

Renal Biopsy in the Transplanted Patient

Closed percutaneous biopsies of the transplanted kidney are undertaken to support evidence of rejection and also to confirm suspicion of recurrent or primary glomerular disease (see Chapter 11). The procedure is similar to the biopsy of the native kidney but more straightforward due to the superficial position of the transplanted kidney. The patient will be placed in a supine position with a pillow beneath the transplant side to move the intra-abdominal contents away from the site. The amount of tissue required in a transplant biopsy will be less than in a native kidney biopsy as fewer tests will be performed.

RADIOGRAPHIC INVESTIGATIONS

Investigations using various radiographic methods are often employed to assist diagnosis and to assess progression of renal disease and its attendant side-effects. The most common techniques are discussed here.

The patient should have adequate explanation prior to entering the department in order to allay any fears they may have on finding themselves in a department full of strange machinery, hazard warnings and unfamiliar staff. If they are aware of the reasons for the investigation and what will be expected of them, the likelihood of an accurate result of the examination will be enhanced. The patient will be asked to sign a consent form for some invasive tests and early information will be of help in the understanding of the procedure.

All investigations involving X-rays must be performed according to the safety regulations in using a potentially hazardous substance, and these techniques must not be used unless the risk to the patient is outweighed by the benefit. Some departments follow the practice that women with reproductive capacity should be only subjected to X-rays and other procedures using ionising radiation during the 10 days following the commencement of the last menstrual period to avoid possible damage of a vulnerable foetus – the so called '10-day rule'. More recently, guidelines have indicated that minimal exposure to a possible foetus must be ensured with the use of shields. Developing foetal organs are at higher risk of radiation damage than mature cells, especially the brain.

Plain Abdominal X-Ray

Plain abdominal X-rays incorporating the kidneys, ureters and bladder (KUB) indicate the size, shape, position and the presence or absence of one or both kidneys, and may be taken before other more complicated radiological procedures in order to provide an overall background picture. The majority of calculi may be seen as they are usually composed of radio-opaque material. KUB X-rays are usually taken from the anterior aspect. A combination of KUB and ultrasound often forms the basic routine screening in renal patients.

Skeletal X-Rays

Skeletal X-rays may be taken in the dialysis patient. This is to detect renal osteodystrophy, which may become apparent in association with impaired glomerular filtration and associated disturbed metabolism of calcium and phosphate. Those bones most likely to show the characteristic abnormalities are the phalanges, skull, pelvis and vertebrae. Pain and deformity will ultimately develop unless imbalances of calcium and phosphate can be corrected and inadequate metabolism of vitamin D can be halted (see Chapter 9).

Intravenous Urogram (IVU)

This procedure is also known as the intravenous pyelogram (IVP). This examination indicates the size and position of the kidneys and the anatomy of the calyces and pelvis. The ureters are also outlined by the progression of the dye containing urine to the bladder, enabling any deformities in these organs to be demonstrated.

Patient preparation

The patient should be told that the investigation will take about an hour to complete – longer if there is renal impairment.

It should be ascertained that the patient is not allergic to iodine and caution should be observed with asthmatics and others who have allergic conditions, as the contrast medium is iodine based. Therefore, it is standard procedure that injections of adrenaline 500–1000 µg i.m., antihistamine (e.g. chlorphreniramine 10–20 mg i.v.) and hydrocortisone should be immediately available to treat anaphylaxis should it occur.

Laxatives should be given to the constipated patient prior to this examination to clear the bowel so that there is no interruption to the view of the urinary system. Adult patients should fast for 3 h, but limited fluid is usually allowed until 1 h before the IVU. After an explanation of the procedure with adequate time to ask questions, the patient may be asked to sign a consent form.

Procedure

The patient wears a gown and lies on the X-ray table, having first emptied the bladder. A radiologist (or radiographer trained in intravenous work) gives the iodine-based radio-opaque contrast medium by intravenous injection into a vein, usually in the antecubital fossa in renal patients. The patient may well feel a hot flush sensation at this point and a metallic taste in the mouth, and should be warned in advance that this may happen and is an expected reaction. The iodine contrast will be excreted entirely by the kidneys and should start to appear in the renal system within minutes. The first image taken is the nephrogram showing the kidney outline, then a series of radiographs will be taken at intervals over the following hour to plot the course of the dye through the system, and illustrating abnormalities as the dye reaches the different areas of the urinary tract. The prior emptying of the bladder is important or the contrast will become overdilute on reaching a full bladder and a poor picture will result.

Following this test, the patient should be encouraged to drink fluids, as he may become dehydrated if fluids were restricted prior to the examination. Nurses should be aware that there is a possibility of acute renal failure following this investigation, so urinary output should be monitored.

The IVU gives little useful information in advanced chronic renal failure and consequently is not the investigation of choice if more than 50% of nephron loss is suspected. If impaired renal function is known and an IVU is indicated, a greater dose than usual of the radio-opaque contrast medium may need to be given – this in itself is nephrotoxic and may exacerbate the renal failure at least temporarily.

Retrograde Pyelogram

In this examination, radio-opaque dye is injected directly into the upper urinary tract, via a catheter inserted through a cystoscope into the ureter. It may be performed on one or both kidneys. This test is useful in outlining stones, calyceal defects and masses in the ureter or renal pelvis and in defining deformities such as hydronephrosis or hydroureter. This investigation is sometimes performed after an IVU or ultrasound (US) has demonstrated a hydronephrosis and more clarification is needed for a diagnosis.

This procedure is carried out under general anaesthetic (or occasionally local anaesthetic) in an operating theatre, with the patient in the lithotomy position. There is minimal risk of allergy to the iodine-based contrast medium as the mode of delivery is not intravenous but directly into the urinary system.

Patient preparation
The patient should be fully informed of the need for the investigation and should have appropriate instructions on fasting if a general anaesthetic is to be given. They should be told that a cystoscope will be passed into their bladder to enable the dye to be infiltrated into the upper urinary tract. Care should be taken to preserve the patient's dignity in what they may feel is an embarrassing situation. Their written consent should be sought.

Patient care after the procedure
Urine should be observed for haematuria and the patient should be watched for signs and symptoms of infection. They should be encouraged to drink copiously to help to avoid infection (antibiotics may be given as a prophylaxis).

Computerised Axial Tomography or Computed Tomography (CT Scan)

This expensive investigation is reserved for the patient who needs staging of a renal mass or a diagnosis when other methods of detection have failed to provide a clear picture. CT is an X-ray technique which uses a computer to reconstruct cross-sectional images of 1 cm slices of the organ targeted. The dose of radiation is about the same as that for an IVU.

Patient information and preparation

A clear bowel is necessary so a suitable laxative may be given 2 days prior to the scan. A light diet should be taken for 2 days before the scan and nothing on the day of examination apart from clear fluids. The patient should be informed that the procedure will take about 20 min to accomplish. Iodine-based contrast dye may be used, so precautions should be taken as in the IVU. The investigation will take place with the patient lying on a table in a specially constructed tunnel, with the scanner taking cross-sectional images. The patient must be able to follow instructions such as when to hold their breath, to be able to lie motionless and not to talk. As the patient is alone in the area of X-ray and has instructions relayed by microphone, the procedure should not be attempted unless the patient can be relied upon to co-operate; therefore, a full explanation must be given beforehand. Written consent should be obtained.

Nuclear Magnetic Resonance or Magnetic Resonance Imaging (MRI)

This form of scanning has recently entered the medical diagnostic arena, involving an application of a strong external magnetic field along with a radiofrequency signal that produces a current in a receiving coil proportional to the density of protons in the body organ being scanned. This signal is processed by computer to create a tomographic slice of the organ similar to a CT scan. In renal medicine a clear picture of tumour invasion into blood vessels can be demonstrated as well as differentiation of tissue character.

The advantage of MRI over CT imaging is that no ionising radiation or contrast media is used and many planes can be visualised. However, this method is three times as expensive as CT imaging.

Patient information

This procedure needs no patient preparation. However, claustrophobia may be a problem as the patient is placed alone in an enclosed compartment – children are usually sedated. It is vitally important that the patient is not wearing any metal object, and it must be ascertained that no internal metal objects are present such as aneurysm clips, screws, pacemakers or shrapnel. Therefore, an X-ray may be taken before the procedure to ensure that no hidden metal objects are within the body.

MRI scans take about 1 h to perform and written consent should be obtained.

ULTRASONOGRAPHY

Ultrasound investigations (US) have replaced some X-ray procedures (especially the IVU) to a large degree, and because this procedure does not carry the hazards associated with radiation this method can be used in women without consideration of the possibility of pregnancy. This is a non-invasive procedure where a transducer (sonar probe) is moved in close contact with the skin over the area of investigation and can be repeated frequently if necessary, unlike X-ray. Ultrasound is especially useful in examinations of the abdominal and pelvic organs. In the renal patient ultrasound is widely used to determine the size and shape of the kidney, its presence and position, and composition of cysts or neoplasms if present, and also in the diagnosis of polycystic kidney disease, but is less useful in providing information about the ureters.

Ultrasound is also used to guide the operator in procedures such as renal biopsy.

Patient preparation

Patients who are to have renal ultrasound scans are usually asked to fast for 8 h (in order to keep pockets of air in the gut to a minimum) except for drinks of clear fluids. The patient should be dressed in a gown to allow for easy access to the abdomen for scanning. The patient should be told to expect the application of an aqueous gel to the abdomen to enable the sonar probe (transducer) to maintain contact with the skin. This procedure is usually performed with the patient in a supine position and takes only about 10 min.

Ultrasound in Renal Transplantation

Ultrasound scanning is an ideal method of examining the transplanted kidney, as it is a simple and non-invasive technique (Nicholson *et al.*, 1990a). The most important and common cause of early transplant dysfunction is acute rejection, which occurs in 10–20% of all patients. This is accompanied by inflammation, which leads to swelling of the kidney and an increase in pressure inside the organ. Ultrasound is used to diagnose the increase in size using diameters relating to the local renal anatomy (Nicholson *et al.*, 1990a). This procedure should be used daily and two size increases on consecutive days would be strongly indicative of acute rejection. However, dysfunction attributed to other causes must be excluded. Infection may be associated with an increase in the kidney size, but this is easily diagnosed by routine testing of mid-stream specimens of urine.

Renal vein thrombosis is a serious complication and will cause a rapid increase in size, possibly resulting in a tear of the kidney substance. If this condition is quickly diagnosed with ultrasound, rapid surgical intervention would be possible and the graft rescued. Renal artery thrombosis may be diagnosed ultrasonically by the observation of lack of vessel pulsation. For greater accuracy, duplex scanning using a combination of imaging and frequency waveform analysis is available.

Early complications following transplantation include urine leaks, usually from the site of the ureteric anastomosis. These are seen ultrasonically as a fluid collection around the graft site. Later complications are obstructive lesions, which are often insidious in onset and lead to deteriorating renal function. Routine scanning of outpatients is a simple and easy method of detecting dilatation and stenoses of the urinary tract, which are then treated surgically.

Needle core biopsy of the transplanted kidney remains the best method of detecting rejection (Nicholson *et al.*, 1990b). Using ultrasound guidance of the biopsy needle a good core of the renal cortex may be safely obtained, carefully avoiding the structures of the renal medulla and damage to the graft.

Ultrasound is therefore a valuable tool in the detection and diagnosis of renal allograft dysfunction, allowing intervention and early treatment of problems.

RADIONUCLIDE STUDIES

Radionuclide studies are performed in the isotope department by staff especially trained in the use of radionuclides, but are described here briefly to enable nursing staff to adequately explain them to their patients. Patients should be informed that a small dose of an isotope will be injected, but that the radioactive effect will disappear in a fairly short time. Normal clothing can be worn but jewellery and other metal objects should be removed, for example coins in pockets. Children undergoing tests in this department may be given a mild sedative to help them remain still and also EMLA cream should be used on any needle site. The strict precautions used in the department are mainly for the protection of staff from overexposure, as they are in day-to-day contact with radioactive materials. Protection of Persons Undergoing Medical Examination and Treatment – Ionising Radiation Regulations 1988 (POPUMET) gives guidance on the use of materials in this area.

Renograms

Renograms calculate percentages of renal function and indicate position of obstruction. This investigation can be used in place of IVU if the patient is allergic to iodine contrast medium, and is also used in transplanted patients. In renal artery stenosis, a renogram may be performed and then repeated incorporating an injection of captopril to outline any response induced.

Patient information

The isotope, usually ^{99m}technetium-labelled diethylene triamine penta-acetic acid (^{99m}Tc DTPA), is injected with the patient in position so that a sequence of pictures can be taken as the isotope concentrates in the renal system. A diuretic may also be given intravenously and the patient should be well hydrated. The procedure takes about 1 h.

Renal Scanning

The isotope ^{99m}technetium-labelled dimercaptosuccinic acid (^{99} ^{m}Tc DMSA) identifies areas of cortical scarring and solid lesions and relative renal function can be calculated during this test.

Patient information

^{99m}Tc DMSA is injected intravenously 2 h before imaging. The patient should empty his/her bladder immediately before scanning. The scan is accomplished with the patient sitting or lying on a couch whilst the gamma camera is positioned close to the patient. The test takes about 30–60 min to accomplish.

SUMMARY

The investigations which have been discussed above are by no means exhaustive. Since renal patients usually have multifactorial disease processes, many other specific investigations may be indicated, especially cardiovascular tests such as electrocardiography (ECG) and echocardiography. The gastrointestinal tract in the renal patient is frequently investigated for bleeding problems using techniques involving endoscopy (e.g. gastroscopy, sigmoidoscopy).

Such is the commercial pressure to exploit the latest technology, it is inevitable that new methods and procedures will enter the renal field in the near future, condemning some present-day tests to redundancy. However, it is hoped that by nurses understanding something of the current techniques used in renal investigations, they will be able to inform and reassure their patients reliably.

REFERENCES

BMA (1990) *A Code of Practice for the Safe Use and Disposal of Sharps.* British Medical Association, London, UK.

BROWN, S.C.W. AND O'REILLY, P.H. (1991) Iohexol clearance for the determination of glomerular filtration rate in clinical practices: evidence for a new gold standard. *J. Urol.,* **146**: 675–9.

DEPARTMENT OF HEALTH (1990) *Guidance for Clinical Health Care Workers, Protection Against Infection with HIV and Hepatitis Viruses: Recommendations of The Expert Advisory Group on AIDS.* HMSO, London.

GREENHALGH REPORT (1994) *The Interface Between Junior Doctors and Nurses.* Greenhalgh, Macclesfield, UK.

MACDOUGALL, I.C., HUTTON, R.D., CAVILL, I., COLES, G.A. AND WILLIAMS, J.D. (1989) Poor response to treatment of renal anaemia with erythropoietin corrected by iron given intravenously. *BMJ,* **299**: 157–8.

NICHOLSON, M.L., WILLIAMS, P.M., BELL, A. *et al.* (1990a) Prospective study of the value of ultrasound measurements in the diagnosis of acute rejection following renal transplantation. *Br. J. Surg.,* **77**: 656–8.

NICHOLSON, M.L., ATTARD, A.R., BELL, A. *et al.* (1990b) Renal transplant biopsy using real time ultrasound guidance. *Br. J. Urol.,* **65**: 564–5.

RAO, S.D., SHIH, M-S. AND MOHINI, R. (1993) Effect of serum parathyroid hormone and bone marrow fibrosis on the response to erythropoietin in uraemia. *N. Engl. J. Med.,* **328**: 171–5.

SUNDAL, E. AND KAESAR, U. (1989) Correction of anaemia of chronic renal failure with recombinant human EPO: safety & efficacy of one year's treatment in a European multicentred study of 150 HD dependent patients. *Nephrol. Dial. Transplant.,* **4**(11): 979–87.

UKCC (1992) *Scope of Professional Practice.* London: UKCC.

VIBERTI, G.C. AND WALKER, J.D. (1992) Pathogenesis of diabetic nephropathy. In *Advanced Renal Medicine* (ed. A.E.G. Raine) Oxford, pp. 83–91. Oxford: Oxford University Press.

FURTHER READING

ANDREW, E.R., BYDDER, G., GRIFFITHS, J., ILES, P. AND STYLES, P. (1990) *Clinical Magnetic Resonance – Imaging and Spectroscopy.* Chichester: Wiley.

CHESNEY, D.N. & M.O (1986) *Care of the Patient in Diagnostic Radiography.* Blackwell, Oxford.

FISCHBACH, F. (1992) *A Manual of Laboratory & Diagnostic Tests.* Lippincoat, Philadelphia, USA.

THORPE, S. (1991) *A Practical Guide to Taking Blood.* Baillière Tindall, London.

CHAPTER 7

HAEMODIALYSIS AND OTHER EXTRACORPOREAL TREATMENTS

INTRODUCTION

Haemodialysis is an area of renal nursing that has, and continues to develop at an incredible rate. Expert practitioners in this field are constantly striving to promote excellence in the application of nursing practice. New developments in medicine and technology impact greatly on the rate of change for nursing the patient on haemodialysis. As a consequence, studies are constantly being performed to ensure evidence based practice.

Terms and Definitions

Haemodialysis, haemofiltration and haemodiafiltration are terms used to describe the removal of waste products and water from the blood through a filter (dialyser). Techniques have become technically advanced and increasingly sophisticated, resulting in a variety of highly efficient methods of clearing waste products that would normally be removed by the healthy kidney.

The process of each of these therapies is dependent on the utilisation of the physiological principles of diffusion or ultrafiltration/convection or both. It is essential to have a clear understanding of how these physiological principles relate to each of the treatments to appreciate fully both the benefits and the limitations of each as a form of renal replacement therapy (RRT).

Diffusion

Diffusion is the term used to describe the movement of molecules from a region of high concentration to a region of low concentration until they are equal. For diffusion to take place a concentration gradient is essential. In RRT a physiological salt solution (dialysate) is passed on the opposite side of the semipermeable membrane to the blood. The dialysate contains essential solutes in similar concentrations to normal serum. The dialysate, however, does not contain waste products such as urea creatinine and so these substances will therefore pass across the membrane from a region of high concentration (the patient's uraemic blood) to region of low concentration (the dialysate).

In addition to the concentration gradient, the rate of removal of waste products by diffusion will depend upon the size of the molecules (measured by molecular weight (MW)) in relation to the size of the pores in the semipermeable membrane, or in other words, the permeability of the membrane. Small molecules will diffuse more readily than larger ones.

Hydrostatic Pressure

As blood is pumped through a filter a positive pressure will be exerted on the membrane. The pressure in the space on the opposite side of the membrane will be lower, whether or not the space is filled with dialysate. As a result of this, fluid from the patient will move from the area of greater pressure across the membrane, to the area of lower pressure.

Ultrafiltration/Convection

As a result of hydrostatic pressure, fluid will move across the semipermeable membrane, and this process is called ultrafiltration. The rate of ultrafiltration will depend on the permeability of the membrane and the hydrostatic pressure exerted upon it. The sum of the positive pressure in the blood compartment and the negative pressure in the dialysate compartment equals the transmembrane pressure (TMP).

The removal of fluid by ultrafiltration also results in the removal of solute, or those molecules dissolved in the water; this process is known as convection or solvent drag. Again, the higher the permeability of the membrane, the higher the removed volume of fluid and contained solute will be.

Haemodialysis

Haemodialysis depends on the utilisation of diffusion for the efficient clearance of waste products. The patient's blood is pumped through the filter (dialyser) on one side of the membrane whilst a physiological dialysis fluid (dialysate) is passed through the dialyser on the opposite side of the membrane. To optimise the concentration gradient the blood and the dialysate flow in opposite directions (counter current flow).

During a conventional haemodialysis treatment some fluid will be removed by ultrafiltration, but this is usually a small amount (2–3 l) and will not provide significant removal of waste products by convection.

Haemofiltration

Haemofiltration relies totally on the principle of ultrafiltration/convection. Blood is pumped through the filter in much the same way as in haemodialysis. However, there is no dialysate on the other side of the membrane, resulting in the absence of diffusion. The membrane is much more permeable to water than a standard dialyser resulting in very high volumes of ultrafiltrate. As such large volumes of plasma water are removed there is significant clearance of waste products by convection. The large volumes of ultrafiltrate require the simultaneous and continuous replacement of fluid to the patient.

Haemodiafiltration

Haemodiafiltration uses the physiological principles of both diffusion and ultrafiltration/convection in approximately equal amounts. Diffusion takes place from the patient's blood to the dialysate and the large volume of ultrafiltrate results in the removal of molecules by convection. As the ultrafiltrate volume is so large, a replacement fluid is given to the patient to compensate. The dialysate is similar to that used for conventional dialysis and the replacement fluid contains physiological levels of sodium, potassium, magnesium calcium and a buffer, preferably bicarbonate.

Haemodialysis has traditionally been the standard form of extracorporeal treatment, with haemofiltration and haemodiafiltration limited to use in acute renal failure and intensive care as continuous therapies. Some centres, however, now routinely use intermittent haemodiafiltration in place of conventional haemodialysis. For the purpose of the chapter, however, the reference is to standard haemodialysis unless otherwise stated.

ACCESS FOR HAEMODIALYSIS

The success of a haemodialysis treatment depends almost entirely on the adequacy of the blood flow through the dialyser. Optimal clearance of waste products depends on dialysate flow rate, membrane permeability, membrane surface area, duration of treatment and most significantly blood flow rate. Dysfunctional access will therefore adversely affect dialysis adequacy and consequently increase patient mortality and morbidity (Butterley and Schwab, 1996).

The nurse has a responsibility to ensure that the prescribed blood flow is achieved. Poor access which fails to deliver the required blood flow is a waste of time for the patient and the resources of the dialysis unit. If access becomes problematic it should be addressed as a priority.

There are a variety of types of access which can be used for haemodialysis which fall broadly into two categories:

1. **Percutaneous Access** including subclavian, femoral and jugular lines which can be either temporary or permanent, and the arteriovenous shunt.
2. **The Arterio-Venous Fistula** (AVF) and arteriovenous grafts.

For patients with end-stage renal disease the AVF is preferred. The creation and maintenance of long term access remains, however, one of the most challenging aspects of caring for renal patients, particularly patients with vascular disease such as the elderly and diabetics.

The Arteriovenous Fistula (AVF)

The AVF is created during a surgical procedure to join together an artery and a vein (Fig. 7.1). Most commonly the radial artery and the cephalic vein are used in the patient's nondominant forearm. Other sites include the upper arm (brachial artery and cephalic vein) and the upper leg.

As a result of the anastamosis, blood from the artery is forced into the vein where it flows in a retrograde direction. The increased blood flow and pressure causes the vein to thicken and dilate. Once established, blood flow of up to 800–1000 ml min^{-1} can be achieved (Anderson et al., 1977).

Ideally the patient should have the fistula created long before the need for dialysis arises. This will ensure that the operation is performed when the patient is well and will allow the fistula time to mature, preventing the need for insertion of temporary access and the associated risk of infection. Many renal centres have a policy that medical and nursing staff avoid phlebotomy or cannulation into the forearms of patients with suspected renal disease. This precaution will help to prevent damage to vessels that may subsequently be required for fistula formation.

Before anastamosis

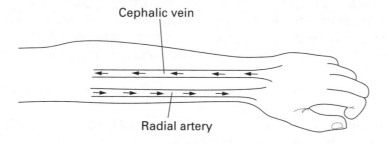

After anastamosis

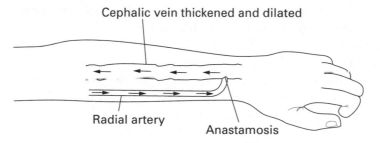

Fig. 7.1 *Arteriovenous fistula.*

Formation of the Arteriovenous Fistula

Preoperative Care

Patients should be given every opportunity to participate in their plan of care and all aspects of treatment should be discussed with them. As part of the patient's predialysis preparation and education a full explanation of the surgical procedure and after care should be given to the patient. The patient may wish to visit and speak with a patient who has a well established functioning fistula to find out what it looks and feels like.

The patient should understand that the fistula will be cannulated each dialysis and the needles that will routinely be used should be available for the patient to see and examine. When the patient reaches end stage renal failure they may feel unwell and anxious at the thought of starting dialysis. Participation from the beginning may help the patient feel more secure and confident.

Postoperative Care

In addition to the routine postoperative care the nurse should ensure that the following specific postoperative care is completed.

- The limb should be kept warm and well supported to help peripheral circulation.
- Blood pressure should be monitored closely and maintained at a minimum of 100 mmHg systolic. If the blood pressure falls below this, peripheral blood flow may be affected, with an increased risk of the fistula clotting.
- The wound site should be examined regularly for signs of excess bleeding or swelling.
- The blood flow through the fistula should be checked regularly by completing the following observations:
  (a) by placing a stethoscope lightly over the incision a buzzing/ whooshing sound should be heard. This is called a bruit. The bruit should be loudest near the incision and gradually becomes softer as the stethoscope is moved further up the vessel.
  (b) by placing a hand lightly over the incision site a buzzing sensation should be felt. This is called the thrill.
- The bruit and thrill should be checked regularly and the patient taught how to perform these observations as soon as s/he is able.
- Prior to discharge the patient should be informed how to care for the fistula and advised to avoid using the fistula arm for carrying heavy loads and to avoid tight or restrictive clothing on the arm. Additionally, the patient must be advised to inform nonrenal doctors and nurses that the arm should never be used for phlebotomy, cannulation or for recording blood pressure, as all of these may result in permanent damage to the fistula. Finally, the patient should be advised to contact the hospital immediately if they notice bleeding, swelling or absence of bruit or thrill.

Complications of Arteriovenous Fistulae

Thrombosis

Thrombosis may occur in the immediate postoperative period or at a later date. Surgical treatment is usually required, but if reported promptly, permanent damage may be avoided.

Aneurysm

Extravasation of blood on removal of fistula needles results in the frequently seen bulging areas of the fistula. The skin eventually becomes much thinner as the aneurysms dilate. Cannulation in the aneurysm should be avoided.

Steal syndrome

The patient may complain of pain, oedema, coldness or pins and needles as blood is 'stolen' from the hand as a result of the fistula. Surgical correction to restore blood supply to the hand is usually required with subsequent loss to the fistula.

Heart failure

The formation of the fistula will result in an increased cardiac output of approximately 6–18% due to increased venous return (Anderson, 1977). If the increase in output exceeds this, heart failure may occur. Brachial fistulae are associated with a higher incidence of heart failure due to increased flow (Nicholls, 1994).

Cannulation of the Arteriovenous Fistula

In the first instance the fistula should be allowed 2–4 months to mature before cannulation is attempted, to allow healing of the anastamosis and some development of the vessels. After this time the fistula can be safely cannulated but the procedure should be undertaken by experienced practitioners only.

New fistulae may be prone to extravasation and clotting which can be painful and distressing for the patient. Therefore, all attempts should be made to minimise trauma during the first few visits. If the patient is anxious a local anaesthetic may be offered. Topical creams are the sensible choice as subcutaneous injections rather defeat the object of pain free cannulation. Prior to each cannulation a thorough physical examination of the fistula should be undertaken to check that there is no evidence of oedema, infection or bruising and that blood flow through the fistula is evident through the presence of the bruit and thrill.

The unit policy for strict asepsis and cleansing of the arm should be adhered to. Universal precautions should be employed, including the wearing of gloves, aprons and a face visor, as blood may splash into the face and eyes during cannulation. A tourniquet may be used prior to cannulation to help engorgement of the vessel but in well established larger fistulae this is often unnecessary.

Cannulation protocols

Many units are now evaluating the use of planned protocols for insertion of fistula needles with the aim of reducing complications and extending the longevity of the fistula. The effect of repeated puncture on fistulae was first described by Kronung (1984).

During each cannulation a small area of vessel tissue is displaced. When the needle is removed this area is filled with a thrombus. Scar tissue is then formed, resulting in increased tissue and subsequent elongation of the vessel wall. Over time this results in a loss of elasticity of the vessel and dilation results in aneurysm formation and adjacent stenosis.

Kronung (1984) described three methods of cannulation and the effects of each (Fig. 7.2). They are:

1. **Rope ladder puncture**   describes the systematic use of the entire length of the vessel. Each needle is inserted at approximately 2 cm above the last site and back again, resulting in a uniform use of the vessel. This demonstrated less aneurysm formation as the punctures per area were reduced.
2. **Area puncture**   This describes the development and use of one or two areas of the fistula which are regularly used. This may result in increased aneurysm formation related to the number of repeated punctures over a small area causing increased tissue elongation and aneurysm formation.
3. **Button hole puncture**   This describes the repeated puncture of exactly the same site at exactly the same angle into exactly the same hole each dialysis. Over time cylindrical scar tissue develops, guiding the needle into the right place. It is suggested that button hole technique results in less aneurysm formation.

Whilst the adoption of protocols may be beneficial and ensure high standards of uniform practice it is acknowledged that additional evaluation is

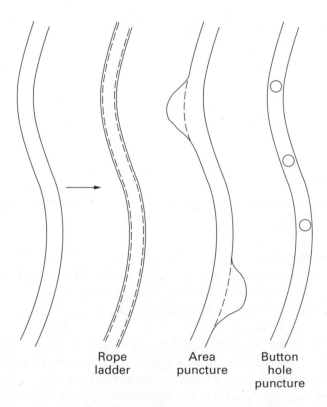

Rope   Area   Button
ladder   puncture   hole
                             puncture

Fig. 7.2 *Needle protocols (Kronung, 1984).*

necessary to provide the evidence for the long-term effects of any of these protocols on the longevity of fistulae.

Needle Sets

The achievable blood flow for many patients is often underestimated. The careful selection of needles will ensure that optimum flows are obtained. Smaller needles (e.g. 16 and 17 gauge) produce a high resistance as the blood pump is increased. This results in a sucking effect of the needles and machine arterial alarms. Larger needles (14 g and 15 g) produce lower resistance and therefore avoids the sucking as the blood pump speed is increased.

Needle tubing also influences the achievable blood flow rate (Greenwood, 1982). The longer tubing results in an increased pressure drop which will adversely affect the blood flow. It is recommended that thin walled larger needles with short tubing are used when high blood flows are required.

Needles should be inserted aseptically at 45° to the skin. The entire needle shaft should be inserted and the butterfly wing secured with tape. On insertion, a syringe should be attached to the end of the needle tubing and blood withdrawn. Any resistance to withdrawal may indicate that the needle position needs adjusting. Often the needle hole is occluded against the side of the vessel wall. This can be corrected by placing a small ball of cotton wool under the butterfly which will lift the needle externally and lower the needle tip internally. If flow is still not obtainable the presence of a clot may be suspected or complete misplacement of the needle. In this event the needle should be removed.

If the needle punctures the wall of the vessel extravasation will occur, resulting in a painful visible swelling around the site. The needle should be removed and firm pressure applied for about 10 min before a further insertion is attempted. On no account should the nurse push and pull the needle blindly hoping that the needle will finally find the vessel. This will result in much pain and discomfort for the patient and will bruise and damage the surrounding tissue which may in turn cause permanent damage to the fistula.

It is also important that nurses, no matter how experienced, recognise their limitations in relation to cannulation. If a cannulation attempt has failed after more than two or three attempts, assistance should be sought from a colleague, as the increased anxiety of the nurse and patient may negatively influence further attempts at successfully siting the needle.

Arteriovenous Grafts (Fig. 7.3)

If the peripheral blood vessels are unsuitable for fistula formation the surgeon may decide to create a graft. Most grafts are created using synthetic materials such as polytetrafluoroethylene (PTFE) and Goretex.

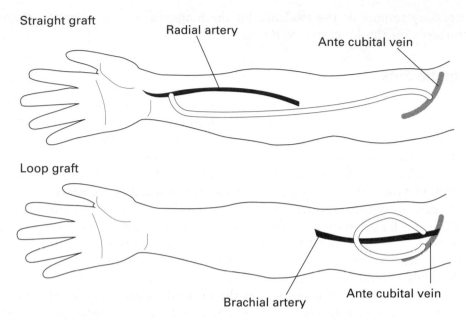

Fig. 7.3 *Arteriovenous graft configuration.*

The graft may be configured in a straight line or in a loop. Grafts are less compliant than fistulae, resulting in a higher pressure through the vessels. Patients should be taught how to care for the graft in the same way as a fistula.

The nurse should perform the same predialysis physical examination prior to cannulation. The arterial needle should be inserted at the arterial end of the graft at least 5 cm from the anastamosis site. The venous needle should be inserted in the venous end with the same considerations. For loop grafts it is important to identify the arterial and venous sides of the graft as incorrect needle placement will result in recirculation.

Percutaneous Access (Fig. 7.4)

Percutaneous access is the term used to describe the insertion of a cannula or catheter into a major vein. Catheters may be inserted as a temporary measure, as in acute renal failure, or for temporary use whilst a fistula matures. Potential sites include the subclavian, femoral and internal jugular veins. The use of the subclavian vein is not recommended in patients with chronic renal failure as this may adversely affect the success of the creation of an AV fistula due to central venous stenosis (Uldall, 1996).

More commonly percutaneous catheters are being inserted as permanent access for patients whose fistulae have either failed or whose vessels are inadequate to attempt AVF creation in the first place. The permanent catheters are cuffed and inserted through the creation of a subcutaneous

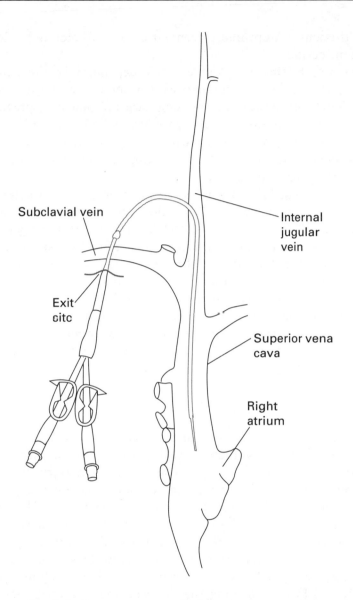

Fig. 7.4 *Permanent tunnelled percutaneous catheter.*

tunnel, as this ensures optimal placement of the catheter and helps reduce the rate of infection.

Catheters may be single or double lumen depending on the unit's policy for single needle or dual needle dialysis. Catheters may be inserted under general or local anaesthetic and nursing care pre and post preoperatively will be the same as for any surgical procedure. Post insertion it is essential that the correct placement of the catheter is checked by X-ray prior to dialysis as postinsertion complications can include pneumothorax and puncture of the adjacent vessels.

The nurse's responsibility includes the maintenance of catheter patency, patient education, prevention of infection and early intervention when infection occurs (Thomas-Hawkins, 1996). Nurses caring for percutaneous access must demonstrate meticulous care as defined by a strict unit policy. The policy should include the need for strict asepsis during any catheter intervention. The exit site should be examined prior to each dialysis and observed for signs of infection such as soreness, redness or the presence of exudate. Exit sites should be dressed with a dry gauze dressing (Conley et al., 1989). Both the catheter exit site and the entire length of the catheter and tips and bungs should be thoroughly cleansed with chlorhexidine 2% (Maki et al., 1991).

Patency

To maintain patency between dialysis treatments a bolus of heparin (5000 iu ml) equal to the volume of each catheter lumen is inserted. This is called the heparin lock. The purpose of the lock is to prevent blood entering the catheter and clotting, not to anticoagulate the patient. For dual lumen catheters the volume for each lumen may be different. It is important that the exact volume of each respective lumen is ascertained to prevent giving a systemic dose of heparin to the patient.

Prior to the next dialysis treatment, the heparin lock should be removed by aspirating the catheter with a syringe and then flushing with 0.9% normal saline before connecting the dialysis lines. Nevertheless, clotting is a common complication. Several attempts may be needed to aspirate a clot in the catheter if resistance is felt. It is vital that any clot is removed and no attempt is made to flush a catheter which cannot be aspirated. In permanent catheters, the administration of a urokinase or streptokinase infusion should dissolve the clot if all other methods have failed.

In dual lumen catheters it is important to use the arterial and venous lumens appropriately. Occasionally flow from the arterial lumen is partially occluded owing to poor positioning of the arterial holes against the side of the vessel wall. The lines may have to be reversed to achieve an acceptable blood flow, but it should be remembered that reversal of the lines will result in increased recirculation (Twardowski et al., 1993).

Arteriovenous Shunt (Fig. 7.5)

Until the early 1980s, the AV shunt was used as a method of access for both chronic and acute haemodialysis. Current use is rare and is generally limited to acute use for patients undergoing continuous arteriovenous haemofiltration (CAVH).

The creation of a shunt involves the surgical cut down of the peripheral vessels of the forearm where the radial artery and cephalic vein are used, or the ankle where the posterior tibial artery and long saphenous vein are used (Uldall, 1996). Teflon tips are inserted into the vessels and silicone tubing attached. The two ends of tubing are then joined together with an additional Teflon connector to form a loop. Blood from the artery exits the body through the tubing and returns through the loop into the vein.

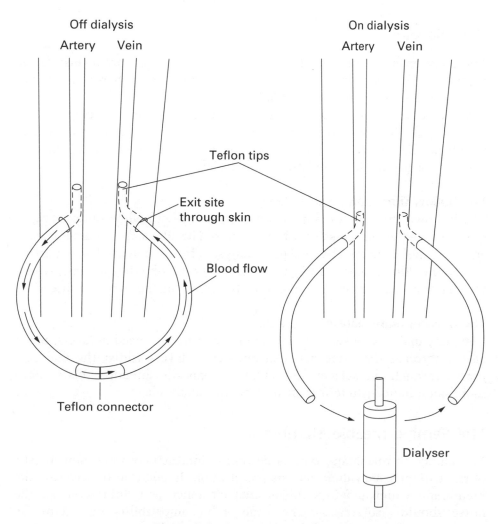

Figure 7.5 *Arteriovenous shunt.*

For dialysis the two ends of the shunt are disconnected and attached to the dialysis lines. Advantages of the shunt include their ease of accessibility and that they produce good blood flows. Disadvantages include that they are prone to clot easily and have a high risk of infection. Arguably, one of the most important disadvantages is the issue of patient safety. The nurse caring for a patient with a shunt *in situ* should be extremely vigilant. The unconscious or confused patient should not be left at any time. Accidental disconnection of the shunt is relatively easy and may result in massive blood loss within seconds, with potentially fatal consequences. A set of clamps should be placed at the patient's bedside for use in an emergency.

HAEMODIALYSIS EQUIPMENT

The Dialyser

The dialyser is the functional unit of the extracorporeal circuit just as the nephron is the functional unit of the kidney, and some patients and nurses refer to the dialyser as the artificial kidney.

Manufacturers have made significant advances in the development of membranes which provide highly efficient clearance of waste products and which are biocompatible for the patient. There are two types of dialyser design, the hollow fibre and the parallel plate.

The hollow fibre dialyser (Fig. 7.6)
The hollow fibre dialyser is made up of thousands of hollow fibres or capillaries about the thickness of a human hair. The fibres are secured at each end of the cylindrically shaped dialyser in a polyurethane potting compound. Blood passes through the centre of each fibre like a straw, whilst the dialysate passes on the outside of the fibres in the opposite direction.

The parallel plate dialyser (Fig. 7.7)
The plate dialyser consists of sheets of membranes arranged in layers. Blood passes through the space between one set of layers whilst the dialysate passes through the adjacent layers in the opposite direction. Plates have more compliance (stretch) than hollow fibre dialysers.

The Semipermeable Membrane

The choice of membrane type is becoming increasingly important as part of the patient's individual dialysis prescription. In addition to selecting the membrane which provides the desired clearance and fluid removal, the nurse should also consider the issue of biocompatibility related to the patient's needs.

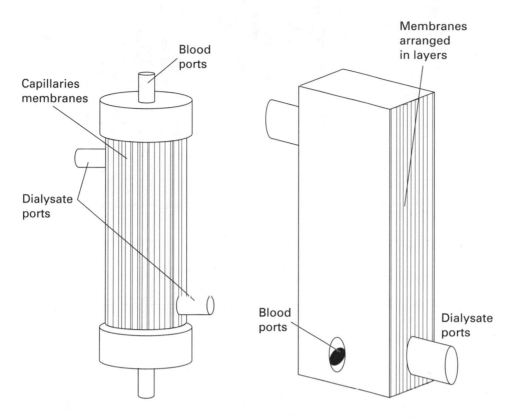

Fig. 7.6 *Hollow fibre dialyser.*   **Fig. 7.7** *Parallel plate dialyser.*

There exists a large and increasing variety of membrane types available, but these fall broadly into three categories, which are:

1. Cellulose membrane (e.g. Cuprophan)
2. Modified cellulose membranes (e.g. Cellulose Acetate, Hemophan)
3. Synthetic membranes (e.g. Polysulfone, Polyacrilnitrile (PAN), Poly-methylmetacrylate (PMMA) and Polyamide (Hoenich, 1992).

The efficiency with which a membrane clears water and solutes is described as its flux properties. Thin membranes with large pores are very permeable to water and large molecules and are called high flux membranes as they have the ability to clear solutes with a molecular weight of up to 30 000. Low flux membranes are less permeable to water and solutes but will provide adequate clearance of solutes up to molecular weight 10 000. The membrane's permeability to water is described as its ultrafiltration co-efficient (Kuf).

High flux membranes have a high Kuf and low flux membranes have a lower Kuf. Details of the properties of each dialyser can be found on the dialyser data sheet which is provided with each box of dialysers (Fig. 7.8).

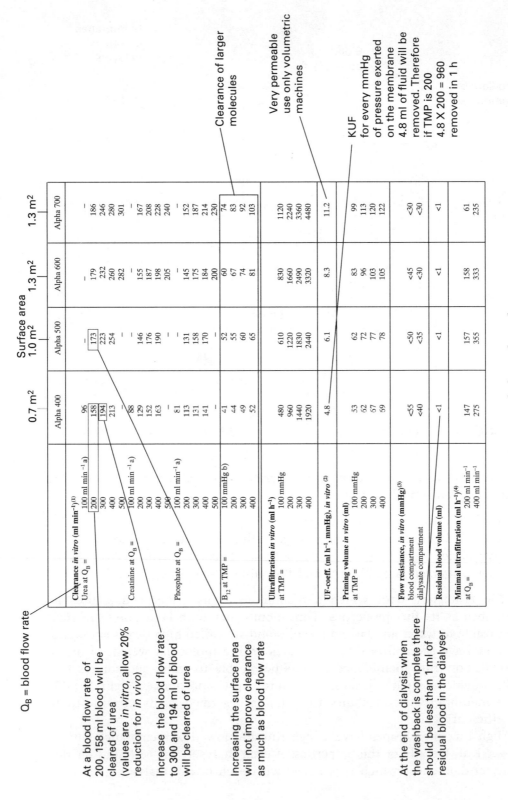

Fig. 7.8 Using a dialyser data sheet.

Table 7.1 Molecular weight

Substance	Molecular weight
Albumin	68 000
Bilirubin	600
Middle molecules	300–2000
Dextrose	180
Uric acid	168
Creatinine	113
Urea	60
Calcium	40
Water	18
Heparin	8000–11 000
Acetate	59
Bicarbonate	61

The nurse should become familiar with the data sheet of the dialysers commonly used in the unit to understand the capabilities of different dialysers.

Table 7.1 gives the molecular weight values for a range of molecules. It can be seen that standard low flux membranes will provide adequate clearance of small molecules such as urea and creatinine. The high flux membranes are chosen for more efficient middle molecule clearance.

Biocompatibility

The process of dialysis requires the repeated exposure of the patient's blood to foreign substances including the dialyser membrane, blood lines, dialysate, chemicals, drugs and water. These components of dialysis may initiate immunological responses which include activation of the complement system and release of cytokines which are involved in the inflammatory process and anaphylactic reactions (Ledebo, 1987).

Haemodialysis is regarded as a sophisticated and safe procedure but the aim of correcting the patient's uraemia to improve quality of life may overshadow the fact that the procedure in itself may be a precipitating factor to many complications. In recognition of this, the issue of biocompatibility is becoming increasingly important. Components of the dialysis process which provoke no or minimal immune response from the patient are considered to be biocompatible, but this may differ from patient to patient. A major biocompatibility issue relates to the use of dialyser membranes. Cellulose membranes are considered to be, arguably, less biocompatible, whilst synthetic membranes may be better tolerated, or more biocompatible.

Methods of sterilisation have been linked to dialyser reactions. Ethylene oxide can cause severe anaphylaxis. This is more common in hollow fibre dialysers than flat plates owing to the retention of ethylene oxide in the potting compound of hollow fibres (Ing and Daugirdas, 1986). The buffer used in dialysis fluid can also affect biocompatibility. The detrimental effects of acetate as a buffer is well documented, causing numerous side effects to the patient such as vasodilatation, nausea, vomiting and dialysis fatigue. Bicarbonate, the body's natural buffer, eliminates the majority of these complications and is therefore considered to be more biocompatible (Ledebo, 1990).

Preparation of the Dialyser

Priming and rinsing of the extracorporeal circuit is a crucial process in the preparation of the dialysis treatment. Manufacturers provide guidelines and recommendations for priming volume and rinsing time and these will vary depending on whether the dialyser is hollow fibre or parallel plate, the membrane type and the dialyser sterilising agent. There are two important aspects to consider:

1. The removal of air. Air must be removed from the blood lines and from all surfaces of the dialyser membranes. Pockets of air retained in the dialyser will result in less available surface area for diffusion to take place. Additionally, the presence of air will promote clotting in the dialyser with loss of surface area and risk to the patient.
2. The removal of any chemicals or sterilising agents used during the dialyser manufacturing process. Of most concern is ethylene oxide (ETO), a gas which is a highly effective sterilent against all micro-organisms. It may, however, have toxic effects and cause hypersensitivity reactions in some patients (see first use syndrome p. 234). Alternative sterilising methods are now routinely used including heat sterilisation and gamma radiation. Careful priming is essential to ensure all traces of ETO are rinsed from the dialyser prior to the patient being connected. Typically a minimum of 1 l of saline is required to remove residual ETO.

If any delay is incurred between the initial priming and the patient commencing dialysis then additional rinsing should take place (Ansorge *et al.*, 1987). This is particularly important for hollow fibre dialysers because higher levels of residual ETO are retained in the potting compound. As plate dialysers do not have potting compound most of the ETO is removed during the initial rinse.

Dialyser Reuse

The majority of dialysers are packaged with a statement from the manufacturers indicating that the dialyser is for single use only. Despite this, many centres reuse dialysers (up to 20 times) with no complications. The most significant advantage to reusing a dialyser is the cost saving achieved and this is often the driving force for commencing a reuse programme. The cost saving allows the selection and use of superior dialysers that are efficient and biocompatible that would be cost prohibitive without a reuse programme.

Reuse can be performed manually but fully automated systems offer benefits such as speed and automatic tests to measure loss of surface area and pressure tests which will prompt the replacement of the dialyser. Chemicals used are an important consideration and strict protocols for the safe handling and storage should be in place. The reprocessing of dialysers is a technical and time-consuming role. If a reuse programme is introduced dedicated technicians should be employed and trained on methods to fulfil the task. This will allow the nurses to focus on the delivery of patient care.

The Dialysate

Dialysate is the term used to describe the fluid which is pumped through the dialyser on the opposite side of the semipermeable membrane to the patient's blood. The purpose of the dialysate is to create a concentration gradient to promote diffusion of waste products from the patient's blood.

Dialysate is produced by mixing a concentrated electrolyte solution (concentrate) with purified water. This is usually mixed as a ratio of one part concentrate to thirty-four parts water (1 : 34). Dialysate composition can be tailored to individual patient requirements but on the whole the solution will be physiological, i.e. resemble normal serum biochemistry with specific deviations (Table 7.2).

Table 7.2 *Concentration of substances in blood and a typical dialysate*

Blood	Solute	Dialysate
133–144	sodium (mmol l^{-1})	140–145
3.3–5.3	potassium (mmol l^{-1})	2.0–4.0
2.5–6.5	urea (mmol l^{-1})	0
60–120	creatinine (μmol l^{-1})	0
2.1–2.6	calcium (mmol l^{-1})	1.25–3.5
0.85	magnesium (mmol l^{-1})	0.5–1.5
4.0–6.6	glucose (g l^{-1})	5–10
22–30	bicarbonate (mmol l^{-1})	30–38

Water

Patients on maintenance haemodialysis are exposed to approximately 400 l of dialysis water per week (Ismail *et al.*, 1996). Because of this level of exposure, water should be considered a drug (Schulman, 1996). Water contains many contaminants which pose a potential risk to the patient. Examples of major contaminants include aluminium (with associated risks of dementia and osteomalacia), chloramines (haemolysis and anaemia), fluoride (osteomalacia, osteoporosis), calcium, magnesium (hard water syndrome), copper (haemolysis and liver damage), zinc (anaemia) and endotoxin (pyrogenic reactions) and organisms.

Methods of water treatment

1. A reverse osmosis (RO) unit uses a semipermeable membrane to filter water and works by rejecting 90–95% of univalent and divalent ions in addition to microbiological contaminants
2. Water softeners remove calcium and magnesium
3. Carbon filters adsorb chlorine and chloramines
4. Sediment filters remove particulate matter (Ismail *et al.*, 1996)

Water should be regularly analysed to measure endotoxin levels and numbers of organisms to ensure that they do not exceed the standard for the dialysis unit.

Dialysate Composition

Sodium

Standard sodium concentrations are set at approximately 140 mmol l^{-1}. Below this level the patient may suffer symptoms such as hypotension, muscle cramps and disequilibrium. Levels higher than this may cause thirst and hypertension. Many machines now offer the option of programming a variable sodium concentration. This sodium profiling allows the nurse to tailor the sodium concentrations to the individual patient's needs. The profile can be set to increase from a low to a high sodium or conversely a decreasing sodium starting off high and finishing lower.

Potassium

Many renal patients present for dialysis with raised potassium levels. The standard dialysate concentration is 2.0 mmol l^{-1} which will allow for steady and efficient removal of potassium from the patient. Patients who routinely present with lower potassium levels should dialyse against a solution containing 3.0 mmol or those patients known to suffer from arrythmias or taking digitalis should dialyse against a higher potassium concentrate (4.0 mmol l^{-1}).

If the patient presents with a dangerously high potassium level some centres dialyse against a zero potassium concentrate to ensure rapid lowering of the serum potassium. These solutions should be used with extreme caution and for a limited time only. Rapid reduction of serum potassium will lead to large potassium shifts in the body with risk of arrhythmia. If the unit does employ the use of these concentrates they should be stored separately and away from the standard dialysis solution to prevent the risk of dialysing patients against the wrong concentrate.

Calcium

Dialysate calcium may be physiological or lower than normal if the patient has hypercalcaemia or if calcium intake is high through the use of calcium containing phosphate binders. Patients who have recently undergone parathyroidectomy should have their calcium level checked prior to dialysis. The calcium can drop suddenly and may result in the need for calcium to be added to the concentrate.

Dextrose

Dextrose should be added to the concentrate of diabetic patients to prevent hypoglycaemia during dialysis. Glucose-free dialysis promotes more efficient removal of potassium by reducing plasma insulin levels and consequent redistribution of potassium enabling removal by dialysis (Ward, 1987).

Buffers (Acetate and Bicarbonate)

Haemodialysis patients tend towards a moderate to severe acidosis. The aim of the buffer in dialysis is to normalise the patient's acid base balance as far as possible. Bicarbonate is the body's major buffer and is the preferred choice to use in the dialysate.

The use of acetate is largely historical and its use presents no feasible argument for use as a first choice. In the early days dialysis bicarbonate was the buffer used but caused many operational problems largely due to dialysate preparation. Dialysate used to be prepared in large tanks with the manual weighing and mixing of the added salts. Unless the pH of the solution is tightly controlled the bicarbonate and calcium salts precipitate. The pH was maintained by pumping carbon dioxide (CO_2) into the tanks. This was time-consuming and laborious.

The 1960s witnessed the advent of acetate as an alternative to bicarbonate. Acetate is an organic ion which generates bicarbonate when metabolised. Metabolism in the body takes place in the muscle cells and the mitochondria of the liver. Acetate dialysis became the norm and was convenient and cheap to use. However, as dialysis techniques have become increasingly efficient the disadvantages of acetate have become apparent. Symptomatic hypotension, nausea and vomiting and dialysis fatigue have all been shown to increase with acetate dialysis and decrease or disappear with bicarbonate dialysis (Graef et al., 1978).

A patient's ability to metabolise acetate is considered critical. It is essential that patients are able to metabolise acetate at a rate equal to the rate at which they lose bicarbonate. Patients who are at risk of poor metabolism include those with reduced muscle mass and those with liver failure (Ledebo, 1990).

The Renal Association (1995) have recommended that all units move towards the universal availability of bicarbonate dialysis.

Anticoagulation

As blood comes into contact with the extra corporeal circuit the clotting cascade will be initiated. Optimal anticoagulation regimes, like all aspects of the dialysis prescription, should be tailored to the needs of the individual patient. Heparin is the most commonly used anticoagulant for haemodialysis with the average patient receiving approximately 1.5 million units per year (Vienken and Bowry, 1993). A baseline clotting time should be recorded before the anticoagulation regime is commenced.

For standard heparinisation a value of 1.5 to 2.0 of the baseline should be aimed for after anticoagulation. On commencing dialysis a bolus dose of heparin is given and then a continuous infusion set at a rate to maintain the clotting times within pre-determined limits.

Minimal heparin should be used for patients who are at risk of bleeding or who are dialysed preoperatively. The clotting time should be monitored very closely.

Heparin free dialysis should be performed for patients who have a bleeding disorder or who are considered to be at risk from bleeding, i.e. postoperatively. Heparin free dialysis requires a rapid blood flow and very close observation of the blood lines and dialyser and additionally requires the frequent flushing (every 15 to 20 min) of the lines with normal saline (the additional saline must be accounted for in the total ultrafiltration volume).

The Haemodialysis Machine (The Monitor)

The haemodialysis machine is simply a monitor to ensure the safe delivery of dialysis to the patient (Fig. 7.9). State of the art machines offer impressive and sophisticated systems capable of assisting the nurse to deliver a wide range of treatment options. Operating the machine for the first time can be a daunting experience for the nurse, but competence is soon mastered. It is important that the nurse ensures that the machine is merely an accessory to the delivery of treatment and that the patient, and not the machine, remains the focal point in all nursing interventions. Despite the huge variances in machines they are all broadly separated into two component parts – the blood monitor and the fluid monitor.

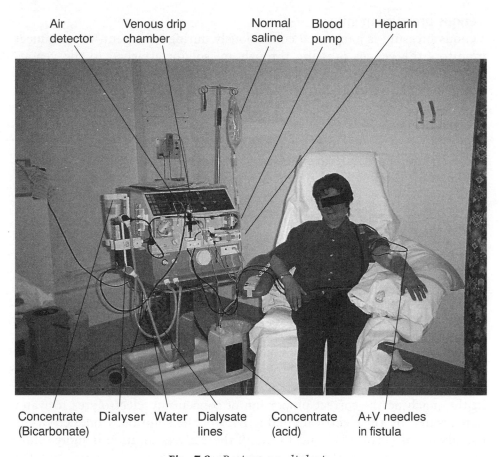

Fig. 7.9 *Patient on dialysis.*

The Blood Monitor

Blood pump
Peristaltic blood pumps are integral to the machine. Blood pumps can be set to deliver blood flow rates of between 0–600 ml min⁻¹.

Air detector
An ultrasonic detector is situated at the venous drip chamber. The detector should detect air bubbles or the lowering of the level within the drip chamber. An audible alarm will sound and the venous line will clamp, preventing the risk of administering air to the patient.

Arterial and venous clamps
These clamps close the respective lines automatically if there is an alarm. They are also used to regulate the blood flow in single needle dialysis.

Venous pressure monitor

Venous pressure is monitored continuously during treatment. A transducer monitors the venous pressure through an isolator attached to the venous drip chamber. Alarm limits can be set to alert the nurse to significant changes in the venous pressure (± 30).

Arterial pressure

This can be monitored either via a transducer the same as the venous pressure or with an arterial sac and a sensor plate. If the arterial flow is reduced the sac will collapse, causing the sensor plate to trigger an alarm.

Fluid Monitor

Temperature

The machine can provide dialysate temperature between 30–40°C. High temperatures increase the risk of haemolysis and hypotension due to vasodilation. Low temperatures result in less efficient dialysis and hypothermia. Within reason the patient can adjust the temperature for comfort. Low temperature dialysis is an efficient way of cooling the patient with pyrexia.

Conductivity

In the machine the correct proportion of concentrate electrolytes to water is measured by the electrical conductivity of the solution. Conductivity is usually set at between 13 and 14 mS. If the dialysis solution is more dilute or concentrated than the set standard the machine will alarm and the dialysate flow will be cut off.

A pH meter will ensure that the correct acid and base concentrates are used, which is important for safety in bicarbonate haemodialysis. For units that use both acetate and bicarbonate concentrates, it is important to be extremely vigilant during concentrate selection. Without a pH meter the conductivity meter may not detect the incorrect use of acetate instead of the acid component for bicarbonate dialysis. The result will be dialysing the patient against the pure bicarbonate solution with acetate, resulting in a base excess and the patient becoming alkalotic.

Blood leak detector

A small leak or larger rupture of the dialyser membrane will result in blood escaping into the dialysate. A detector on the dialysate outflow line will sense this and the machine will alarm. The detector may be set on high or low sensitivity. Small leaks often resolve and dialysis can safely be continued. Larger leaks are more serious, with risk of dialysate entering the patient's blood. In this instance dialysis should be discontinued without returning the blood to the patient.

Bypass valve

If there is an alarm related to the dialysate, e.g. a blood leak, conductivity alarm or temperature alarm, the dialysate flow will be diverted from the dialyser via the bypass valve. This enables the patient to remain on the dialysis machine without risk whilst the problem is rectified.

Ultrafiltration Control

The machine can control the ultrafiltration by either pressure control or volume control.

Pressure control

Transmembrane pressure (TMP) is calculated by the machine as the difference between the pressure in the dialyser blood compartment and the dialysate compartment. For example, if the venous pressure is 50 mmHg and the dialysate pressure is 150 mmHg, the TMP will equal 200 mmHg. TMP is a fairly reliable method of monitoring ultrafiltration but does not account for deviations in the treatment such as an obstruction in the dialyser which would result in an increased pressure drop in the dialyser with a subsequent increase in the ultrafiltration rate. The actual TMP may not be affected and therefore the increase in ultrafiltration rate may also go undetected.

Volume control

Machines that measure ultrafiltration by volume control can respond to pressure drops in the dialyser and compensate for them. If there is an increase in the ultrafiltration rate the machine will compensate by increasing the pressure of the dialysate compartment to prevent excess fluid removal.

Single Needle Dialysis

When two needles are used for dialysis there are, in effect, two separate blood pathways – one removing blood from the patient and the second returning blood to the patient. Single needle dialysis is ideally used for those patients with good established access. The use of single needle dialysis for patients with failing access should be discouraged (Aldridge, 1991). If, however, access is a problem, single needle dialysis can be considered as a temporary measure to enable the patient to dialyse (albeit inadequately) if only one needle can be inserted, if the patient has a single lumen catheter, or if one lumen of a dual lumen catheter is blocked.

To facilitate the treatment a 'Y' connector is attached to the single source of access. Once the blood flow has been established through the circuit the single needle mode is activated. This initiates the alternate clamping of the arterial and venous lines to control the blood flow through the dialyser. Blood is removed from the patient with the venous line on the machine clamped. This will cause the venous pressure to rise. When the pressure reaches a predetermined limit the pump will stop, the arterial clamp will close and the venous clamp will open allowing the blood to return to the patient under pressure by gravity. During single needle dialysis, some plate dialysers are compliant enough to accommodate the extra volume of blood in the extracorporeal circuit. Hollow fibre dialysers are not, and therefore a compliance chamber must be added to the circuit to prevent rupture of the dialyser membrane. During a 4 h treatment there will be a reduction in the total volume of blood processed through the dialyser in comparison with dual needle dialysis. In addition, there will be recirculation of dialysed blood around the 'Y' connector and catheter, resulting in a further reduction of dialysed blood volume. The use of a second pump in the circuit increases the total volume of blood processed through the dialyser.

PRESCRIBING THE DIALYSIS DOSE

For many years patients have been given dialysis treatments based entirely on subjective evaluation of blood biochemistry along with a general assessment of perceived patient well-being. Patients themselves have been held responsible for the success of their treatment in relation to these parameters by being instructed to comply with restricted diets aimed at maintaining biochemistry within acceptable limits. Limited resources and lack of understanding have compounded this philosophy over time.

More recently there have been attempts to provide a more objective and scientific method of assessing dialysis adequacy. The aims of nursing care, utilizing the dose of dialysis and nutritional parameters, should be to measure dialysis adequacy as well as encouraging patients to eat well.

Urea Kinetic Modelling

The direct relationship between dialysis dose and long-term patient survival has been demonstrated (Lowrie et al., 1981). It is therefore essential that dialysis prescription is aimed at preventing or reducing the mortality and morbidity of patients receiving haemodialysis. High levels of urea clearance are correlated with improved patient outcomes.

One method of determining the dose is by the use of Kt/v. Kt/v is estimated by measuring pre- and postdialysis urea concentrations. K equals the dialyser clearance of urea, t equals the treatment time and v equals the amount of urea distributed in the body water.

To complete the equation it is necessary to know the clearance of urea through the dialyser. This is estimated by pre : post dialysis urea ratio. To ensure an accurate assessment of (v) the nutritional status of the patient must be optimised, ensuring that the patient has an adequate protein intake. The patient's weight, height and sex are included in the calculation to estimate the percentage of body weight that is water (usually 55% in women and 65% in men).

For accurate assessment of K it is essential to calculate the pre- and post-dialysis urea ratio. The dialyser data sheet may be cautiously used to estimate the dialyser clearance but it is wise to assume a 10–20% reduction on the manufacturers' *in vitro* values. An approximate example is given but more precise information is essential (i.e. the patient's height, etc.) for accurate calculation. For example:

A woman weighs 60 kg, therefore, an approximate estimation of v = 33l

K = 150 ml min^{-1}, t = 4 h, k × t = 36l, divided by v = 36/33 = 1.09.

Therefore Kt/v = 1.09

Measuring the urea reduction ratio (URR) is possibly the simplest method of determining dialysis adequacy (Lowrie and Lew, 1991). This is expressed as a percentage reduction.

URR = 100.(1 – Ct/Co)

Ct = post dialysis urea and Co = pre dialysis urea

These parameters can now provide an acceptable standard for dialysis dose. The Renal Association 1995 recommend the following:

A URR of 55% or a Kt/v of greater than 1 in patients dialysing three times per week.

A URR of 85% or Kt/v of 1.8 for patients dialysing twice a week.

The mathematical concepts of urea kinetic modelling (UKM) can be complicated but nurses should not feel inadequate if they do not have a clear grasp of these principles. There are many computer software packages available to complete the calculations and to advise on corrective measures to achieve the desired Kt/v. What is vital is a clear understanding of the need for highly accurate sampling of pre and post blood specimens and the comprehensive dietary support of the patient.

Another significant role of the nurse is to ensure the delivery of the prescribed dialysis and to understand the effect of deviations in treatment on the dialysis dose and the subsequent effect this may have on the patient's well-being.

Prescribed dialysis dose versus delivered dialysis dose The dialysis prescription may be affected by a number of events that will effectively reduce the dialysis dose.

Errors of time (t) patient starts dialysis late, machine in bypass due to concentrate running out, other machine fault or isolated ultrafiltration, patient comes off dialysis early.

Errors of clearance (K) blood flow reduced, wrong dialyser selected, recirculation.

Errors of volume (v) residual renal function increasing or decreasing, excessive or inadequate protein intake, incorrect sampling.

High flux/high efficiency dialysis by Kt/v measurement and the use of high flux membranes dialysis treatment time can be shortened with use of rapid blood and dialysate flow rates. The benefits for the patient of less time on dialysis may be outweighed by the potential complications such as increased hypotensive episodes. The use of short high efficiency treatments is controversial – the long-term survival of patients has been correlated with longer treatment times (Charra *et al.*, 1996).

THE HAEMODIALYSIS PATIENT

The period of time from diagnosis to commencement of renal replacement therapy can be sudden, but often there is a period of time from a few months to several years when the patient will have time to adjust his lifestyle and prepare for whichever form of dialysis is appropriate. The need for predialysis care, including psychological support as well as clinical monitoring of the progression of the renal failure, cannot be over emphasised.

Patients have a right to be informed of all treatments available, including the advantages and disadvantages of each, and to refuse treatment if they wish. An important role of the nurse is to ensure that patients with chronic renal failure should have the opportunity to experience a supportive process of information, education and counselling before reaching end-stage renal failure and the need for dialysis.

Unfortunately many patients in the UK may still present for haemodialysis with little or no preparation regarding their treatment. Patients may be unaware of alternative treatments and lack knowledge and insight into the permanency of dialysis and the impact of the treatment on their lives both now and in the future. The sudden presentation of patients at end stage presents a challenge for the nurse in both providing the highest standard of clinical care to the patient and additionally in ensuring patients are armed with the necessary information to enable them to make informed choices and feel included in decision making about their treatment. It should be a goal of multidisciplinary care teams to enable patients to maintain their independence as far as possible. The aim should be to rehabilitate the patient and promote health to sustain or improve quality of life. The judgement of quality of life should always be the patient's judgement and not that of the health care professionals or other family members.

When to Start Dialysis

Patients who present with severe symptoms of renal failure supported by the clinical confirmation of uraemia will need to commence dialysis immediately. Patients with progressive but controlled renal disease may be reviewed regularly in clinics by nephrologists and nephrology nurses.

Creatinine clearance is monitored and should not fall below 10 ml min^{-1} (15 ml min^{-1} for diabetics) (Schulman and Hakim, 1996) without dialysis being initiated, but if the patient is very symptomatic before this then dialysis should be started sooner. Dietary protein restriction may alleviate uraemic symptoms but does not slow progression of renal disease and may lead to malnutrition.

For the patient on maintenance haemodialysis there are a number of options to be considered related to the location of the haemodialysis treatment.

In-centre haemodialysis

Regional dialysis centres may provide both an acute and chronic haemodialysis service. In-centre haemodialysis may be offered, but the service may be overstretched in terms of available dialysis space. For this reason the options of home haemodialysis or satellite haemodialysis should be explored for the patient who chooses or requires maintenance haemodialysis .

Home haemodialysis

The patient who expresses a desire to take the home haemodialysis treatment option should receive support and encouragement from the multidisciplinary team. The patient, once established and familiar with the dialysis regime, may want to learn the technique quickly in order to be selfsupporting at home at the earliest possible time. With support and co-operation a training programme can be completed in 6 weeks if the patient is well and has no other complications such as poor access, but most training programmes aim to get the patient home within 12 weeks.

To optimise training and learning opportunities the patient can be encouraged to come to the unit on nondialysis days to practise lining and priming the machine. Partners should be encouraged to attend as often as they can, but will need to negotiate a minimum amount of time with the nurse to learn emergency procedures. It should be emphasised to the patient and partner that the overall management of the treatment (setting up, monitoring and discontinuing of the treatment) is primarily the responsibility of the patient. The partner is there to provide support and help, not to accept complete responsibility for the procedure.

Satellite haemodialysis

The availability of satellite dialysis is increasing within the UK. Satellite centres provide an ideal setting for patient on maintenance haemodialysis.

The centres are community based, closer to the patient's home, making them more convenient and accessible. Satellite centres are essentially nurse managed and led. A nephrologist will oversee patient dialysis prescription and consultation, but day-to-day dialysis management is the responsibility of the nurse.

ASSESSMENT OF THE PATIENT (Fig. 7.10)

Weight

Regular assessment of dry weight is essential to enable the nurse and patient to determine the amount of fluid removal required during dialysis. One kilogram is equal to 1l of fluid, meaning that patient weight is a simple and accurate method of assessing fluid gain or loss between dialysis treatments. The term dry weight (ideal body weight, target weight) refers to the weight at which there is no clinical evidence of oedema, shortness of breath, increased jugular venous pressure or hypo/hypertension.

The initial determination of dry weight should involve the expertise of the doctor and dietician. On a day-to-day basis this remains the responsibility of the nurse. Many nurses are now trained in the routine clinical skills of fluid assessment and this is wholly appropriate.

The aim of dialysis will be to remove the excess volume of fluid to ensure that the patient comes off dialysis at the dry weight. To calculate this the following formula is required:

Actual weight	68.5 kg
Dry weight	66 kg
Weight gain	2.5 kg
Add any additional fluid intake during treatment	400 ml washback
Total fluid to be removed	$2.9 \div 4$ h
Divide by total number of hours = Ultrafiltration rate	0.721 per h

Blood Pressure

Blood pressure should be recorded predialysis to provide a baseline from which to measure any significant changes during treatment. If a patient is overloaded prior to dialysis, blood pressure may be raised due to an increased circulating volume. Patients who are hypertensive as a result of their underlying renal disease may be prescribed antihypertensives. If these patients become hypotensive on dialysis it may be necessary to omit the dose prior to or nearest to the next dialysis session.

Temperature

The patient's temperature should be routinely recorded predialysis. Pyrexia prior to dialysis should be investigated immediately to eliminate the possibility of infection.

Pulse

Pulse should be recorded on patients with known arrythmias or who present with very high or low potassium levels.

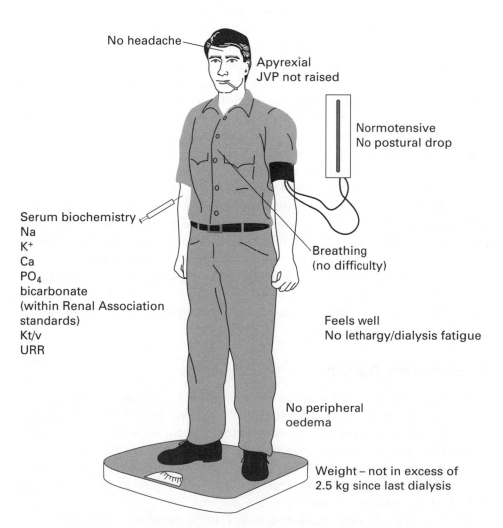

No headache

Apyrexial
JVP not raised

Normotensive
No postural drop

Serum biochemistry
Na
K^+
Ca
PO_4
bicarbonate
(within Renal Association
standards)
Kt/v
URR

Breathing
(no difficulty)

Feels well
No lethargy/dialysis fatigue

No peripheral
oedema

Weight – not in excess of
2.5 kg since last dialysis

Fig. 7.10 *Predialysis assessment and post dialysis evaluation.*

Serum Biochemistry and Haematology

Blood tests are routinely done monthly but more frequent tests may be ordered as necessary. The nurse must ensure that serum levels meet the required unit standards and alert the physician to any significant problems.

Infection Control

The Rossenheim report (1972) set standards for infection control in relation to hepatitis B in renal units. Over 25 years later patients and staff within renal units must acknowledge daily the risks associated, not just with hepatitis B, but other blood-borne viruses (BBV) such as hepatitis C and HIV. A review of the Rossenheim report is currently in progress. Early indications are that recommendations are likely to suggest the use of tight precautionary measures based on the identification and isolation of all patients with BBV including HIV (Gower, 1996).

The practicalities of providing isolation for every patient with BBV will need to be explored along with the desired philosophy of care towards patients with BBV. Whilst the identification of patients with hepatitis is, on the whole, accepted, the screening of patients for HIV will be controversial and nurses must ensure that they advocate for patients and are satisfied that the rationale for testing is in the patient's interests and is only carried out with informed consent.

Universal precautions should be used as standard practice in the haemodialysis unit for the protection of the patient(s) and the staff. Universal precautions require that body fluids of *all* patients are treated as potentially infectious and therefore protocols for handwashing, protective clothing, eyewear, and disinfection of machinery should be strictly adhered to prior to nursing interventions with all patients. When universal precautions are used effectively the isolation of patients should be unnecessary unless it is to protect the immunocompromised patient from opportunistic infections.

Commencing Dialysis

On completion of the predialysis assessment and preparation of the access the nurse should complete an additional machine check before connecting the patient to the machine. On connection, careful attention must be paid to both the patient and the extracorporeal circuit at this vital time. As the blood passes through the lines the nurse should monitor the passage, ensuring there are no obstructions to flow, no air visible in the line and that all connections are secure.

Dialysis centres vary as to the policy for commencing dialysis. Some centres connect both lines directly to the access, resulting in the patient receiving the volume of saline in the lines, while others bleed out by only connecting the venous line when the lines are filled with blood. If the policy is to connect up both lines together then the additional fluid will have to be accounted for. It is also necessary to ensure that the priming and rinsing has been optimal and that additional rinsing is completed if the machine has been left to stand. If it is preferred to bleed out the venous line should be placed in a sterile container to avoid contamination and infection risk to the patient.

Patients connected to the dialysis machine for the first time may be alarmed at the sight of their blood travelling through the circuit and should be reassured.

Blood Flow Through the Extracorporeal Circuit

Blood is pulled from the patient by the blood pump through the arterial line by negative pressure. Once the blood has passed the occluding pump rollers the pressure then becomes positive and the blood is then pushed through the circuit. Heparin is infused on the positive pressure side to prevent heparin, or air, or both, being sucked into the circuit.

The blood is pumped through the arterial end (top) of the dialyser and leaves the dialyser at the venous end (bottom). The blood then passes through the venous bubble trap and returns to the patient via the venous access.

Flow Through the Fluid Monitor

Purified water is taken into the machine via the water inlet port at the back of the machine. It is then heated, degassed and mixed with the concentrated electrolyte solution to make the dialysate. The machine will measure the correct proportioning of the solution through the conductivity meter. Dialysate enters the dialyser at the venous end (bottom) and leaves the dialyser at the arterial end (top) to maintain counter current flow between the blood and the dialysate. The dialysate is pulled through the circuit by a pump situated at the out flow line, resulting in negative pressure in the machine dialysate circuit.

Completing dialysis

Prior to completing the dialysis the nurse must make sure that the prescribed dose has been delivered and that time has been added for any nondiffusion time during treatment. The total ultrafiltrate volume should be checked. Postdialysis blood samples should be taken if required from the arterial access with the venous line clamped prior to washback with saline. The blood pump should be stopped and the arterial and venous lines clamped. The arterial line is then disconnected from the arterial needle and connected to a bag of 0.9% normal saline. Once connected, the clamps on both lines are removed and the pump is restored, allowing the saline to push the blood through the circuit back to the patient. When the lines are clear (rose from the venous bubble trap) the pump can be stopped and the lines clamped. The lines can be disconnected and the machine stripped and put into disinfect mode. The needles can then be removed or, if percutaneous access, the catheter flushed and the heparin lock installed.

Postdialysis the clinical observation of blood pressure and weight are completed to check that the patient has lost the desired weight and is not hypo/hypertensive. Blood results will provide information to fully evaluate treatment effectiveness to facilitate further treatment plans.

HAEMODIALYSIS COMPLICATIONS

Continuous and progressive development of equipment and expertise has ensured that haemodialysis is a safe procedure and if prescribed and monitored correctly serious complications should be rare. The treatment should only be carried out under the supervision of an expert practitioner. The aim of nursing care should be to prevent the occurrence of complications through comprehensive assessment and planning. Nevertheless, unplanned events will happen and the role of the nurse is then to ensure early recognition and prompt intervention to protect the patient from harm. A summary of the complications is given in Table 7.3.

Hypotension

Hypotension will occur if the rate of fluid removal in the dialyser exceeds the plasma refilling rate in the patient. Some measures can help to limit the risk of hypotension, including advising the patient to ensure that interdialytic weight gains are not excessive. Intake of fluid remains a difficult aspect of treatment for patients to control. In addition to beverages, fluid contained in food will need to be accounted for. Time and patience must be afforded to patients in attempting to grasp the principles and realise the consequences of poor fluid control. If the predialysis weight gain is excessive the treatment time may be extended to allow gentle fluid removal or isolated ultrafiltration can be used. Greater volumes of fluid can be removed by this method as isolated ultrafiltration increases peripheral resistance thereby reducing the risk of hypotension (Baldemus, 1981).

Another method of potentially reducing the risk of hypotension related to slow plasma refilling is the use of the haematocrit and blood volume monitor. Some machines have this device as an integral part of the machine, but a separate monitor can be used. Changes in blood volume are measured through the haematocrit and oxygen saturation of the blood. The monitor will alarm when the patient is at risk of hypotension.

Nausea and Vomiting

Nausea and vomiting may be associated with hypotension. This may either be prior to a hypotensive episode, i.e. the patient has nausea, vomits and then becomes hypotensive, or conversely the patient is hypotensive first, is revived with IV saline and then vomits subsequently. Some patients who dialyse against acetate suffer from nausea and vomiting which disappears when they are dialysed against bicarbonate. Finally, some patients who are dialysing for the first time or who are relatively new to dialysis may vomit due to anxiety. In this case reassurance and understanding will help the patient to relax.

Cramp

Cramp is another common side effect of haemodialysis. Cramps, as with hypotension, may be caused by the ultrafiltration rate being set too high, causing rapid fluid shifts. Infusion of saline helps alleviate the symptoms but if fluid is a problem a smaller volume of hypertonic glucose can be given with effect. For the patient who suffers regularly with cramp, the prophylactic use of quinine sulphate tablets may help. These should be given 2 h prior to dialysis to ensure that peak concentrations coincide with peak risk time on dialysis.

Patients with cramp in the leg or foot may wish to stand up and push their foot against the floor to help relieve the pain. This should be avoided where possible as simultaneous hypotension will result in the patient falling to the floor. Pressure can be applied to the foot by allowing the patient to push their foot against the nurse. The use of a heat pad and/or vigorously rubbing the painful area may also help.

Disequilibrium

Dialysis relies upon the diffusion of solute across the semipermeable membrane of the dialyser. At the same time diffusion will be taking place across the semipermeable membranes between all body compartments from the intracellular, interstitial and intravascular compartments. The rate of diffusion should be equal to maintain equilibrium. If diffusion in the dialyser is highly efficient the result will be a disequilibrium in the body compartments. Rapid urea removal will result in the plasma in the intravascular compartment being hypotonic to the fluid in the cells. This will result in osmotic shifts of fluid from a region of low concentration to a region of high concentration. This is particularly significant in the cerebrospinal fluid and brain cells. Additionally, rapid changes in the pH of the cerebrospinal fluid may predispose to disequilibrium (Bregman *et al.*, 1994).

Symptoms of disequilibrium can be mild or severe. Mild symptoms may include headache, dizziness, nausea and vomiting, or disorientation. Severe symptoms include fits, coma and potentially death.

Patients who are acutely ill, have a very high urea predialysis or who are dialysed for the first time, are considered most at risk of disequilibrium. However, it may still occur in patients who are well established on dialysis. For those considered at risk the nurse must ensure that the dialysis prescription aims at a gentle reduction in serum biochemistry – the golden rule is 'little and often'. There is no urea in the dialysate so diffusion will take place freely, but the rate and efficiency of diffusion can be influenced by the nurse by ensuring the following:

Blood flow rates should not exceed 150 ml min^{-1}
Dialysers with low surface area should be used
Treatment time limited to approximately 2 h.

This type of prescription may need to be performed daily until the patient is considered stable and risk of disequilibrium is reduced. Despite these preventative measures it is possible that disequilibrium may still occur. If disequilibrium is suspected the dialysis should be discontinued. The infusion of hypertonic solutions such as mannitol may help to correct the fluid shifts.

Dialyser Reactions (Membrane Reaction/First Use Syndrome)

Allergic responses may occur as the patient's blood is exposed to foreign materials. Some examples include the dialyser membrane, the chemical sterilising agents such as ETO, and bacteria or endotoxin (Hoenich and van Holder, 1993). Allergic reactions can be type A or type B (Daugirdas and Ing, 1994). Type A is a severe anaphylactic reaction usually occurring within the first 5 min of dialysis. Symptoms can begin with a rash itching and become severe, including dyspnoea and a burning sensation throughout the body. There may be laryngeal oedema and possibly cardiac arrest.

Treatment necessitates the immediate discontinuation of dialysis; the blood should not be returned to the patient. Maintenance of the airway is paramount and the administration of oxygen is required. The administration of adrenaline, chlorpheniramine and hydrocortisone may be necessary.

Patients who have suffered this type of reaction should be dialysed against synthetic membranes which have been steam sterilised. Extra rinsing of the dialysis circuit may also be advised.

Type B reactions are less severe and include chest pain, and may occur up to 1 h after dialysis is commenced. The cause is unknown but it is suggested that the use of synthetic membrane and/or reuse is beneficial (Bregman et al., 1994).

Dysrrhythmias

Many patients with end-stage renal failure have associated heart disease. Patients with heart disease are more susceptible to dysrrhythmias which may be precipitated during dialysis by hypertension, hypotension, and fluid and electrolyte shifts, particularly potassium. Patients taking digitalis should be dialysed against solutions containing higher levels of potassium to minimise potassium shifts and prevent the serum potassium level falling below 3.5 mmol l^{-1} (Nicholls, 1994).

Haemolysis

Haemolysis is the damage or rupture of red blood cells. As most of the body's potassium is contained within the cells, massive haemolysis can quickly lead to hyperkalaemia and cardiac arrest. Haemolysis may be caused by dialysing against dialysate that is too hot or dialysing against water or hypotonic dialysate. An error in concentration selection and checking may result in a patient dialysing against bleach or formalin, as these will not necessarily cause a conductivity alarm.

Modern blood pumps have low shearing stresses and should not cause haemolysis but if wrongly adjusted, the rollers of the blood pump may cause damage to cells. The high venous pressure resulting from occluded or obstructed (kinked) venous access/blood lines may also damage red blood cells. The patient will complain of chest pain and dyspnoea and may be in a state of collapse. If haemolysis is suspected the dialysis should immediately be discontinued and the blood should not be returned to the patient. Another machine should be prepared as a standby, as emergency dialysis may be needed to treat hyperkalaemia.

Air Embolism

Modern monitoring equipment with integral ultrasonic air detectors provides some assurance to patients and nurses for the prevention of air embolism. But the equipment is only as good as its user and strict adherence to alarm and safety checks prior to initiating each treatment is essential.

Extreme care should be taken during the priming procedure and when connecting the patient to the extracorporeal circuit. The air detector should be activated during the priming procedure, and any problems with false alarms resolved prior to the patient commencing dialysis. An air detector which persistently/intermittently alarms with no obvious cause should not be accepted as troublesome or oversensitive. The machine should not be used, and sent to the technicians for service.

If the patient requires intravenous infusions during dialysis, they should

Table 7.3 *Complications of haemodialysis (summary)*

Complication	Cause	Prevention	Treatment
Hypotension	Dry weight too low Excessive UFR Antihypertensive drugs Acetate	Regular assessment of dry weight Correct UFR calculation Bicarbonate dialysis	0.9% NaCl Lay patient flat Reduce UFR and recalculate fluid loss
Cramp	Excessive UFR	Correct UFR calculations Quinine sulphate 2 h prior to HD	0.9% NaCl or hypertonic solution Heat pad/massage
Disequilibration	Too efficient dialysis	Small surface area dialyser $< 1.0\,m^2$ Reduce blood flow rate $< 150\,ml\,min^{-1}$ Reduces time $< 2\,h$ maximum Daily dialysis until biochemistry satisfactory Bicarbonate dialysis	Discontinue dialysis I.V. mannitol
Arrythmias	Underlying hypertension Coronary artery disease Excessive potassium shifts Digoxin	Dialyse against dialysate with minimum 4.0 mmol potassium	Monitor
Membrane reaction	Complement activation on exposure to membrane and/or ETO	Use synthetic membranes that have not been sterilised with ETO for patients at risk or with known allergies Correct rinsing and preparation of dialyser	Stop dialysis Do not return blood to patient Treat as anaphylaxis I.V. adrenalin/hydro-cortisone/piriton
Air embolus	Air entry to venous end of extracorporeal circuit	Ensure all lines secure Ensure correct use of air detector Observe lines	Stop treatment Lay patient on left side Give 100% oxygen
Haemolysis	Damage to red blood cells through pump or kinked lines Dialysate temperature too high	Low shearing pumps Ensure venous pressure is not high Set temperature gauge	Give oxygen ?Give blood Test for high potassium from damaged red cells Dialysis
Clotting of blood lines	Inadequate anticoagulation Air in the dialyser	Review anticoagulation regime Review priming procedure Ensure airtight connections	Stop treatment Discard dialyser and lines Review anticoagulation before resuming treatment
Blood leak	A tear or rupture in the membrane within the dialyser	Careful handling of the dialyser Keep pressures within limits	Stop dialysis Discard extracorporeal blood

ETO, ethylene oxide; HD, haemodialysis; UFR, ultrafiltration rate.

be given as intermittent bolus doses by the nurse, as an infusion left to run continuously presents a greater risk of air entering the circuit.

Before connection, the entire length of the venous line from the bubble trap end should be visually examined for presence of air and/or micro-bubbles. On completion of dialysis, the blood in the extracorporeal circuit should be returned to the patient with saline (or other solution). The approximate volume of the washback is 200–250 ml. This is usually accounted for at the beginning of treatment and therefore causes no problem. Some centres, however, aim to reduce all additional fluid given to patients and advocate the use of air to return blood to the patient. Whilst hesitantly accepting that this practice may be acceptable in special circumstances under the observation of an expert practitioner, this practice by nurses in a busy haemodialysis unit is considered neither justified nor safe.

In the event of a patient receiving an air embolus the nurse must stop dialysis and lay the patient on their left side with the head lower than the rest of the body. This will force air in the circulation into the ventricle which is said to act as a bubble trap (Daugirdas, 1994). Immediate medical assistance must be sought and emergency resuscitative measures commenced. Outcome may be related to the volume of air infused.

Clotting of the Blood Lines and Dialyser

Clotting of the circuit will occur if anticoagulation is inadequate, if blood flow is inadequate and if there is air in the circuit.

Signs and symptoms
A change in the pressure of the circuit will occur as a result of clotting. If the dialyser has clotted there will be a decrease in the venous pressure and possibly a rise in the arterial pressure. Clotting of the bubble trap will result in a raised venous pressure. If clotting occurs the treatment should be discontinued without returning the blood to the patient. The cause should be investigated, i.e. anticoagulation regime, access or dialyser preparation.

Blood Leak

A tear or rupture in the dialyser membrane will result in blood escaping across the membrane into the dialysate compartment. This will be detected by a sensor causing the machine to alarm and the blood and dialysate pump to stop. A small tear may resolve and although treatment must be discontinued, the blood can be returned to the patient as the machine will allow the alarm to override. A large tear or rupture will present a risk to the patient and treatment should be discontinued. The blood should not be returned to the patient. Some centres test the dialysate with a lab stick to confirm the presence of blood in the dialysate. If machines are serviced and cleaned regularly this should be unnecessary with the technology of the sensors on the machine.

Continuous Renal Replacement Therapy (CRRT)

The use of CRRT has developed enormously during recent years. The first therapy of this type was continuous arteriovenous haemofiltration described by Kramer *et al.* in 1982. This became a popular method of managing fluid and electrolyte balance of patients in the ITU with acute renal failure. Patients who required more efficient fluid and electrolyte clearance remained dependent on intermittent haemodialysis treatments performed by renal nurses.

The 1990s has witnessed both an evolution of the treatments with a concomitant devolution of the responsibility of prescribing and monitoring of RRT. The nurses in the ITU have developed their skills to take on the additional responsibilities which were once the domain of the renal nurse. It is recognised that intermittent haemodialysis may be contraindicated in patients with acute renal failure who are critically ill. Complications such as cardiovascular instability, sepsis and multiorgan failure may make conventional treatments difficult.

There are a large variety of treatment options available and actual choice will depend on physician preference, nurse expertise and availability of resources such as machinery and disposable equipment.

Today the options fall broadly into three categories, which are continuous haemodialysis, continuous haemofiltration and continuous haemodia-filtration. The use of arterial access is becoming outmoded (Bellomo, 1996) as the relative superiority of pumped techniques is recognised.

A full description of each method will be given to enable the nurse new to CRRT to understand how the treatments have evolved.

Continuous Arteriovenous Haemofiltration (CAVH)

CAVH has been performed in the ITU setting since the early 1980s (Fig. 7.11). (Kramer *et al.*, 1982). CAVH provides a simple method of removing fluid from the patient and at the same time, convective removal of solutes. Access to the arterial circulation is essential as CAVH relies on the patient's own blood pressure to push the blood through the filter. This is provided in the form of an arterial catheter or an arteriovenous shunt. Adequate blood flow through the filter is dependent on the patient's blood pressure which in turn has a linear correlation with the rate of ultrafiltration. The ultrafiltrate is replaced by a physiological electrolyte solution. The main

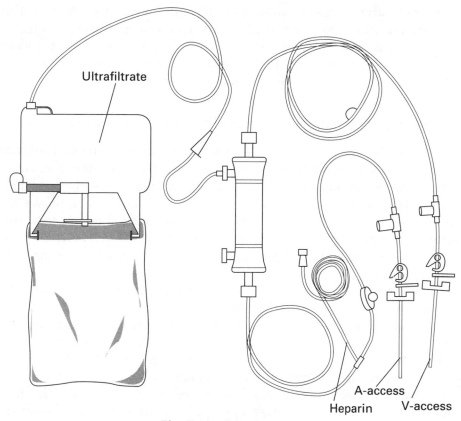

Fig. 7.11 *CAVH circuit.*

benefits of CAVH are its relative simplicity to use in as much as no technical equipment is required. It is a satisfactory method of removing fluid with convective solute removal. However, the rate of solute removal is often limited and therefore may not be an adequate method of RRT in the patient with severe electrolyte disturbances.

Continuous Arteriovenous Haemodiafiltration (CAVHD)

If the blood flows with CAVH are satisfactory but clearance of urea is inadequate the addition of dialysate will provide a concentration gradient and increase the clearance of small molecules by diffusion. A pump will be needed to deliver the dialysate at the required flow rates which results in the relative simplicity of CAVH becoming a more complicated procedure.

Continuous Venovenous Haemofiltration (CVVH)

The addition of a blood pump to the circuit removes the necessity for arterial access and provides a more reliable and controllable method of delivering treatment. Larger volumes of ultrafiltrate can be achieved (1l/h) and therefore increased removal of solutes by convection can be achieved with venous access. The initiation of CVVH requires the use of a blood pump which in turn requires the addition of safety monitoring equipment such as a venous pressure monitor and an air detector.

Continuous Venovenous Haemodiafiltration (CVVHD)

To increase the efficiency of small molecule clearance a dialysis solution is continuously pumped through the filter in a counter current direction to the blood. Small molecule (urea) clearance by diffusion is more efficient.

In the ITU setting many centres use a standard blood monitor for the extracorporeal circuit and then employ the use of infusion pumps to administer dialysate and replacement fluid. Fortunately, the development of fully automated systems for CRRT provide a preferable means of delivering treatment to patients.

From the nursing perspective the use of fully automated systems provides a reliable and easy to use method of monitoring fluid balance of patients who are critically ill. This allows more time for the nurse to dedicate to direct patient care. Described is the Gambro Haemofiltration monitor (HFM), which provides a reliable and timesaving method of CVVH (Fig. 7.12). The machine comprises a basic blood module with blood pump, venous and arterial pressure monitoring and an air detector. The fluid monitor has two additional integral pumps – one to remove fluid from the filter and the second to pump replacement fluid to the patient. The replacement fluid and the ultrafiltrate are suspended on a weigh scale. Fluid on the scale is accurately measured from the scale via a microprocessor which calculates and controls a predetermined linear patient weight.

With such accurate fluid control the nurse does not need to constantly measure and record fluid loss and replacement as with CAVH and CAVHD. Ultrafiltrate can be removed at a rate of between 15 and 100 ml min^{-1}. Standard therapies aim to remove 25–30 ml min^{-1} exchanging approximately 35–40 l in 24 h. The replacement fluid is a physiological solution with either lactate or bicarbonate as a buffer. With this continuous therapy hypokalaemia may develop and therefore extra potassium may be added to the replacement fluid.

Clotting time should be assessed daily and ACT measurement taken regularly to ensure adequate anticoagulation. Anticoagulation regimes will depend on unit policy by using heparin or prostacycline or both. The patency of the blood line will depend on the adequacy of anticoagulation. The filter may continue to be effective for some days. Warning signs that the filter is clotting include a drop in the ultrafiltration rate with a subsequent need to increase the TMP, a drop in the venous pressure and visible signs of clotting in the circuit.

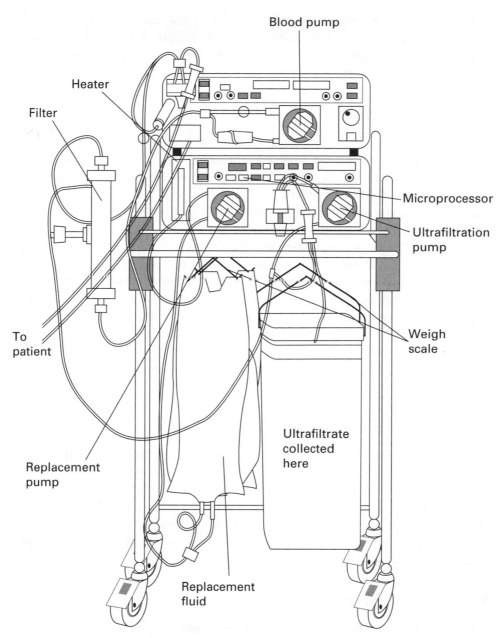

Fig. 7.12 *Gambro haemofiltration monitor (GHF).*

Feeding is of vital importance and usually TPN runs concurrently with CVVH. Extra volumes of fluid can be accommodated with relative ease. As the filter is so permeable it is important to account for the possibility of certain vital vitamins and drugs passing through the filter.

Plasma Exchange

Plasma exchange is an intensive treatment used to treat a variety of immunological and nonimmunological disorders. Examples include Goodpasture's disease, Guillain Barré, Wegner's granulomatosus and anti GBM disease. Blood is pumped through a special plasma filter which separates the plasma containing antibodies and immune complexes whilst retaining the red blood cells. A colloid substitute such as human albumin solution is infused into the patient to replace the plasma removed. As vital clotting factors are simultaneously removed, these too need to be replaced at the end of the treatment. Regimes for plasma exchange vary depending on physician preference and clinical need. The patient may be treated daily with a 2–3 l exchange for up to 10 days. Cyclophosphamide or other immunosuppressive drugs are often given in conjunction with plasma exchange for some disorders. Plasma exchange can be carried out using the Gambro HFM. The colloid replacement fluid is warmed and measured before being delivered to the patient. A 3 l exchange takes about 2 h.

Charcoal Perfusion

The extracorporeal circuit can be engaged in a variety of configurations and settings to perform similar treatments. In the event of drug overdose the dialyser can be replaced by a charcoal filter. The charcoal adsorbs the drugs, particularly drugs such as theophilline, and salicylates. This method is highly effective, but clotting times should be monitored regularly as the charcoal also absorbs plasma protein and platelets and can cause idiosyncrasies with the patient's clotting mechanisms.

Immunoadsorption

Immunoadsorption is a therapy which involves the use of an adsorption column which has the ability to bind antibodies, particularly Immunoglobulin G (IgG). HLA antibodies bind successfully and this treatment has therefore been used to treat patients who are highly sensitised and unable to be transplanted.

A programme of treatments is prescribed on an individual basis. The treatment is usually carried out three times per week for up to 3 months. During this time the patient is cross-matched for a potential donor kidney. Combined with immunosuppressive therapy, the patient who is potentially untransplantable has an increased chance of successful transplantation.

SUMMARY

The patient on maintenance haemodialysis should have a named nurse who is responsible for the planning, delivery and evaluation of the highest standards of individual care. Patients should have the opportunity to participate in decision making related to all aspects of their care. Patients have a right to be cared for by nurses who are competent in all aspects of haemodialysis treatments. Ideally this competence should be assessed in a formal and structured training programme. Finally, the skills needed to provide comprehensive nursing care to patients on haemodialysis cannot be measured solely by a nurse's competence to set up and use a haemodialysis machine or by the ability to insert a pair of fistula needles first time. The haemodialysis nurse is constantly demanding access to the skills and knowledge which tacitly underlie the rapidly expanding scope of professional practice. There is a professional expectation of all nurses to ensure continuous learning and development in order to keep abreast of new research findings, new technology and the ever-increasing needs and demands of the patient.

The nurse working within the haemodialysis unit is faced on a day-to-day basis with a practical dichotomy. On the one hand, the working environment is highly technical and the delivery of optimal treatment a cognitive challenge. On the other hand, the nursing focus must acknowledge the very special affective skills required in providing support, counselling and rehabilitative interventions to patients with chronic ill-health. Although units will function with nurses whose strength or preference lies in one or other domain, it is the careful combination of the skills, knowledge and attitudes of both aspects that result in the advanced and expert practice of the nurse on the haemodialysis unit.

REFERENCES

ALDRIDGE, C. (1991) The use and management of arterio venous fistulae: fact and fiction. *EDTNA Journal*, **17**: 29–35.

ANDERSON, C.B., ETHERIDGE, E., HARTER, H.R., CODD, J.E. AND NEWTON, W.Y. (1977) Blood flow measurements in arterio venous fistulae. *Surgery*, **81**: 459–61.

ANSORGE, W., PELGER, M., DIETRICH, W. AND BAURMEISTER, U. (1987) Ethylene oxide in dialyser rinsing fluid. Effect of rinsing technique, dialyser storage time and potting compound. *Artif Organs*, **11**: 118–22.

BALDEMUS, C.A. (1981) Cited in dialysis haemodynamics dialysis quality an issue for the nurse educational session presented at EDTNA conference Hamburg 1992 Gambro Lund.

BELLOMO, R. (1996) Choosing a therapeutic modality haemofiltration vs. haemodialysis vs. haemodiafiltration. *Seminars in Dialysis*, **9**: 88–92.

BREGMAN, H., DAUGIRDAS, J.T. AND ING, T.S. (1994) Complications during haemodialysis handbook of dialysis pp 149–68 (2nd edition) New York: Little Brown and Company.

BUTTERLEY, D.W. AND SCHWAB, S.J. (1996) Haemodialysis vascular access. Effect on Urea kinetics and the dialysis prescription. *Am Journal Nephrol.* **16**: 45–51.

CHARRA, B., CALEMARD, E. AND LAURENT, G. (1996) Importance of treatment time and blood pressure control in achieving long term survival on dialysis. *Am J Nephrol*, **16**: 35–44.

CONLEY, J., GRIEVES, K. AND PETERS, B. (1989) A prospective study comparing transparent and dry gauze dressings for central venous catheters. *Journal of Infectious Diseases*, **159**: 310–19.

DAUGIRDAS, J.T. AND ING, T.S. (1994) *Handbook of Dialysis* (2nd edn.). New York: Little, Brown and Company.

GREENWOOD, R.N., LAMBOURNE, L. A., PAVITT, L. AND CATTELL, W.R. (1982) Selection of arterio venous needle sets for haemodialysis. *Dialysis and Transplantation* **11**(4).

GOWER, P. (1996) Presentation on the recommendations for the Rossenheim review. British Renal Symposium Eastbourne 1996.

HOENICH, N.A. (1992) Membranes for renal replacement therapy. *EDTNA/ERCA Journal*, **18**: 2–4.

HOENICH, N. AND VAN HOLDER, R. (1993) Allergic reactions associated with haemodialysis: biocompatibility monograph, *EDTNA/ERCA*. 3–6.

ISMAIL, N., BECKER, B.N. AND HAKIM, R.M. (1996) Water treatment for haemodialysis. *AJN*, **16**: 60–72.

ING, T.S. AND DAUGIRDAS, J.T. (1986) Extractable Ethylene oxide from Cuprammonium Cellulose plate dialysers importance of potting compound.

KRAMER, P., BOHLER, J., KEHR, A., GRONE, H.J., SCHRADER, J., MATTHAEI, D. AND SCHLER, F. (1982) Intensive care potential of CAVH. *Trans. Am. Soc. Artif. Organs*, **28**: 28.

KRONUNG, G. (1984) Plastic deformation of Cimino fistulae by repeated puncture. *Dialysis and Transplantation*, **10**.

LEDEBO, I. (1990) Acetate vs. Bicarbonate in Everyday Dialysis. Lund Gambro.

LOPOT, F. (1990) Urea kinetic modelling. *EDTNA/ERCA*, **4**.

LOWRIE, E.G., LAIRD, N.M., PAKER, T.F., SARGENT, J.A. (1981) Effect of the haemodialysis prescription of patient morbidity. Report from the National Co-operative Dialysis study. *New England Journal Med.*, **305**: 1176–81.

LOWRIE, E.G. AND LEW, N.L. (1991) The urea reduction ratio (URR). *Contemp. Dail. Nephrol.*, **Feb**: 11–20.

MAKI, D.G., RINGER, M., ALVARADO, C.J. (1991) Prospective randomised trial of povidine iodine alcohol and chlorhexidine for prevention of infection associated with central venous and arterial catheters. *Lancet*, **338**: 339–43.

NICHOLLS, A.J. (1994) Heart and Circulation Handbook of Dialysis Daugirdas Ing op cit.

SCHULMAN, G. AND HAKIM, C.M. (1996) Improving outcomes in chronic haemodialysis patients: should dialysis be initiated earlier? *Seminars in Dialysis*, **9**(3): 225–9.

SCHULMAN, G. (1996) Dialysis prescription: Introduction. *American Journal of nephrology*, **16**: 5–6.

THOMAS-HAWKINS, C. (1996) Nursing interventions related to vascular access infections. *Advances in Renal Replacement Therapy*, **3**(3):

TWARDOWSKI, Z.J., VAN STONE, J.C., JONES, M.R.E., KLUSMEYER, M.E., HAYNIE, J.D. Blood recirculation in intravenous catheters for haemodialysis. *J. Am. Soc. Nephrol.*, 1993 **3**: 218–21.

ULDALL, R. (1994) Subclavian cannulation for haemodialysis access in patients with end stage renal failure is no longer necessary or justified. *Seminars in Dialysis*, **7**: 161–4.

ULDALL, R. (1996) Vascular access for continuous renal replacement therapy. *Seminars in Dialysis*, **9**(2). 93–7.

VIENKEN, J. AND BOWRY, S. (1993) Optimisation in anti coagulation. *EDTNA Journal*, **19**(2).

WARD (1987) Cited in Ledebo (1990) Bicarbonate vs. acetate in everyday dialysis op cit. Renal Association Standards Document 1995.

CHAPTER 8

PERITONEAL DIALYSIS

INTRODUCTION

Peritoneal dialysis (PD) as a treatment for end-stage renal disease (ESRD) is a relatively simple and very effective technique. As such, it has been successfully developed as the preferred method of home dialysis.

From its introduction in the late 1970s, PD has been refined and developed into a flexible and adaptable therapy which is the treatment of choice for many patients. It has been found to be most effective if performed as a continuous treatment, either by the patient during the day (continuous ambulatory peritoneal dialysis or CAPD) or by a machine, usually whilst the patient sleeps (automated peritoneal dialysis or APD). Owing to its continuous nature, patients who are treated by this therapy tend to have a more stable biochemical and fluid profile. Its flexible nature makes it suitable for most types of ESRD patients.

This chapter discusses the importance of having an individualised treatment for each patient which is structured around both their clinical and lifestyle needs. The chapter starts with an overview of the anatomy and physiology of the peritoneum. Practical aspects of the therapy such as catheter insertion techniques and care, problem solving and infectious complications are discussed in detail. The different therapy options PD can offer are discussed and included in the chapter is a section on patient selection. Other aspects of PD such as adequacy of dialysis, solution formulation, PD in the diabetic patient and education and training of patients are all covered in a practical and readable format.

The chapter is primarily aimed at nurses working within the field of PD, whose role has changed markedly over the last decade (Kelman, 1995). However, it should prove an equally useful chapter to other health care professionals such as social workers, dietitians and physiotherapists caring for these patients.

As the therapy is performed by the patients themselves, in the community, the main focus is on providing these patients with not only an individualised treatment, but also adequate psychological and nursing care which are essential elements for the successful treatment of these patients and their families.

PHYSIOLOGY OF PERITONEAL DIALYSIS

The peritoneal membrane, so called because it covers the abdominal cavity and is derived from the Greek word 'peritonaion' meaning to stretch around, has a surface area of up to 2 m^2. The peritoneal cavity is the potential space between the parietal membrane (which lines the abdominal cavity) and the visceral membrane (the inner layer which closely covers the organs and includes the mesenteries). Under normal circumstances this cavity contains between 50 and 100 ml of fluid which acts as a lubricant (Fig. 8.1).

During PD, physiological solution or dialysis fluid is instilled into the peritoneal cavity. Uraemic toxins and solutes move across the membrane by the process of diffusion, from the blood stream into the dialysis fluid, or vice versa, depending on the concentration gradient. The composition of the dialysis fluid is near to that of normal extracellular fluid.

Fluid removal takes place by osmosis. The dialysis fluid is made hypertonic to plasma by the addition of osmotic agent, usually glucose.

The membrane is made up of three layers (Fig. 8.2):

- *The mesothelium*. Underneath this lies the connective tissue. The luminal side of the mesothelium is covered with numerous microvilli

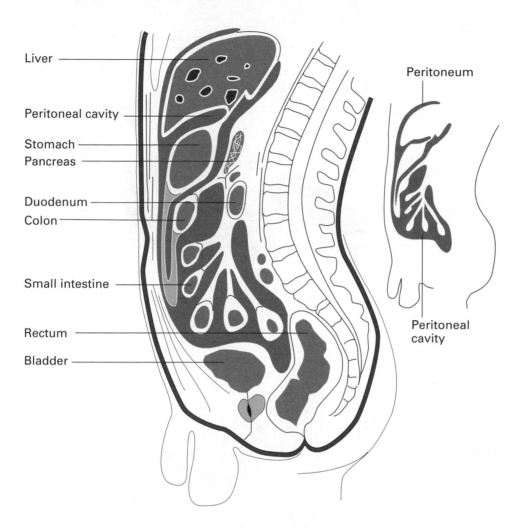

Fig. 8.1 *Location of the peritoneal cavity.*

which are believed to increase the surface area of the peritoneum to up
to 40 m² in a healthy individual. During PD the density of these
microvilli appears to be reduced (Dobbie, 1989).

- *The peritoneal interstitium.* This is composed of fibres and bundles of
  collagen.
- *The capillary endothelium.* This forms a complex branching system.

Blood Supply

The visceral peritoneum is supplied by the superior mesenteric artery. The
parietal peritoneum is supplied by the intercostal, epigastric and lumbar
arteries. Venous return from the visceral peritoneum is to the portal circulation whereas that from the parietal peritoneum goes into the caval

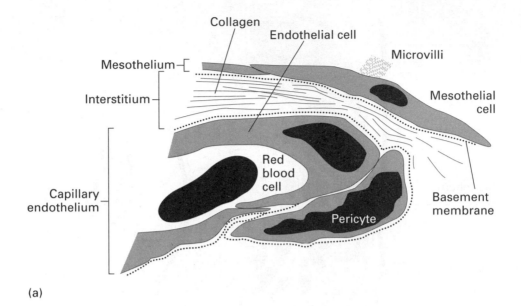

(a)

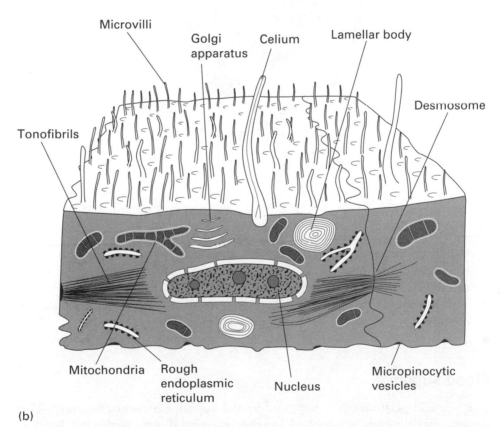

(b)

Fig. 8.2 *(a) The three layers of the peritoneal membrane. (b) Diagrammatic representation of a normal mesothelial cell.*

circulation. This is important because it means that any drugs administered via the peritoneum will be transported to the liver, the normal route.

Lymphatic Drainage

Lymphatic drainage from the peritoneal cavity returns excess fluid and proteins into the systemic circulation. Its other function is to remove foreign bodies from the peritoneal cavity. Lymphatic drainage is a one-way system, the flow rate of which may be affected by respiratory rate, intraperitoneal hydrostatic pressure, posture or peritonitis.

Peritoneal Membrane Transport Characteristics

The peritoneal membrane is semipermeable and allows the passage of both water and solutes.

During PD three processes are involved in removing fluid and wastes from the blood stream and balancing electrolytes. These are osmosis, diffusion and convection.

Osmosis

This is the movement of water through a semipermeable membrane from a solution of low concentration into a solution with a higher concentration. The solution into which the water moves in PD contains an osmotic agent, usually glucose (other osmotic agents are discussed later in this chapter). The higher the glucose concentration, the more the osmotic effect will be, so removing more water from the patient's blood stream (Fig. 8.3).

Diffusion

This is solute exchange between two solutions separated by a semipermeable membrane. The solutes will travel in either direction across the membrane until equilibrium is achieved. The direction and speed at which the solutes flow depends on the concentration gradient. Solutes will flow from the stronger solution into the weaker solution (Fig. 8.4). Therefore, solutes can pass in either direction across the peritoneal membrane.

Other factors that affect diffusion rate are molecular weight and membrane resistance.

Molecular weight Diffusion is a spontaneous process whereby solutes move randomly. Lighter, smaller molecules will move quicker than larger, heavier molecules. Urea (which has a molecular weight of 60 Da) diffuses from blood to dialysate more rapidly than creatinine (molecular weight of 113 Da) or vitamin B12 (molecular weight of 1352 Da). Unlike haemodialysis, where the membrane pore size is controlled, the peritoneal membrane allows transport of large molecules and even proteins. Protein transport

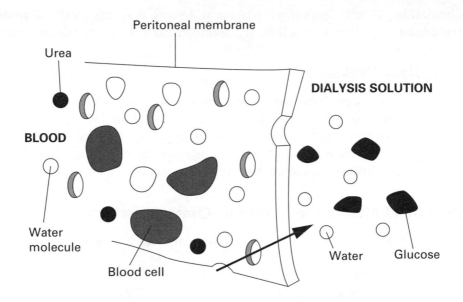

Fig. 8.3 *Osmotic ultrafiltration across the peritoneal membrane with a glucose dialysis solution in the peritoneal cavity.*

into the dialysate is unfortunate as this is an essential nutrient, particularly in dialysis patients who may be catabolic.

Membrane resistance   The permeability of the individual's membrane is an important factor controlling diffusion of solutes. Measurement of this is discussed later in this section.

A patient's peritoneal permeability may be changed during illness. Acute episodes of peritonitis appear to increase greatly the membrane permeability to both solutes and water. However, fibrotic thickening of the membrane, also due to peritonitis, may lead to a severe reduction in its permeability (Davis *et al.*, 1993).

Convection

Owing to the large amount of osmotic ultrafiltration that takes place during PD, connective flow transports or 'drags' water and solutes across the membrane. This occurs at a much faster rate than that which may be accounted for by diffusion alone.

The ability of glucose to exert an effective osmotic pressure depends on its ability to stay in solution in the dialysate. If the peritoneal membrane were perfectly semipermeable (i.e. only permeable to water), the osmotic pressure would be maximised. However, the peritoneum is permeable to solutes as well as water, and therefore allows the glucose through. The osmotic gradient is therefore maximal at the beginning of the exchange.

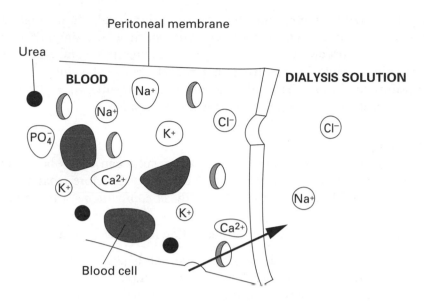

Fig. 8.4 *The peritoneum acts as a semipermeable membrane, allowing small solutes and water to diffuse through, but retains large particles such as proteins and blood cells.*

The ultrafiltration will decrease during the dwell time as glucose is absorbed into the blood stream. It is estimated (Diaz-Buxo, 1984) that the ultrafiltration volume peaks at a dwell time of around 2–3 h, when the ultrafiltration equals reabsorption. The total dialysate and ultrafiltrate volume continues to decrease after this point due to lymphatic absorption.

Measurement of Peritoneal Permeability

The peritoneal equilibration test (PET)

Twardowski *et al.* (1987) and Twardowski (1989) developed a standardised test to measure the equilibration rates of various solutes during a 4-h dwell of PD. Based on his findings, an individual's peritoneal equilibration rate can be categorised as low, low average, high average or high. Twardowski standardised the tests to measure the equilibration rates of creatinine and glucose, therefore allowing measurement of the membranes solute and fluid transport rates.

A patient with a membrane of low transport characteristics (low transporter) will equilibrate creatinine and glucose slowly. Although solutes take a long time to cross this type of membrane, glucose also travels across slowly, maintaining osmotic pressure. Patients whose membranes have very low transport characteristics therefore obtain maximum dialysis with long dwells of dialysis fluid.

A patient with a membrane that, on the other hand, shows high transport characteristics (high transporter) will optimise the amount of their dialysis with short dwells. This is because both creatinine and glucose cross the membrane quickly, resulting in rapid clearance of solutes and rapid absorption of glucose. This glucose absorption results in a decrease in osmotic pressure and therefore poor ultrafiltration.

Performing a PET
The test has been standardised so that the results can easily be compared over time and between patients. It is important, therefore, that the steps of the test are followed exactly so that these comparisons are accurate.

Sampling   This should be performed following a dwell of at least 8 h.

(1) Prepare a 2000 ml medium glucose strength (2.27% or 2.5%) bag of dialysis fluid by warming to body temperature.
(2) Drain out the patient's overnight dwell of dialysate over 20 min. The patient must be vertical, either sitting or standing. Measure and record the drained fluid volume.
(3) Infuse the new solution at a rate of 400 ml 2 min^{-1} (i.e. total infusion time = 10 min). The patient must be supine and should roll from side to side every 2 min to ensure solution mixing. Zero dwell time is the time at completion of infusion.
(4) Collect dialysate samples at zero and 2 h dwell time:

    (a) Drain approximately 200 ml into the drainage bag and invert the bag to mix solution.
    (b) Disinfect the sample port.
    (c) Withdraw 10 ml via the sample port and reinfuse remaining 190 ml.
    (d) Transfer the sample to the appropriately labelled collection tube.

(5) Draw a venous blood sample at 2 h dwell time. Transfer to an appropriately labelled collection tube.
(6) At 4 h dwell time drain dialysate over 20 min with the patient vertical.
(7) Mix the sample by inverting the bag. Withdraw 10 ml. Transfer to the appropriately labelled tube.
(8) Weigh and record drain volume, adding sample volumes to give total drain volume.

Calculating results   Creatinine and glucose values should be obtained on the three dialysate samples and the serum sample.

Corrected creatinine   Owing to glucose interference with creatinine assays, corrected creatinine values may need to be determined. A corrected creatinine result may be provided by individual laboratories, depending on the

Peritoneal Equilibration Test (PET)

1. Collect patient samples

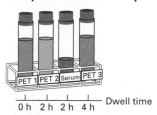

Name patient:
Date:
Completed by:

2. Calculations

a. Creatinine (D/P)

$$D/P = \frac{\text{dialysate concentration of corrected creatinine}}{\text{serum concentration of corrected creatinine}}$$

$$\frac{PET\ 1\ ....}{Serum\ ....} = A\ ....\ value\ (0\ h)$$

$$\frac{PET\ 2\ ....}{Serum\ ....} = B\ ....\ value\ (2\ h)$$

$$\frac{PET\ 3\ ....}{Serum\ ....} = C\ ....\ value\ (4\ h)$$

b. Glucose (D/DO)

$$D/O = \frac{\text{dialysate concentration of glucose at 2/4 h}}{\text{dialysate concentration of glucose at 0 h}}$$

$$\frac{PET\ 2\ ....}{PET\ 1..................} = D\ ....\ value\ (2\ h)$$

$$\frac{PET\ 3\ ....}{PET\ 1\ ....} = E\ ....\ value\ (4\ h)$$

3. Plot to graph

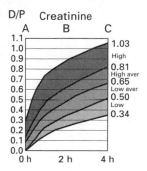

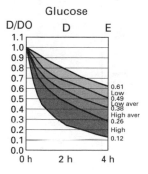

4. Diagnosis

Baseline PET prognostic value			
Solute transport	Predicted response to CAPD		Preferred dialysis
	UF	Dialysis	
High	Poor	Adequate	CCPD dry day CAPD dry night
High average	Poor-medium	Adequate	Standard CAPD or APD
Low average	Good	Adequate Inadequate	StandardCAPD High dose PD APD
Low	Very good	Inadequate	High dose PD Haemodialysis

Fig. 8.5 *Peritoneal equilibration test (PET).*

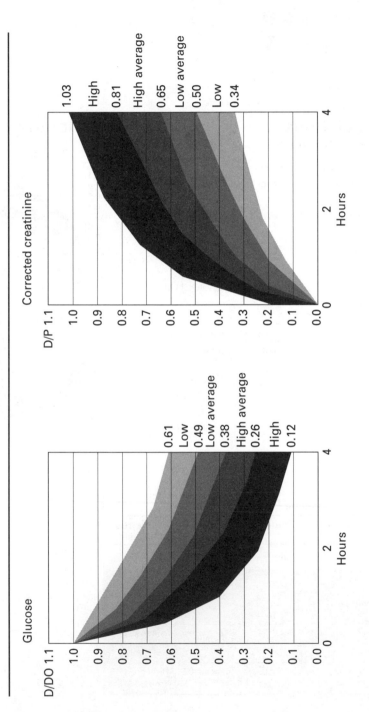

Fig. 8.6 *Peritoneal equilibration test (PET) curves.*

type of laboratory test used. Enzymatic tests do not require correction. Analysis of samples must always be carried out on the same analyser to avoid erroneous results. If corrected creatinine is not available the standard creatinine results should be used throughout (Baxter Healthcare, 1992).

Dialysate to plasma ratio (D/P) for creatinine and dialysate to dialysate at zero hours ratio (D/DO) for glucose can be calculated by using the worksheet (Fig. 8.5). When the results have been calculated, they should be plotted on the PET curve graph shown in more detail in Figure 8.6, enabling membrane characteristic categorisation (Fig. 8.6). For a quick guide to the membrane transport characteristics it is possible to look at the dialysate to plasma ratio (D/P) at 4 h. The closer this number is to 1, the higher the patient's membrane transport characteristics.

Analysis of results   The numbers themselves are not necessarily the most important feature of the test. Some significance can be attached to the shape of the curves on the graph and the position of individual patients within each of the bands.

It has been suggested (Davis *et al.*, 1993) that repeat tests should be routinely performed once a year or if problems arise such as an apparent loss of ultrafiltration. Changes over time in the test results can then be related to clinical performance and treatment regimens may be altered accordingly.

Recommendations for optimal use of the PET
Patients should be in optimum health when the PET is performed. The catheter should be functioning well, the patient should not be constipated and should have no infection. Ideally the patient should not be fluid overloaded.

Patients who normally have overnight automated PD should start their programme earlier in the evening before the day of the test. Their treatment should finish earlier in the morning with a last bag fill of 2000 ml. This can then be drained at lunch time (following an 8-h dwell) for a test that afternoon. In this way a CAPD situation can be mimicked.

When interpreting the results, an abnormal PET curve on the graph may be due to an error in the way the test was performed or a clinical problem with the patient. It may also be due to a mathematical or laboratory error.

PERITONEAL DIALYSIS ACCESS AND EXIT SITE CARE

It is widely agreed that the key to successful PD is good, permanent and safe access to the peritoneal cavity. Up to 20% of transfers from PD to haemodialysis are directly related to catheter problems (Gokal *et al.*, 1993).

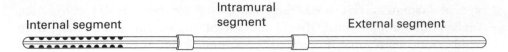

Fig. 8.7 *Straight Tenckhoff catheter.*

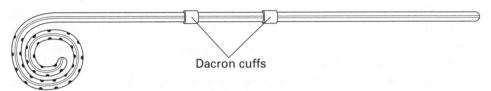

Fig. 8.8 *Curled Tenckhoff catheter.*

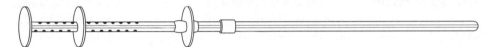

Fig. 8.9 *Toronto Western catheter.*

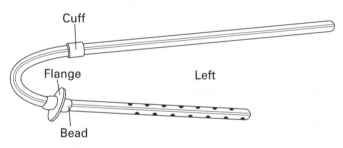

Fig. 8.10 *Swan-neck (Missouri) catheter.*

It is therefore essential that good catheter and exit site practices are maintained by all those involved in the care of these patients.

Types of Catheters

The design of a peritoneal catheter needs to be such that it gives the patient the maximum inflow and outflow rates as well as discouraging infection.

The very early peritoneal catheters which were used in the 1960s for acute PD were rigid, made from polyvinyl chloride. Developments in the late 1960s led to the introduction of a flexible silicone rubber (silastic) catheter, much more suited to chronic PD. There are currently four main types of permanent peritoneal dialysis catheter in use:

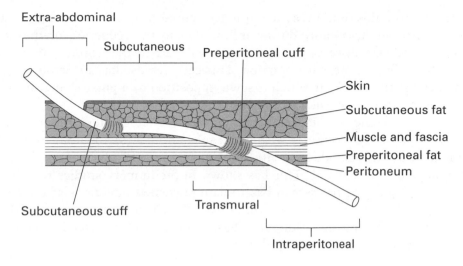

Fig. 8.11 *Functional parts of the peritoneal catheter.*

- Straight Tenckhoff (Fig. 8.7)
- Curled Tenckhoff (Fig. 8.8)
- Toronto Western (Fig. 8.9)
- Swan-neck (Missouri) (Fig. 8.10).

When implanted, the catheter has three functioning segments (Fig. 8.11):

- The outer part which connects via an adapter (usually titanium metal) to the solution transfer set.
- An intramural part which has either one or two Dacron cuffs. These cuffs are spaced about 8 cm apart. They create an inflammatory response which then progresses to form thick fibrous tissue which fixes the catheter cuff in position. This anchors the catheter, helps to minimise leakage of dialysate and acts as a barrier to infection by preventing bacteria entering the catheter 'tunnel'.
- The intraperitoneal part, which has many small holes up the side, is situated inside the peritoneal cavity for the in and out flow of the solution.

The choice of catheter used is generally of local preference. The most widely used catheter is the Straight Tenckhoff catheter. It is easily inserted under local or general anaesthetic. The Swan-neck, Curled and Toronto Western catheters were all developed to aid outflow of the dialysate. The Swan-neck, because of its two downward pointing segments, serves to aid outflow, as migration of this type of catheter is rare. It is also thought to prevent infections at the exit site as this segment of the catheter also points downwards, thus preventing accumulation of sweat and pus. The coil catheter also aids outflow as it too is less prone to migration. It may also reduce patient discomfort during inflow due to the reduction of the 'jet effect'. The two discs at the intraperitoneal part of the Toronto Western catheter help it to prevent migration. This catheter also has a Dacron flange and bead at the deep cuff which is sewn in position by a purse string suture, so helping to reduce leaks at the exit site.

There are some new PD catheters currently under review. Moncrief *et al.* (1996) describe a catheter with a cuff made from a microporous material which passes through the exit site and allows microvascular in-growth into the pores of the material. This has shown in preliminary studies to create a bacteriological barrier which has to date prevented infections at the exit site. The silver-coated catheter which was thought to contribute to a 50% reduction in exit site infection rates (Vas, 1996) has so far proved ineffective, possibly due to manufacturing difficulties.

Preinsertion Preparation of the Patient

The catheter exit site should be determined before the catheter is inserted. The preferred site should first be discussed with the patient to help promote participation in and an understanding of the therapy. The following points should be followed when determining the exit site of the patient's catheter:

- The site should be determined whilst the patient is in a relaxed sitting position.
- It should be either above or below the belt line, whichever the patient prefers.
- Skin folds and abdominal scars should be avoided.
- The catheter exit site should be located where the patient can effectively carry out exit site care.
- Once the exit site has been determined, it should be marked clearly with a skin marker.

Preoperative Care of the Patient

Skin preparation
The removal of abdominal hair may be performed if this is common practice within the hospital or renal unit.

Surgical skin preparation, for example bathing with chlorhexidine soap, may also be performed if practised within the unit.

Bowel preparation
The bowel should be empty before the catheter is inserted. This may need to be achieved by the administration of an enema.

It is also important that the patient ensures an empty bladder before the insertion procedure takes place.

Staphylococcus aureus screening

There is recent evidence (Coles *et al.*, 1994) that patients who have nasal carriage of *Staphylococcus aureus* have an increased risk of exit site infection and peritonitis. Results of a multicentre trial on the use of Mupirocin nasal cream to prevent such infections show that using it amongst *Staphylococcus aureus* nasal carriers reduced exit site infections from 1 episode in 28 patient months to 1 episode in 99 patient months (Coles *et al.*, 1994). It was concluded from this trial that intermittent use of intra-nasal Mupirocin is effective in significantly reducing *Staphylococcus aureus* infection in CAPD patients. There have been fears, however, that the use of such antibiotics may cause the emergence of resistant strains of bacterium.

Prophylactic antibiotics

There is no hard evidence to suggest that administration of antibiotics prior to catheter insertion will reduce the incidence of infection (Gokal *et al.*, 1993). Many physicians and surgeons do administer them, as with other current practices associated with implantation of foreign bodies.

Psychological preparation of the patient

This is of absolute importance for the new PD patient and is discussed in detail in Chapter 3.

Insertion Techniques

PD is a life-maintaining therapy. Access to the peritoneal cavity, the PD catheter, is therefore particularly important in ensuring its success (Fig. 8.12). The insertion technique should be treated as a skill acquired by experienced surgeons and physicians only, rather like implantation of a pacemaker or similar device. A team approach is essential and nurse involvement most important. The nurse's role in insertion of PD catheters starts with the preoperative preparation described above, all of which can be carried out by the nurse. In many centres the PD nurse accompanies the patient to the operating theatre to ensure correct procedures are carried out and that the catheter is functioning well before final wound closure is made.

The three most frequently performed methods of catheter insertion include:

- *Simple trochar insertion technique.* The catheters which are inserted using this technique have a high incidence of leakage and herniation. It may also be difficult for the surgeon to create the exit site at the preferred site.

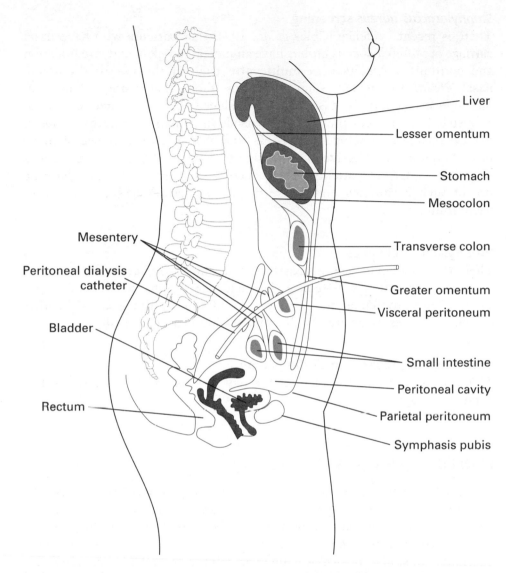

Fig. 8.12 *The position of a peritoneal dialysis (PD) catheter in the abdomen.*

- *Mini laparotomy with lateral incision*. This technique is effective and popular with nephrologists. During this technique it is possible for the surgeon to perform an omentectomy. It is generally performed under local anaesthetic.
- *Formal laparotomy*. This technique is used mostly by surgeons and may be performed using a laprascope. This technique makes it difficult to anchor the catheter in the peritoneal cavity.

Another implantation technique which has recently been described was the prolonged subcutaneous implantation of the catheter for up to 6 weeks before being brought to the surface and used. This technique has shown in preliminary studies to reduce the rate of infections (Park *et al.*, 1996).

Postoperative Care of the Patient

Ideally the exit site should be undisturbed for 7–10 days following insertion of the catheter. The patient may be discharged home during this period. If, during the first 10 days, the dressing becomes soiled, it should be redressed by a nurse. If it merely becomes dislodged, it should simply be replaced with a fresh sterile dressing. During this period, the catheter tubing must be immobilised by securely taping it to the patient's abdomen.

Before discharge from hospital, during this resting of the patient's catheter, clear instructions must be given as to the correct procedures for caring for the catheter at home. It may be appropriate to involve the community district nursing team if no specific community PD nurse is available. In this case, adequate training and support must be provided for the nursing team.

Directly following insertion of the catheter, it may be flushed with 500–1500 ml of PD fluid until the fluid is clear on outflow. It may then be 'capped off' using a small 'locking cap' on the titanium adapter and left covered until PD commences. Ideally, PD should not be started until healing of the exit site and tissue in-growth into the catheter's Dacron cuffs has taken place, usually after 10 days. If dialysis is necessary before this time, and if haemodialysis is inappropriate or unavailable, automated PD would be the preferred method. This is because this treatment will help to minimise the risk of leakage of PD fluid by allowing the patient to be treated using small fill volumes of fluid in a supine position. It is worth noting that the patient's healing mechanisms may be altered in those who are uraemic or who have diabetes mellitus.

Long-term Care of the Exit Site

As with any wound, care is aimed at keeping the site clear of exudate or debris which could encourage bacterial growth. A method of exit site care which best fits in with the patient's lifestyle is most likely to encourage full participation in the treatment, and therefore reduce the risk of complications. A number of studies have been undertaken to attempt to ascertain which particular method of exit site care is preferred. Various protocols do exist, for example cleansing with soap and water (Prowant *et al.*, 1988; Khanna and Twardowski, 1989) or cleaning with povidone iodine (Starzomski, 1984; Piraino *et al.*, 1986) or cleaning with chlorhexidine gluconate (Fuchs *et al.*, 1990); however, there is to date no consensus on which method will reduce the incidence of infection. Research suggests that chlorhexidine may be the agent of choice (Maki, 1991).

Whichever solution is chosen, the following points should be considered:

- Harsh solutions should be avoided as they have the potential to cause skin damage, which may predispose to bacterial colonisation.
- Different agents may be preferred in different circumstances. In an immunosuppressed patient the normal skin flora may represent an infection risk; in this case an antiseptic solution may be preferred.
- Whichever method is used, it is important to ensure that the exit site is carefully dried to avoid skin maceration which could predispose the site to bacterial colonisation.

There is also some debate as to whether it is necessary to keep the catheter exit site covered. The use of no dressing and a simple exit site care routine for a well-healed exit site would appeal to many; however, most centres do use some kind of cover (Uttley and Gokal, 1986).

Catheter Immobilisation

From the moment the catheter is inserted, it should always be securely anchored to the patient's skin to avoid torque movements at the exit site. This has been shown to reduce the risk of exit site infections (Gokal *et al.*, 1993) and can be achieved by using tape or a commercially available immobilisation device or tube holder.

Swimming and Bathing

According to a consensus of opinions of leading nephrologists (Gokal *et al.*, 1993), PD patients may swim following healing of the catheter, usually 4–8 weeks following insertion. The exit site may be covered with either clear occlusive dressing or a colostomy bag. Diving should be avoided as this may put tension on the catheter at the exit site. Following swimming the patient should shower, clean and dry the exit site and cover it with the usual dressing.

Soaking the exit site, for example in a tub bath, is not recommended (Gokal *et al.*, 1993).

Indications for Catheter Removal

A PD catheter is the patient's only access to the therapy. It is therefore designed to be a permanent access device, removal of which should not be routine.

Catheters may have to be removed under the following conditions:

- if they are no longer needed;
- recurrent peritonitis without an identifiable cause;
- peritonitis due to an exit site and/or tunnel infection;
- unusual causative organism of peritonitis, e.g. fungal, tuberculosis;
- bowel perforation accompanied by peritonitis;
- persistent and severe pain due either to the catheter impinging on internal organs or during solution inflow;
- Dacron cuff erosion and infection.

PERITONEAL DIALYSIS THERAPY OPTIONS

Dialysis should be prescribed according to each individual patient's need. The dose of PD can be increased or decreased by adjusting any one of the following parameters:

- dialysis fluid fill volume per exchange;
- number of dialysis fluid exchanges;
- length of dialysis fluid dwell time;
- osmotic strength of the dialysis fluid.

By using the PET each patient's membrane characteristics can be determined, therefore allowing optimisation of the therapy according to each patient's clinical and lifestyle needs.

There are two general methods of performing peritoneal dialysis: CAPD and APD.

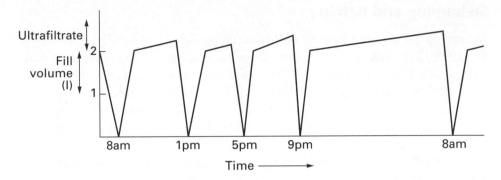

Fig. 8.13 *Continuous ambulatory peritoneal dialysis (CAPD).*

Continuous Ambulatory Peritoneal Dialysis (CAPD)

CAPD (Fig. 8.13) is carried out during the day time, manually by the patients themselves. Dialysis fluid is infused into the peritoneal cavity and left to dwell for between 3 and 10 h. After this time the dialysate is drained from the cavity, fresh solution is infused and the whole process starts again. Patients usually perform four 'exchanges' of PD fluid each day (some patients may perform five, depending on the prescription), fitting them in as appropriately as possible with their normal lifestyle. For example, exchanges may be performed at breakfast, lunch and supper times with the last exchange of the day being carried out at bedtime. Each exchange takes about 20 min to complete.

CAPD is most suited to those patients whose membranes transport solutes at a slow to average rate (i.e. low, low average and high average 'transporters') as it provides the opportunity for longer dwell times. This long dwell period is best achieved during the night time whilst the patient sleeps. Those patients whose membranes transport solutes quickly ('high transporters') may need to have a 'dry night'; that is, the dialysate is drained from the peritoneal cavity at bedtime and not replaced until the following morning. This will avoid dialysate absorption which would occur in these patients during long dwell periods. It is important to remember, though, that utilising a 'dry night' may result in lower solute clearances and therefore the possible risk of underdialysis.

Automated Peritoneal Dialysis (APD)

APD is the fastest growing therapy modality (Baxter Healthcare Survey, ongoing). It has many advantages for patients, both clinical and lifestyle, mainly due to its flexibility. An APD machine automatically controls the fill volume, dwell time and length of treatment the patient receives. APD is most often carried out at home whilst the patient sleeps, but it may also be carried out in the hospital dialysis unit. The dose of dialysis can easily be increased during APD as it is easy and convenient to alter any of the parameters of the treatment. Dialysis fluid fill volumes can be safely increased due to the reduction in intra-abdominal pressure achieved whilst the patient is supine. This not only decreases the risk of problems associated with high intra-abdominal pressure such as leaks around the catheter exit site, abdominal hernias and back pain, but it also increases the amount of dialysis the patient can achieve, particularly in patients whose membranes transport solutes quickly. The length of the dwell time and the number of 'exchanges' can effectively be altered without disruption to the patient's lifestyle. This is a major advantage to 'high transporters'. Performing frequent exchanges is essential for these patients to achieve adequate dialysis but this can be inconvenient if the patient is on CAPD. APD provides an effective and convenient alternative by enabling rapid exchanges of dialysis fluid whilst the patient sleeps. This increases clearances of solutes whilst maintaining maximum ultrafiltration. As with CAPD, the osmotic strength of the fluid can be altered according to each patient's need. The reduction in intra-abdominal pressure achieved during APD may also aid an increase in appetite.

APD is particularly suitable for those patients needing to be free from daytime CAPD exchanges. Patients who work or who are studying can benefit from this treatment, as the preparation time for the treatment is short and the dialysis takes place whilst they sleep, leaving them free during the day. APD is also suitable for those patients who rely on a carer to perform their dialysis, for example children, the elderly or the infirm. The carer simply prepares the machine, connects the patient to the machine at bedtime and disconnects them the following morning. APD is therefore an effective therapy option for those patients who require more dialysis and/or freedom during the daytime.

There are four different types of APD (APD being the term used to describe PD performed by a machine):

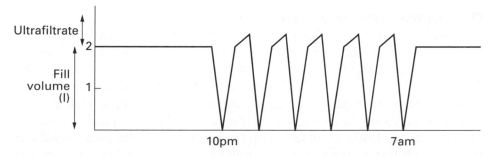

Fig. 8.14 *Continuous cycling peritoneal dialysis (CCPD).*

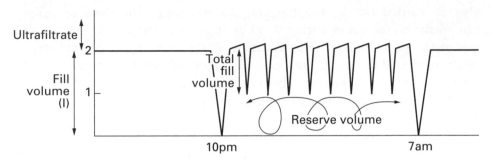

Fig. 8.15 *Tidal peritoneal dialysis.*

- CCPD – continuous cycling peritoneal dialysis
- Tidal peritoneal dialysis
- OCPD – optimised cycling peritoneal dialysis
- IPD – intermittent peritoneal dialysis.

Continuous cycling peritoneal dialysis (CCPD) (Fig. 8.14)

CCPD is performed overnight whilst the patient is asleep supine in bed. The 'continuous' part of the acronym is derived from the fact that the patient has dialysis fluid in constant contact with the peritoneal membrane. There are typically between five and seven exchanges of fluid with relatively short dwell periods, so maximizing the ultrafiltration and clearance capabilities of those patients whose membrane transports solutes quickly. The treatment regimen can be programmed to end with a 'fill', giving the patient a 'wet' day (the fluid would be left inside the peritoneal cavity during the day and drained when the patient next starts treatment on the machine at bedtime).

The treatment may end following the 'drain', giving the patient a 'dry day'. This may help to prevent absorption of the PD fluid in 'high transporters'. It should be noted, though, that utilising a 'dry day' will result in reduced clearances and possible underdialysis. A solution designed for long dwells such as icodextrin could be used in this circumstance.

Tidal peritoneal dialysis (Fig. 8.15)

This regime is usually performed by a machine in the patient's own home at night. It can also be performed in the dialysis centre incorporated within an IPD regime (see IPD below). The dialysis fluid fill volume is only partly drained, so leaving a designated 'reserve' volume in contact with the peritoneal membrane at all times. The tidal fill volume brings fresh fluid to mix with part of the reserve volume on each cycle. As a result of dialysis fluid constantly being in contact with the membrane, some patients achieve improved clearance of up to 20%, compared to standard PD (Twardowski, 1990). This means that patients can achieve the same clearances as CCPD

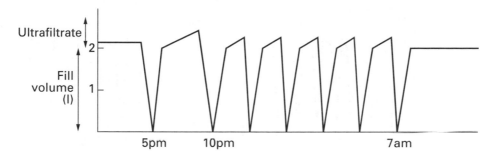

Fig. 8.16 *Optimised cycling peritoneal dialysis (OCPD).*

in less time, or more clearance in the same time. Tidal PD can be used with a 'wet day' or a 'dry day' as discussed above. An additional benefit of tidal PD is that some patients experience less pain whilst draining out, since the peritoneal cavity is not totally emptied after each exchange. For a patient dialysing at night this may be extremely important in terms of comfortable, unbroken sleep.

Optimised cycling peritoneal dialysis (OCPD) (Fig. 8.16)
OCPD provides another way to individualise the patient's treatment. It allow the delivery of more dialysis as residual renal function declines. During OCPD the patient performs overnight CCPD or tidal as well as adding up to nine daytime exchanges of PD fluid. Some APD machines are designed so that the patient can perform both the night and day exchanges using the same disposable equipment and solution bags. The longer dwell of fluid during the daytime will optimise clearance opportunities and the shorter dwells of the night time dialysis will help to achieve ultrafiltration goals.

Intermittent peritoneal dialysis (IPD) (Fig. 8.17)
This form of APD is performed with the patient in a supine position. It is generally carried out in the dialysis centre in sessions of between 12 and 20 h, two or three times each week. Large volumes (20–40 l) of dialysis fluid are cycled each session with short dwell times and fill volumes of between 2 and 3 l per cycle. If the patient spends sufficient time on the treatment with large enough fluid volumes per session, adequate dialysis can be achieved. However, for patients with little or no residual renal function, IPD often fails to provide adequate dialysis in the long term.

This treatment is most appropriate for elderly people, unable to dialyse at home and who are unsuitable for other therapies (i.e. haemodialysis or transplantation). These patients may gain from the regular social occasion, particularly if several people are treated in the same centre at the same time. IPD may also be used to treat acute patients or for catheter

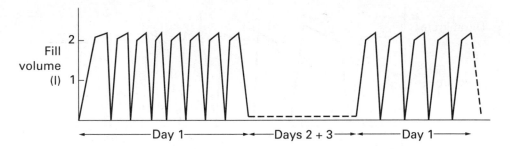

Fig. 8.17 *Intermittent peritoneal dialysis (IPD).*

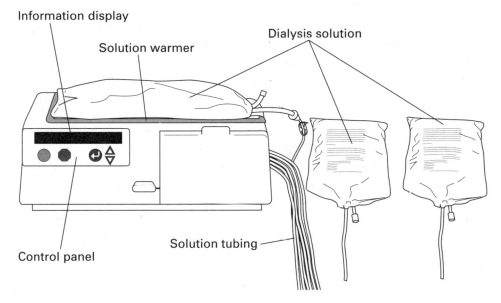

Fig. 8.18 *Baxter Healthcare Ltd HomeChoice APD machine.*

conditioning (following the insertion of the catheter) when dialysis fill volumes can be gradually increased.

Whichever method of PD is chosen for the patient at any particular time, it should provide a balance between both their clinical and lifestyle needs.

Figure 8.18 shows an example of an automated peritoneal dialysis machine.

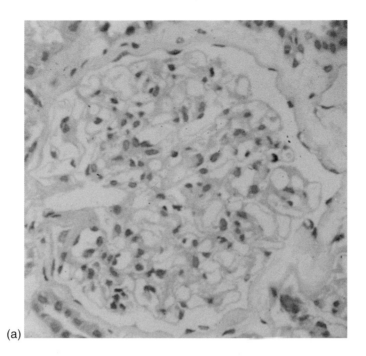

(a)

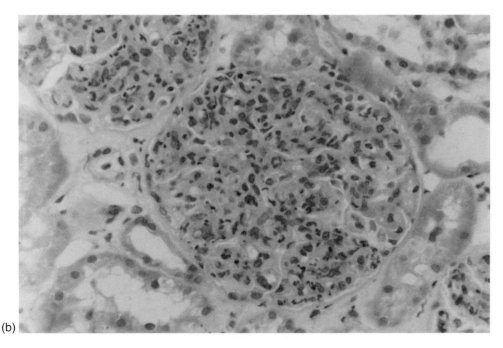

(b)

Plate 1. Renal histology from biopsy specimen (light micrographs). (a) A normal glomerulus. (b) A glomerulus from a patient with a diffuse proliferative (post-streptococcal) glomerulonephritis. Note how 'full' the glomerulus appears with a great increase in the number of cells due to inflammation. (See Chapter 6)

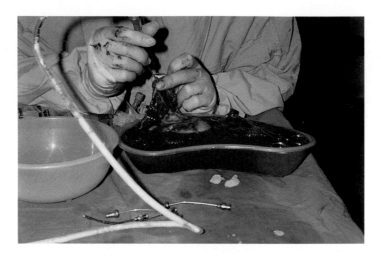

Plate 2. Kidney undergoing perfusion (in ice) immediately after harvesting. (See Chapter 11)

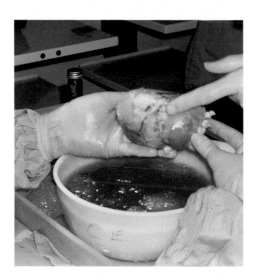

Plate 3. Cooled kidney in surgical glove, ready for transplantation. (See Chapter 11)

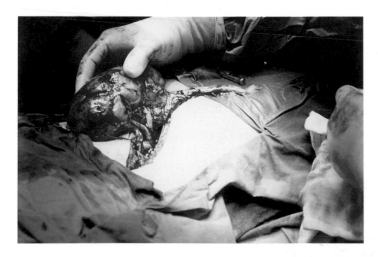

Plate 4. Transplanted kidney after removal of clamps showing 'pinking up' and urine formation. (See Chapter 11)

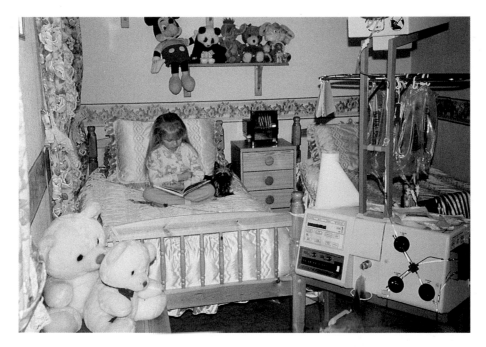

Plate 5. A child at home receiving peritoneal dialysis. (See Chapter 10)

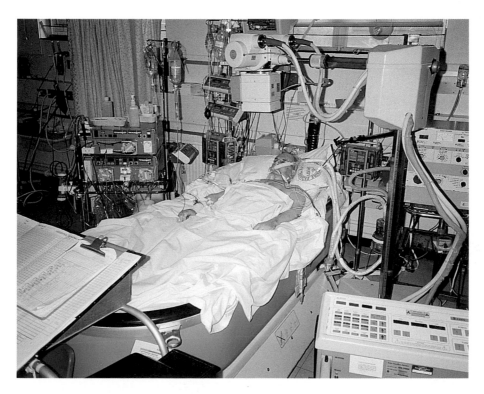

Plate 6. A typical scene of a patient with acute renal failure in an intensive therapy unit (See Chapter 4).

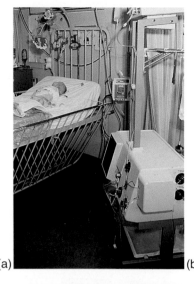

(a)

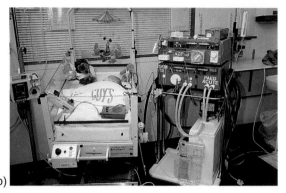

(b)

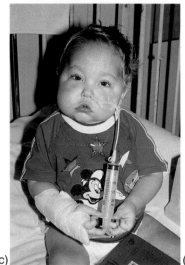

(c)

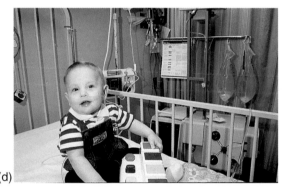

(d)

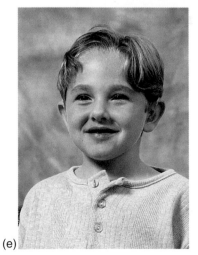

(e)

Plate 7. The story of Matthew. (a) on peritoneal dialysis at 3 months; (b) on haemodialysis at 3 months; (c) feeding himself with a nasogastric tube; (d) on peritoneal dialysis at an older age and (e) transplanted, aged 5 years. (see chapter 10)

***Table* 8.1** *Patients who are suited to continuous ambulatory peritoneal dialysis (CAPD) or automated peritoneal dialysis (APD)*

Suited to CAPD	Suited to either CAPD or APD	Suited to APD
Patients whose membranes transport solutes slowly or at an average speed	Promotion of home dialysis Patients with complicating cardiovascular disease Children with small body size Patients with poor vascular access Diabetic patients Patients with severe hypertension Anaemic patients Patients who wish to travel	Patients who seek daytime freedom to attend work or school Patients at risk of complications associated with raised intra-abdominal pressure Patients who require a carer to perform their dialysis Patients with chronic back ache Patients who require enhanced dialysis, i.e. those without residual renal function

***Table* 8.2** *Patients who are unsuitable for continuous ambulatory peritoneal dialysis (CAPD) or automated peritoneal dialysis (APD)*

Unsuitable for CAPD	Unsuitable for either CAPD or APD	Unsuitable for APD
Patients with chronic back pain Patients at risk of complications associated with raised intra-abdominal pressure	Patients with chronic obstructive lung disease Patients with diverticular disease Patients who are unable to care for themselves and do not have the assistance of a full time carer	

PATIENT SELECTION

An important consideration when developing a successful PD programme is good patient selection. Treating the most appropriate patients with PD will avoid the patient being subjected to increased risk of morbidity and mortality. In the early years of PD, selection was mainly based on the patient's inability to have haemodialysis – for example, those patients with poor or no vascular access, poor biochemical control on HD with high predialysis serum levels of creatinine, those patients with serve anaemia (i.e. haemoglobin of $< 5\,g\,dl^{-1}$) with a need for frequent blood transfusions, those patients with poorly controlled hypertension, excessive fluid gain between dialysis sessions and those who had progressive metabolic and neurological complications. Although these criteria do recommend patients for PD, positive selection criteria are now preferred as PD has proven to be a successful viable alternative to haemodialysis as a treatment for chronic renal disease.

As there are two different therapy modes within the broad title of PD (i.e. CAPD and APD), the selection criteria for each are seen to be slightly different with many overlaps. Tables 8.1 and 8.2 indicate which patients are more suited to APD and those who are more suited to CAPD.

PERITONEAL DIALYSIS IN THE DIABETIC

Diabetes mellitus can cause damage to many organs. The eyes, bladder, bowel, nervous system and kidneys can all be affected. If diabetic patients are given an intermittent form of dialysis, such as haemodialysis, rapid fluctuations occur in their blood chemistry and fluid status. This may cause episodes of hypertension, thereby increasing the risk of cardiac or cerebrovascular events. Hypertension may worsen peripheral vascular disease.

Access required for haemodialysis may prove difficult to achieve in the diabetic due to poor vascular condition, whereas PD access is much easier to establish. There are considerations to take account of before using PD in diabetic patients:

● blood sugar control
● blood pressure control
● fluid and electrolyte control
● access.

Blood Sugar Control

Although glucose is used as an osmotic agent in PD, this does not deter from the therapy's ability to achieve good results in the diabetic patient. An average PD patient will absorb between 100 and 150 g of glucose per day from the dialysis fluid and this has led to some problems in the past such as hyperinsulinaemia and premature arteriosclerosis. Searches for alternative osmotic agents are promising. New solutions which utilise larger molecules of glucose (Icodextrin) are an advantage to diabetics as there is a marked reduction in the amount of glucose absorbed by the patient. Other solutions which use amino acids as the osmotic agent are glucose free as well as having the advantage of providing the patient with a nutritional supplement.

There are a number of alternative methods of blood sugar control for the diabetic PD patient. These include subcutaneous or intraperitoneal insulin, oral agents or dietary control. Any combination of these methods can be used. No single method has been shown to be more suitable than another for all patients.

Intraperitoneal insulin

The normal route for insulin from the pancreas is via the portal vein to the liver, before it reaches the systemic circulation. Insulin administered intraperitoneally (i.p.) is partly absorbed by diffusion across the peritoneum into the portal venous circulation. This closely mimics the physiological secretion of insulin.

If insulin is administered via the peritoneum it promotes blood sugar control throughout the dwell time – i.p. insulin is absorbed along with the glucose from the dialysis fluid. Approximately 50% of insulin injected i.p. is absorbed after 8 h dwell time.

Insulin which is administered through the peritoneal membrane has a similar effect to physiologically administered insulin. This means that glycaemic control during PD is more physiological than during haemodialysis. Such an advantage should impact on the overall long-term progression of diabetic complications in patients on dialysis.

Insulin should be added to the bag of dialysis fluid before it is connected to the patient. In this way, the bag may be discarded if accidentally contaminated or punctured by the needle. Strict aseptic technique must be followed when adding the insulin, which is usually done through the specially designed medication port. Diabetics who also have poor eyesight due to retinopathy may need a community nurse to add the insulin to each bag of dialysis fluid. This will involve a daily visit when the nurse injects insulin into the dialysis fluid in the normal way but through a small hole made in the over-pouch of the bags. All bags should be inverted several times before the fluid is drained into the patient to ensure thorough mixing of the insulin.

Several protocols of blood sugar control with i.p. insulin have been published (Khanna *et al.*, 1986; Routtembourg, 1988; Lameire *et al.*, 1993). There are no studies which compare the effectiveness of different methods; however, they all appear to be effective in achieving metabolic control of blood sugar. Most patients require more than 100% of their usual pre-CAPD subcutaneous insulin dose divided between four exchanges. A reduced dose should be added to the overnight dwell to prevent hypoglycaemia during the night. Higher levels of insulin may need to be added to hypertonic glucose dialysis fluid. The exact amount varies between patients but may be assessed at onset by using a sliding scale of insulin with finger prick blood sugar test results.

Intraperitoneal insulin in automated peritoneal dialysis (APD)

Good blood sugar control can be achieved in APD patients with insulin being administered either subcutaneously or intraperitoneally or both subcutaneously and intraperitoneally. The amount of insulin administered needs to be adjusted according to individual requirements. During the day patients are given the daily dose of insulin, usually long acting, by subcutaneous injection. Additional insulin can also be administered either intraperitoneally or subcutaneously at the start of the APD therapy.

Blood Pressure Control

Blood pressure can be well controlled in the diabetic treated by PD due to the continuous fluid and sodium removal during dialysis (Young *et al.*, 1984).

Fluid and Electrolyte Control

This is achieved by the continuous nature of PD and has advantages for diabetic patients in prevention of cardiovascular stress due to fluid overload or hyperkalaemia.

Access

One of the advantages of PD in the diabetic patient is the ease with which the peritoneum can be accessed. The techniques involved in PD catheter insertion in the diabetic are similar to those for other patients. There does not seem to be any higher incidence of either infectious or non-infectious catheter complications for the diabetic patient treated with PD (Linbald *et al.*, 1989).

SOLUTION FORMULATION

The most commonly prescribed and, up until the early 1990s, the most widely available osmotic agent used in PD is glucose. Dialysis fluid comes in three glucose strengths (either 1.36%, 2.27% and 3.86% or 1.5%, 2.5% and 4.25% monohydrate glucose). The strong (hypertonic) solutions provide the greater osmotic strength. Patients would use 1.36% glucose most often whilst their weight is within 0.5 kg of their 'dry' or 'target' weight. Hypertonic solutions should be used when the patient has fluid overload. Most patients ultrafiltrate an extra 200–600 ml by using a 2000-ml medium (2.27%) glucose solution bag and an extra 400–1000 ml by using a 2000 ml strong (3.86%) glucose solution bag. Patients should be taught to record their body weight on a daily basis and choose the appropriate solution strengths for that day.

Ultrafiltration by hypertonic solutions is maintained for approximately 8 h in most patients (Fig. 8.25). After this time some reabsorption of fluid may occur. In those patients whose membranes transport solutes quickly (high transporters) reabsorption may occur sooner than 8 h, giving rise to the need to use other solution formulation exchanges for the longer dwell times (i.e. the overnight dwell in CAPD or the daytime dwell in APD).

The solution is presented in sterile plastic bags with a protective over-pouch in volumes of 500 ml, 750 ml, 1000 ml, 1500 ml, 2000 ml, 2500 ml and 3000 ml. There are bags of 5000 ml available for use with APD machines.

The electrolyte concentration of dialysis fluid is similar to that of normal serum, with lactate acting as a bicarbonate generating agent to combat metabolic acidosis, common amongst ESRD patients.

Electrolyte composition of the dialysis fluid has been changed several times over the years. A major challenge when treating ESRD patients has been effective phosphate control. Consequently, dialysis fluid does not contain any phosphate, and patients are given oral phosphate-binding agents to help eliminate dietary phosphate intake from the body. In the past, these phosphate-binding agents were aluminium based. However, these were implicated in aluminium-related bone disease which many patients experienced (Armstrong and Cunningham, 1994). Aluminium toxicity may also cause microcytic anaemia and encephalopathy and so its use as a phosphate-binding agent in the present day has been reduced (Armstrong and Cunningham, 1994). The alternative ingredient for an effective phosphate binder is calcium given in the form of calcium carbonate or calcium acetate. These binders have their problems too, leading in some patients to raised serum calcium levels, particularly if the patient is also having vitamin D therapy. This relatively recent complication of PD has led to the manufacture of a dialysis fluid containing physiological levels of ionised calcium and this solution (a) is compared to the original solution (b) in Table 8.3.

Table 8.3 *Comparison of dialysis fluid contains ionised calcium (a) with original solution (b)*

	a (mmol l^{-1})	b (mmol l^{-})
Sodium (Na)	132	132
Chloride (Cl)	95	95
Lactate	40	35
Magnesium (Mg)	0.25	0.75
Calcium (Ca)	1.25	1.75

Bicarbonate-Based Peritoneal Dialysis Solutions

Although a bicarbonate-containing solution is the ideal agent for the correction of acidosis in dialysis patients, problems in manufacturing and storage have limited its use in the past. Bicarbonate-based PD fluids have a series of advantages compared to solutions containing only lactate, such as less cytotoxicity, more physiological correction of acidosis and reduced incidence of pain on infusion. Therefore, bicarbonate-containing solutions for PD have been developed. These fluids are presented in a two-chambered bag. Just before use, the contents of both chambers are mixed resulting in the ready to use solution. These solutions have been tested in *in-vitro* studies and in clinical trials.

In the mid 1990s a new fluid with a physiologic level of bicarbonate was introduced. This innovative formulation was chosen in order to provide the most physiologic environment for the peritoneum. *In vitro*, 'bicarbonate concentrations of more than 25 mEq/l were associated with reduced cellular function' (Shambye *et al.*, 1993). In addition to the physiologic 25 mEq/l of bicarbonate, this solution includes 15 mEq/l of lactate. This is thought necessary to provide a total buffer level sufficient to correct the metabolic acidosis associated with uraemic patients. This solution is presented with a neutral pH (7.0–7.4). It is expected that the neutral pH will reduce the risk of pain on infusion experienced by a few patients due to the acidity of current solutions and improve biocompatibility.

The Effect of Dialysis Solution Containing Glucose on the Peritoneum

There has been some concern that long-term effects of glucose on the peritoneal membrane could be damaging. This has led to the search for an alternative osmotic agent.

Dobbie (1989) examined numerous biopsies of peritoneums which showed that PD patients with a normal functioning peritoneum could have a number of related physical changes which would be the adaptive response of the peritoneum's cellular lining to constant immersion in dialysis fluid. These changes consist of increased cell turnover, loss of microvilli, formation of cell vacuoles, reduplication of the basement membrane and hyperplasia of the rough endoplastic reticulum.

These changes, however, are not thought to be damaging. Hutchison (1992) believes that in a PD patient the mesothelial layer of the peritoneum protects the underlying stoma from the high intraperitoneal glucose concentration and only if this layer is removed (i.e. by an episode of peritonitis) will irreversible damage occur.

Krediet *et al.* (1986) performed a study on 38 patients and showed that maximal ultrafiltration capacity did decrease with duration of time on PD;

however, the period of time varied. Krediet *et al.* thought that this decrease in ultrafiltration was caused by increases in both the effective peritoneal surface area and the peritoneal permeability. This could lead to increased glucose absorption which would lead to a decrease in duration of the osmotic gradient. Studies in France (Verger, 1989) have suggested that peritonitis has an effect on the ultrafiltration capacity of the peritoneum. The work that Verger performed showed a thickening of the peritoneum submesothelial tissue following an episode of peritonitis, but the number of episodes did not correlate with the amount of damage. Work published by Davis *et al.* (1993) shows that it is the number of episodes of peritonitis a patient has which damages the membrane, rather than the causative organism.

Using Glucose Polymer as an Osmotic Agent

The search for alternative osmotic agents to glucose is on-going. Problems associated with the use of glucose as an osmotic agent, such as hyperglycaemia and hyperlipidaemia, may prove to be an issue in the management of PD patients. Patients who have poor ultrafiltration provide the greatest challenge in this area, and efforts have concentrated so far on developing a solution with prolonged ultrafiltration properties.

Icodextrin 7.5% is a new formulation of a large molecular weight glucose polymer which is a more biocompatable solution as it is approximately iso-osmolar with serum. The use of this larger molecule means that less glucose is available for absorption through the peritoneal membrane. Its long-acting ultrafiltration performance (up to 12 h) is combined with low carbohydrate absorption. Its formulation is presented as a 7.5% solution of icodexrtin. Icodextrin produces less than 50% of the calorie load of glucose per unit volume of ultrafiltrate and appears to be an effective osmotic agent (Mistry *et al.*, 1987).

The large multicentre MIDAS study (Gokal and the MIDAS group, 1994) demonstrated that icodextrin solution is well tolerated and is as effective as 3.86% glucose over long dwell exchanges. Peers *et al.* (1995) demonstrated that, in patients who are failing on glucose-based CAPD, icodextrin can extend technique survival by an average of at least 1 year when included in the dialysis prescription.

Cooper *et al.* (1995) agreed that overnight APD could be further improved by a prolonged daytime dwell using icodextrin. To achieve this, icodextrin was compared with an empty peritoneum during the day in eight patients and the authors suggested that icodextrin can be useful to increase clearances in APD.

Icodextrin solution (7.5%) is of particular value in patients with ultrafiltration failure, defined by Mactier in 1991 as 'Clinical evidence of fluid overload which persists despite restriction of fluid intake and the use of three or more hypertonic exchanges per day'.

Table 8.4 *The electrolyte formulation of intraperitoneal amino acid solution*

Sodium	132 mmol l^{-1}
Chloride	95 mmol l^{-1}
Lactate	40 mmol l^{-1}
Magnesium	0.25 mmol l^{-1}
Calcium	1.25 mmol l^{-1}

In summary, this solution has been demonstrated to be effective as a long dwell solution both for CAPD and APD patients, resulting in more effective ultrafiltration and improved clearances.

Using Amino Acids as an Osmotic Agent

Forty per cent of PD patients suffer from protein malnutrition (Young *et al.*, 1991) and so it is therefore important to be able to provide additional nutritional supplement to the patient's normal daily intake. There are a number of different methods of administering these supplements, namely oral, enteral, parenteral and intraperitoneal. These are discussed further in Chapter 9.

The traditional forms of supplementing these patients' diets all have shortcomings with regard to compliance, palatability and formulation. Administering amino acids via the peritoneal membrane has many advantages for PD patients in that the solution is specifically formulated for ESRD patients:

- there is no increased phosphate load;
- there is no increased fluid load;
- it reduces the daily glucose load PD patients receive;
- as it is used as a normal dialysis exchange, compliance is not an issue.

Intraperitoneal amino acid solution (IPAA) contains 15 amino acids. Eight are essential amino acids, two are considered essential to ESRD patients and five are non-essential. The electrolyte formulation is shown in Table 8.4. The osmotic agent glucose is replaced by 1.1% amino acids, which have the comparative ultrafiltration capability of 1.36% glucose solution. After a 4–6 h dwell, 65–95% of the amino acids are absorbed, the equivalent to about 18 g (from a 2000-ml bag containing 22 g of amino acids) or 0.3 g kg^{-1} day^{-1} in a 70 kg patient. This is approximately 25% of the daily protein requirement for a PD patient.

IPAA is administered in the same way as other PD solutions. It is prescribed for one exchange per day, replacing one of the usual glucose dialysis solution bags. It should be given either at a main meal or with a high calorie snack, as this will ensure that the amino acids are used in the anabolic process to generate protein rather than being expended as an energy source. Its optimal dwell time is 4–6 h as described above. It is important to note that the solution should only be administered if the patient is receiving adequate dialysis, acidosis has been corrected and the energy intake of the patient is at least 35 kcal kg⁻¹ day⁻¹. These conditions optimise protein synthesis.

The 'Perfect' Peritoneal Dialysis Solution

Hutchison (1992) described the characteristics of the ideal PD solution as being:

- predictable, sustained solute clearance and ultrafiltration capability;
- able to supply deficient solutes and remove uraemic toxins;
- able to supply part of the patient's nutritional needs without promoting metabolic complications;
- iso-osmolar solution at physiological pH, and containing a bicarbonate buffer to correct acidosis;
- minimal absorption of a non-toxic osmotic agent and providing an ultra-filtration of around 2000 ml daily;
- able to inhibit bacterial and fungal growth, but without toxicity to the peritoneal membrane or host defences.

He suggested that a PD solution, probably buffered with bicarbonate, containing an osmotic agent with both nutritional value from amino acids and the sustained ultrafiltration characteristics of glucose polymer, but with the ionic concentration tailored to individual patients' requirements, certainly seems possible in the near future.

ASSESSING PERITONEAL DIALYSIS ADEQUACY

Dialysis has shown over the years to be able to prolong the lives of many patients with ESRD. It would therefore follow that dialysis patients should not die from 'uraemia' (Burkart, 1993).

Unfortunately, there is increasing evidence that inadequacies in dialysis dose or underdelivery of a prescribed dose of dialysis are contributing to high mortality rates amongst dialysis patients. Data compiled by the US Health Care Financing Administration (HCFA) and analysed by the US Renal Data System have shown that the gross mortality rate for the US ESRD population in 1990 was 24%. This means that whilst the average US citizen aged 40 years has an additional added life expectancy of 37.4

years, the average 40-year-old ESRD patient has an additional added life expectancy of only 9.3 years (Burkart, 1993).

Prolonged periods of inadequate dialysis can result in irreversible or slow reversible uraemia which can influence morbidity and mortality. Inadequate dialysis can be defined as the inadequate removal of waste material, clinical symptoms of which include itching, nausea, anorexia and uraemic smell, and inadequate ultrafiltration, clinical symptoms of which include weight gain, oedema and hypertension.

The goals of PD are to prolong life, reverse the symptoms of uraemia, maintain patients in positive nitrogen balance, have an adequate energy intake and have their maximum level of quality of life in a way that is least disruptive to their lifestyle. This can be summarised by saying that a well-dialysed patient is one who feels well enough to eat a sufficient diet rich in protein and who experiences a minimum of complications to his/her treatment.

There are a number of ways in which dialysis adequacy can be measured; however, there is no one measure which is more accurate nor more valuable than another and so it is important, when assessing the level of dialysis a patient achieves, to take all parameters into consideration. These parameters are:

- creatinine clearance – a solute-removal test based on body surface area;
- Kt/V – a urca index relating urea clearance to the volume of urea distributed in the body (see below);
- protein nutrition;
- general 'well-being'.

A number of studies have linked a decrease in creatinine clearance and Kt/V to an increased risk of morbidity and mortality. Teehan et al. (1990) found that Kt/V was linked to clinical outcome. For example, both death on CAPD and transfusion requirements are partially predicted by the level of Kt/V. Blake et al. (1992) came to the same conclusion using creatinine clearance as a predictor of outcome.

The largest study of PD patients was conducted in 14 centres across the US and Canada. The CANUSA study (Churchill et al., 1996) investigated the impact of demographic, nutritional and adequacy parameters on morbidity and mortality and defined adequate PD according to estimates of solute clearance (e.g. urea and creatinine). The United States Renal Data System (USRDS) data show that there is no difference in survival for non-diabetic patients (all age groups) or for diabetic patients under 58 years. The CANUSA study shows that estimates of patients' nutritional status and dialysis adequacy had clinically important and statistically significant associations with patients' survival, technique survival and hospitalisation. This study also indicated that increasing creatinine clearance and Kt/V will lead to higher survival rates. Churchill et al. (1996) also stated that total creatinine clearance and Kt/V decreased during the trial period because loss of residual renal function was not compensated for by increasing the dialysis dose. Churchill *et al.* (1996) also defined 'optimum dialysis' as the dialysis dose at which the clinical gain is not worth the increased patient effort or cost. The adequate dialysis dose should be the minimum target.

In summary, what the CANUSA study tells us is that more dialysis is better. Giving the patient a dialysis prescription which increases Kt/V and creatinine clearance will make the patient feel better and increase survival rate. It is also important to monitor nutritional status since this will influence survival. The risk of death increases with increased age, the presence of insulin-dependent diabetes mellitus (IDDM) and a past history of cardiovascular disease.

Targets for adequate dialysis continue to be re-evaluated. Currently, a weekly creatinine clearance of > 70 l week^{-1}/1.73 m^2 body surface area (BSA) and a Kt/V of > 2.1 week^{-1} are deemed satisfactory so long as the patient's nutritional status and general well-being are also assessed as being satisfactory (Churchill *et al.*, 1996).

There are a number of computer programs available on the market which will calculate the patient's Kt/V, creatinine clearance and nutritional status. Some of these programs will also model the patient's treatment, allowing the nurse or physician to look at a wide range of PD therapy options for the optimal regimen that meets the adequacy needs of each individual patient. This enables the clinician to eliminate the trial and error process of prescribing PD, takes away the need to perform manual calculations, and provides the renal unit with a database of their patients' quality of dialysis. The measures are all calculable manually and the following gives an account of what each measure means and how it is calculated.

Creatinine as a Measure of Dialysis Adequacy

Creatinine is a metabolic product from the breakdown of muscle. Patients who have a larger muscle mass therefore tend to have higher serum creatinine levels. Creatinine, with a molecular weight of 113 Da, will equilibrate more slowly across the peritoneal membrane than urea (molecular weight 60 Da).

When calculating creatinine clearance three values must be considered.

- solute generation rate
- residual renal clearance
- dialysis efficiency.

The consensus amongst dialysis care professionals suggests a minimum target of 70 l week^{-1}/1.73 m^2 BSA. A normalised BSA (Table 8.5) of 1.73 m^2 is used to enable an assumption of the creatinine generation rate based on a patient's size, provided that the patient is infection free and in nitrogen balance. Creatinine clearance for both the patient's dialysis regime and residual renal function can be calculated by using the worksheet (Fig. 8.19).

Table 8.5 *Body surface area (m²)*

Weight (kg)	120	125	130	135	140	145	150	155	160	165	170	175	180	185	190	195	200
36	1.06	1.09	1.12	1.15	1.19	1.22	1.25	1.28	1.31	1.33	1.36	1.39	1.42	1.45	1.48	1.51	1.53
38	1.08	1.12	1.15	1.18	1.21	1.24	1.27	1.31	1.34	1.37	1.40	1.43	1.45	1.48	1.51	1.54	1.57
40	1.11	1.14	1.17	1.21	1.24	1.27	1.30	1.33	1.37	1.40	1.43	1.46	1.49	1.52	1.55	1.58	1.61
42	1.13	1.17	1.20	1.23	1.27	1.30	1.33	1.36	1.39	1.43	1.46	1.49	1.52	1.55	1.58	1.61	1.64
44	1.15	1.19	1.22	1.26	1.29	1.32	1.36	1.39	1.42	1.45	1.49	1.52	1.55	1.58	1.61	1.64	1.67
46	1.18	1.21	1.25	1.28	1.32	1.35	1.38	1.42	1.45	1.48	1.51	1.55	1.58	1.61	1.64	1.67	1.70
48	1.20	1.23	1.27	1.30	1.34	1.37	1.41	1.44	1.48	1.51	1.54	1.57	1.61	1.64	1.67	1.70	1.73
50	1.22	1.26	1.29	1.33	1.36	1.40	1.43	1.47	1.50	1.53	1.57	1.60	1.63	1.67	1.70	1.73	1.76
52	1.24	1.28	1.31	1.35	1.39	1.42	1.46	1.49	1.53	1.56	1.59	1.63	1.66	1.70	1.73	1.76	1.79
54	1.26	1.30	1.33	1.37	1.41	1.44	1.48	1.52	1.55	1.59	1.62	1.66	1.69	1.72	1.76	1.79	1.82
56	1.28	1.32	1.36	1.39	1.43	1.47	1.50	1.54	1.58	1.61	1.65	1.68	1.72	1.75	1.78	1.82	1.85
58	1.30	1.34	1.38	1.41	1.45	1.49	1.53	1.56	1.60	1.63	1.67	1.71	1.74	1.78	1.81	1.85	1.88
60	1.32	1.36	1.40	1.43	1.47	1.51	1.55	1.59	1.62	1.66	1.69	1.73	1.77	1.80	1.84	1.87	1.91
62	1.34	1.38	1.41	1.45	1.49	1.53	1.57	1.61	1.64	1.68	1.72	1.76	1.79	1.83	1.86	1.90	1.93
64	1.35	1.39	1.43	1.47	1.51	1.55	1.59	1.63	1.67	1.70	1.74	1.78	1.82	1.85	1.89	1.92	1.96
66	1.37	1.41	1.45	1.49	1.53	1.57	1.61	1.65	1.69	1.73	1.77	1.80	1.84	1.88	1.91	1.95	1.99
68	1.39	1.43	1.47	1.51	1.55	1.59	1.63	1.67	1.71	1.75	1.79	1.83	1.86	1.90	1.94	1.97	2.01
70	1.41	1.45	1.49	1.53	1.57	1.61	1.65	1.69	1.73	1.77	1.81	1.85	1.89	1.92	1.96	2.00	2.04
72	1.42	1.47	1.51	1.55	1.59	1.63	1.67	1.71	1.75	1.79	1.83	1.87	1.91	1.95	1.99	2.02	2.06
74	1.44	1.48	1.53	1.57	1.61	1.65	1.69	1.73	1.77	1.81	1.85	1.89	1.93	1.97	2.01	2.05	2.08
76	1.46	1.50	1.54	1.59	1.63	1.67	1.71	1.75	1.79	1.83	1.87	1.91	1.95	1.99	2.03	2.07	2.11
78	1.47	1.52	1.56	1.60	1.65	1.69	1.73	1.77	1.81	1.85	1.89	1.94	1.98	2.01	2.05	2.09	2.13
80	1.49	1.53	1.58	1.62	1.66	1.71	1.75	1.79	1.83	1.87	1.92	1.96	2.00	2.04	2.08	2.12	2.15
82	1.50	1.55	1.59	1.64	1.68	1.72	1.77	1.81	1.85	1.89	1.94	1.98	2.02	2.06	2.10	2.14	2.18
84	1.52	1.56	1.61	1.65	1.70	1.74	1.79	1.83	1.87	1.91	1.96	2.00	2.04	2.08	2.12	2.16	2.20
86	1.53	1.58	1.63	1.67	1.72	1.76	1.80	1.85	1.89	1.93	1.98	2.02	2.06	2.10	2.14	2.18	2.22
88	1.55	1.60	1.64	1.69	1.73	1.78	1.82	1.87	1.91	1.95	1.99	2.04	2.08	2.12	2.16	2.20	2.24
90	1.56	1.61	1.66	1.70	1.75	1.79	1.84	1.88	1.93	1.97	2.01	2.06	2.10	2.14	2.18	2.22	2.27
92	1.58	1.63	1.67	1.72	1.77	1.81	1.86	1.90	1.95	1.99	2.03	2.08	2.12	2.16	2.20	2.25	2.29
94	1.59	1.64	1.69	1.74	1.78	1.83	1.87	1.92	1.96	2.01	2.05	2.09	2.14	2.18	2.22	2.27	2.31
96	1.61	1.66	1.70	1.75	1.80	1.84	1.89	1.94	1.98	2.03	2.07	2.11	2.16	2.20	2.24	2.29	2.33
98	1.62	1.67	1.72	1.77	1.81	1.86	1.91	1.95	2.00	2.04	2.09	2.13	2.18	2.22	2.26	2.31	2.35
100	1.64	1.69	1.73	1.78	1.83	1.88	1.92	1.97	2.02	2.06	2.11	2.15	2.20	2.24	2.28	2.33	2.37
102	1.65	1.70	1.75	1.80	1.84	1.89	1.94	1.99	2.03	2.08	2.12	2.17	2.21	2.26	2.30	2.35	2.39
104	1.66	1.71	1.76	1.81	1.86	1.91	1.96	2.00	2.05	2.10	2.14	2.19	2.23	2.28	2.32	2.37	2.41
106	1.68	1.73	1.78	1.83	1.88	1.92	1.97	2.02	2.07	2.11	2.16	2.20	2.25	2.30	2.34	2.38	2.43
108	1.69	1.74	1.79	1.84	1.89	1.94	1.99	2.03	2.08	2.13	2.18	2.22	2.27	2.31	2.36	2.40	2.45
110	1.70	1.75	1.81	1.86	1.91	1.95	2.00	2.05	2.10	2.15	2.19	2.24	2.29	2.33	2.38	2.42	2.47
112	1.72	1.77	1.82	1.87	1.92	1.97	2.02	2.07	2.11	2.16	2.21	2.26	2.30	2.35	2.40	2.44	2.49
114	1.73	1.78	1.83	1.88	1.93	1.98	2.03	2.08	2.13	2.18	2.23	2.27	2.32	2.37	2.41	2.46	2.50

Calculated by the formula:
Body surface area = $0.007184 \times$ (patient's height, cm)$^{0.725} \times$ (patient's weight, kg)$^{0.425}$
From Dubois & Dubois, 1916.

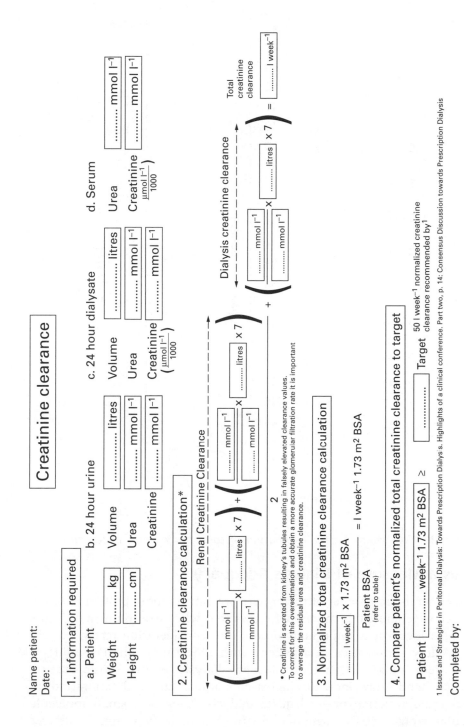

Fig. 8.19 Creatine clearance.

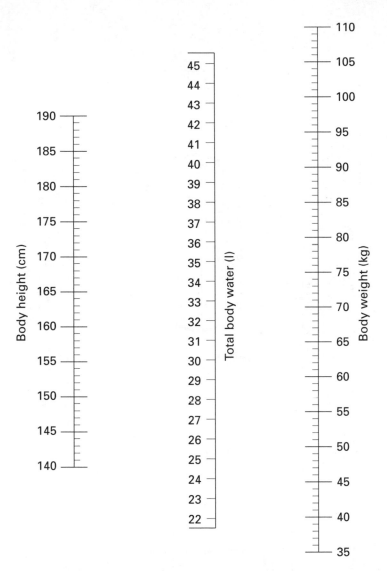

Fig. 8.20 *Nomogram for the estimation of total body water in females.*

Urea as a Measure of Dialysis Adequacy

Urea is a metabolic product of the protein we eat. As more protein is eaten, more urea is generated. It therefore follows that when examining a patient's serum urea levels it is important to take into consideration recent protein intake. A low serum urea in a patient with ESRD may simply be due to a low protein intake, rather than adequate dialysis. A high serum urea on the other hand may indicate increased catabolism, a deterioration in residual renal function or inadequate dialysis. Urea is a small molecule (molecular weight 60 Da) which is distributed in body water. It diffuses readily and is therefore easily removed from the blood.

The prescription index Kt/V was developed by Gotch *et al.* (1983) and Gotch and Sargent (1985) in the National Co-operative Dialysis Study of haemodialysis patients. Kt/V is an index of urea removal, which is patient specific as it looks at urea removal achieved over time (K multiplied by t) and measurement of urea in the body water (V) for each patient. Therefore:

K = clearance
t = time
V = volume of body water in which urea is distributed
(Figs 8.20 and 8.21).

The index does not account for dietary protein intake, protein catabolic rate or urea generation rate. It is just as important to measure residual renal Kt/V as it is to measure dialysis Kt/V. The two should be added together to give a total weekly Kt/V value. Kt/V for both the patient's dialysis regime and their residual renal function can be calculated by using the worksheet in Fig. 8.22.

Currently, a weekly Kt/V of at least 2 is deemed adequate for PD patients, providing their nutrition and general well-being are also assessed as satisfactory. The weekly goal for Kt/V for haemodialysis patients is 3.0–3.2 a week. The reason that this level is higher than for PD patients is explained by the peak concentration hypothesis proposed by Keshaviah *et al.* (1989) (Fig. 8.23). Kt/V for haemodialysis patients has to be increased to equate the peak urea concentrations reached in between dialysis sessions.

Protein Nutrition

'Over 40% of peritoneal dialysis patients are undernourished' (Young *et al.*, 1991). Various terms have been used to identify a patient's nutritional status; these include serum albumin level, dietary protein intake (DPI), protein catabolic rate (PCR) and subjective global assessment (SGA). A patient's nutritional status is an important factor in assessing a patient's dialysis adequacy, but, as with all measures, it should not be taken in isolation.

Proteins are compounds of hydrogen, oxygen and nitrogen and are essential in the make-up of cells. Protein is therefore vital in the diet for growth and repair. When a person is said to be in nitrogen balance they have a balance between the nitrogen content of protein eaten and the amount of nitrogen excreted in the form of urea.

Serum albumin
Albumin is a plasma protein found in both the intra- and extravascular compartments of the body. It is at a higher concentration in the vascular compartment and excretes considerable oncotic pressure, thereby helping to maintain vascular volume. The normal range for serum albumin

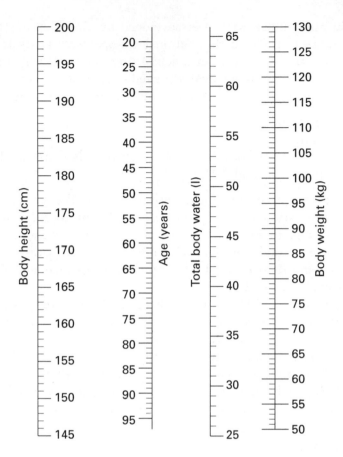

Fig. 8.21 *Nomogram for the estimation of total body water in males.*

$(35–50 \, \text{g} \, \text{dl}^{-1})$ is a powerful predictor of morbidity in PD patients. There are problems inherent within many methods of assessing nutritional status. The main problems associated with using albumin are that it has a half-life of 20 days and therefore cannot be used as an immediate predictor of a patient's nutritional status and that the body will attempt to maintain serum levels of albumin by removing it from other areas, for example the muscle tissues. It is, however, helpful in showing an overall long-term view of a patient's protein intake. Increasingly, pre-albumin is being used as a measure of nutritional status, as it has a shorter half-life than albumin.

Dietary protein intake (DPI)

DPI represents the amount of protein eaten in a 24-h period expressed as grams per kilogram of body weight per day $(\text{g} \, \text{kg}^{-1} \, \text{day}^{-1})$. It is usually calculated by asking the patient to record their dietary intake over a 3-day period and then averaging this for 24 h. Owing to different perceptions of the size of portions of food this may be an inaccurate way of measuring DPI. The normal recommended level of DPI for a healthy individual is 0.7 g kg^{-1} day^{-1}. In PD patients this figure rises to a minimum of 1.2 g kg^{-1} day^{-1} due to loss of protein through the peritoneal membrane during dialysis.

Protein catabolic rate (PCR)

PCR relates the loss of urea nitrogen to the nitrogen content of protein eaten. It is expressed in the same way as DPI (i.e. g kg^{-1} day^{-1}) and a healthy individual should have a PCR which is equal to their DPI (i.e. the patient is in nitrogen balance). As such, the aim for a PD patient is to have a PCR of at least 1.2 g kg^{-1} day^{-1}.

The most commonly used method of calculating PCRs is one that was developed by Randerson *et al.* (1989).

Subjective global assessment (SGA)

SGA of the nutritional status of patients is a simple and reliable tool which is increasingly being used in the diagnosis of malnutrition amongst ESRD patients. The method is based on history and physical examination as described by Detsky *et al.* (1987). The history focuses on gastrointestinal symptoms (anorexia, nausea, vomiting, diarrhoea) and weight loss in the preceding 6 months. The physical examination focuses on loss of sub-cutaneous fat over the triceps and mid-axillary line of the lateral chest wall, muscle wasting in the deltoids and quadriceps, and the presence of ankle oedema. These features are classified as:

0 = normal
1 = mild
2 – moderate and
3 = severe.

On the basis of a subjective weighting of data for history and physical examination, the patient can then be classified into one of three groups: 1, good nutrition; 2, moderate malnutrition; 3, severe malnutrition. This method of assessment can easily be performed by the nurse, dietitian or physician. A study performed by Enia *et al.* (1993) showed that SGA of nutrition is a clinically adequate method of assessing nutritional status in dialysis patients. The CANUSA study (Keshaviah *et al.*, 1996) found that a lower SGA score was associated with an increased relative risk of death.

General Well-Being

Despite the efficacy of a combination of the above physical parameters for measuring adequacy of dialysis, there can be no doubt that the ultimate gauge of success of the treatment must increasingly become the overall

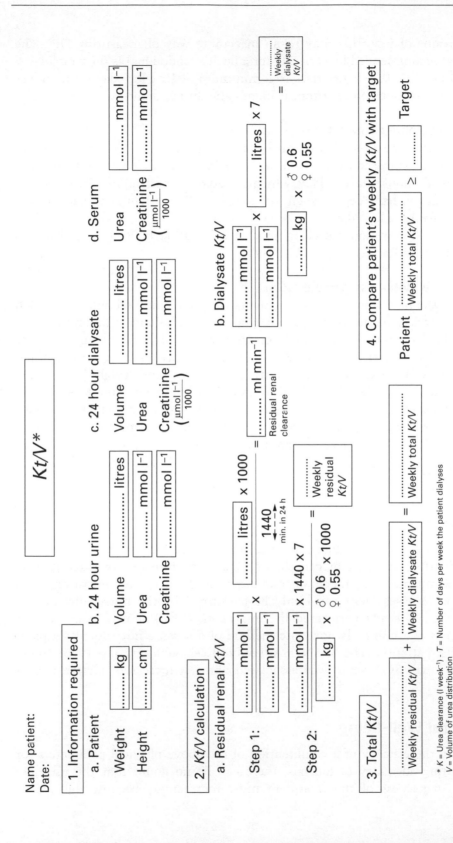

Fig. 8.22 Kt/V worksheet.

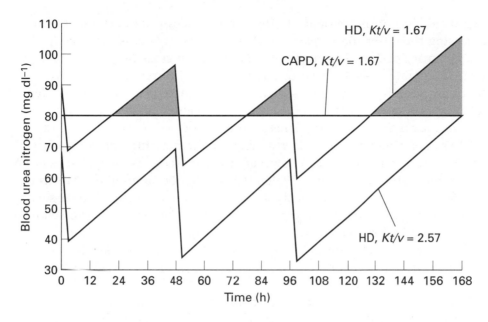

Fig. 8.23 *Keshaviah's peak concentration hypothesis. HD, haemodialysis; CAPD, continuous ambulatory peritoneal dialysis.*

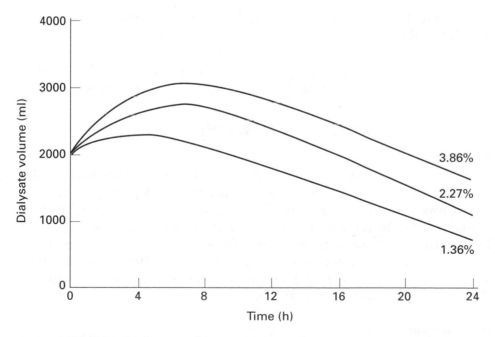

Fig. 8.24 *Dialysate volume versus time (approximate averages).*

quality of life of the patient. There is now widespread agreement that in assessing the effects of a treatment it is essential to assess both the quality and quantity of life. Health care purchasers are increasingly under pressure to demonstrate cost-effective utilisation of the limited resources available to them. Quality of life assessment is a key outcome measure in determining this cost effectiveness, but its multidimensional and subjective nature means that it is problematic to measure.

There are a number of tools available for the measurement of quality of life amongst renal patients; however, to date there is no consensus on which measure is best to use. Welch (1994) describes a number of measures which have been used previously and may be of use in the clinical setting to measure quality of life and general well-being. These include the Sickness Impact Profile (Bergner et al., 1976), the Nottingham Health Profile (Hunt and McEwan, 1983), the SF36 (Ware and Shelbourne, 1992), the Dialysis Stress Scale (Burton et al., 1986) and The Index of Well-being (Campbell, 1976).

What most health care professionals do agree upon, however, is that assessment should become a routine that is systematically incorporated into the on-going evaluation of patients.

PROBLEM-SOLVING IN PERITONEAL DIALYSIS

Complications of PD can be divided into two main groups – those related to ESRD, and those problems directly associated with PD itself.

ESRD-related Problems in PD Patients

Anaemia
Anaemia in PD patients is less severe than in haemodialysis patients due to the absence of blood loss during dialysis. Many PD patients experience an improvement in their anaemia; the reason for this is unknown, although it may be due to the removal of a toxic substance which suppresses the bone marrow's response to erythropoietin secreted by the patient. If PD patients do experience anaemia caused by lack of erythropoietin secretion, subcutaneous recombinant human erythropoietin may be administered. This is discussed fully in Chapter 6.

Hypertension
In many PD patients hypertension can be controlled by reducing total body sodium and correcting fluid overload.

Malignant hypertension should be treated with the appropriate anti-hypertension drug therapy (see Appendix One).

Renal osteodystrophy

Many PD patients have evidence of some bone disease when they start dialysis. In order to prevent worsening of this problem and to correct bone abnormalities it is important to maintain serum ionised calcium levels within the normal range. Many PD patients (up to 30%) experience hyper-calcaemia partly due to the use of calcium carbonate or acetate as a phosphate-binding agent (Armstrong and Cunningham 1994). This can be corrected by using physiological calcium PD solutions (i.e. 1.25 µmol l⁻¹). Phosphate-binding agents are essential as PD alone cannot normalise serum phosphate levels (Armstrong and Cunningham, 1994). This subject is further discussed in Appendix One.

Cardiovascular and cerebrovascular

The incidence of cardiovascular and cerebrovascular problems amongst PD patients is high. The most common problems are recurrent angina, arrhyth-mias, acute myocardial infarction, transient ischaemic attacks and cerebrovascular accident (Khanna *et al.*, 1993).

As yet, there is no clear indication of the relationship between PD and the increased incidence of these diseases. It may be due to hypertriglycer-idaemia-related atherosclerosis; however, many of the patients treated with PD tend to be elderly and therefore be more prone to these complications.

Endocrine function

High levels of prolactin are often found in PD patients and this has been identified as one of the many causes of infertility and sexual dysfunction amongst these patients. Some male PD patients have lower than normal levels of testosterone. Women can have normal menstruation with ovu-lating cycles and some have become pregnant whilst on PD (Hou, 1990).

Dialysis-Related Problems of PD Patients

Protein loss

Protein is lost through the peritoneal membrane at a rate of 6–12 g day⁻¹ in stable patients. To compensate for this loss, PD patients need to eat between 1.0 and 1.2 g kg⁻¹ of body weight day⁻¹ of dietary protein.

This loss is increased during peritonitis, when a patient can lose up to 20 g per day. An alternative method of compensating for this loss is by the use of intraperitoneal amino acid solution (this is fully discussed on p. 280).

Hyperlipidaemia

Patients experience raised levels of cholesterol and triglycerides within the first year on PD. This is mainly due to the glucose absorbed from PD fluid. Several studies have shown that these changes are not long lasting and peak levels usually are reached within 3–12 months of starting dialysis.

The levels often fall after this period back to pretreatment levels (Khanna *et al.*, 1983; Lindholm *et al.*, 1983; Ramos *et al.*, 1983). In fact serum lipid levels in patients after 1 year on PD appear to be the same as in haemodialysis patients (Norbeck and Lindholm, 1982).

Raised intra-abdominal pressure problems in PD patients

Raised intra-abdominal pressure is caused by the pressure of high volumes of fluid in the peritoneal cavity. This pressure is further increased when the patient carries out strenuous exercise. Continuous raised intra-abdominal pressure can increase the risk of abdominal hernias such as inguinal, incisional, diaphragmatic or umbilical and of dialysate leakage around the catheter exit site.

Oedema of labia in females and the scrotum and penis in males is a distressing complication caused by dialysate leakage through soft tissues. It is usually easily rectified by stopping PD for a short period (usually up to 1 week). Hernias and persistent leaks require surgical repair along with stopping PD for a time to allow the site to heal. If haemodialysis is not an alternative form of treatment for the patient during this temporary interruption to treatment, PD may be continued so long as the patient is lying down therefore decreasing the intra-abdominal pressure (i.e. by using some form of APD).

In the event of dialysate leakage at the exit site, PD must be ceased immediately as the presence of a glucose-rich solution at a wound site gives rise to a marked increased risk of infection. Leakage can be identified by using urine test sticks or blood glucose reagent strips at the exit site. The normal healing time for dialysate leakage is 1 week, but this may be increased in diabetic, severely uraemic or malnourished patients.

CAPD patients with previous vertebral disease may experience back pain due to the raised intra-abdominal pressure incurred in an upright position. In this situation APD may be the preferred therapy.

Drainage Problems

These usually have a minor cause which with proper patient training and education can be rectified by the patients themselves at home. Reasons for poor inflow or outflow of dialysis fluid and their treatment are outlined below.

Kinks in the tubing

The most common cause of poor drainage or inflow of PD fluid is tubing kinks or closed clamps. Patients should be taught to check the tubing for kinks and closed clamps as a first line of action in the event of poor in or out flow of dialysis fluid. Catheter kinks sometimes occur due to malpositioning during its surgical insertion. This will become apparent shortly after insertion if not during the insertion procedure, and can be confirmed by X-ray (the PD catheter has a radio-opaque stripe along its length). This problem is usually rectified by surgical intervention; however, it can occasionally be improved if the patient has a bowel motion.

Constipation

Constipation should be avoided in PD patients, not only because it causes problems with dialysate outflow but also because diverticulosis of the colon increases the risk of peritonitis. Constipation prevention is achieved by encouraging the patient to take a diet high in fibre along with a mild laxative if appropriate. If constipation does occur, treatment can be with laxatives, glycerine suppositories or a saline enema. The use of phosphate-containing enemas should be avoided due to the absorption of phosphate through the bowel during their administration. For the same reason the use of magnesium-containing laxatives should also be avoided.

Fibrin formation

Fibrin strands or plugs (a protein formed from fibrinogen in blood plasma in the process of clotting) in dialysate effluent is a common cause of poor drainage. The blockage, usually in the catheter or tubing, can normally be removed by 'milking' the tubing. Heparin may be added to the dialysis fluid (200–500 units l^{-1}) as a prophylactic measure, as it prevents the formation of fibrin.

If 'milking' the tubing does not remove the obstruction a fibrolytic agent can be used. Both streptokinase (250 000 i.u.) and urokinase (5000 i.u.) in 2–3 ml sodium chloride 0.9% for intravenous injection are available and should be infused into the catheter under aseptic conditions; the catheter should then be clamped and the drug left to infuse for 2 h. The catheter can then be checked for patency.

Malpositioned catheter

If catheter obstruction is not relieved by any of the above techniques, the problem may be due to obstruction caused by omentum attached to the catheter tip. The omental attachment usually causes the catheter to migrate out of the pelvic cavity. In such cases it often proves difficult to resolve this problem without surgery.

It is possible to remove omentum from the catheter whilst leaving it in place during surgical procedure. It is common for the surgeon to perform a local omentectomy at the same time to prevent further obstructions by omentum.

If it proves impossible to rectify the obstruction or position of the catheter by surgical methods the final option is to remove the catheter completely and replace it with a new one.

Shoulder Pain

Occasionally, patients complain of shoulder pain following the infusion of fresh dialysis solution. This is thought to be a referred pain caused by intra-abdominal pressure or air under the diaphragm (Uttley and Gokal, 1986). Although it usually resolves within 10–20 min from onset, the patient may find relief by taking a mild analgesia such as paracetamol 1 g.

Blood-Stained Effluent

This is a comparatively rare complication occurring most commonly in menstruating females. It may be due to endometriosis or retrograde bleeding through the fallopian tubes. The bleeding is usually mild and self-rectifies within a day or two without specific intervention.

More severe intraperitoneal bleeding causing darkly blood-stained fluid can be caused by haemorrhage. This could be due to the patient straining whilst lifting a heavy object or suffering trauma to the abdomen.

Membrane Failure

Membrane failure (also referred to as ultrafiltration failure) has been described by Mactier (1991) as 'Clinical evidence of fluid overload which persists despite restriction of intake and the use of three or more hypertonic exchanges per day'. Three different types of membrane failure have since been identified:

- Type I. *Hyperpermeable peritoneum*. These patients have high peritoneal solute transport rates which result in a rapid dialysis fluid and glucose absorption.
- Type II. *Hypopermeable peritoneum*. These patients have low peritoneal solute transport rates.
- Type III. These patients suffer from ultrafiltration failure due to high lymphatic drainage.

A patient's individual peritoneal membrane permeability is determined at birth and under normal circumstances cannot be altered. There is, however, some evidence to suggest that repeated episodes of peritonitis will change the permeability of the patient's membrane irreversibly (Davis *et al.*, 1993). Those patients who suffer from type I membrane failure may be those whose membranes naturally transport solutes across the membrane quickly (i.e. high transporters) or they could have sustained an insult to the peritoneum that prevents mesothelium regeneration. Those patients with type II membrane failure have most likely sustained severe irreversible damage to the membrane such as sclerosing peritonitis (Routtembourg *et al.*, 1985; Verger and Celicont, 1985) or peritoneal adhesions.

Over 80% of cases of total loss of ultrafiltration cited in literature have been associated with the use of PD fluid with acetate buffer (Faller and Marichal, 1984; Nolph *et al.*, 1984). This effect develops over a period of 12 months or more. Dialysis solutions now use lactate buffers and work is currently underway into the use of bicarbonate-based solutions.

Treatment of membrane failure

Verger (1986) has suggested that loss of ultrafiltration with mesothelial cell damage, hypervascularisation and submesothelial fibrotic changes (type I) can be reversible provided PD is stopped early enough. A period of 1 month on haemodialysis would therefore be recommended.

Fleming *et al.* (1985) and Wolfish (1983) have suggested that stopping overnight exchanges in CAPD patients can increase ultrafiltration towards normal; however, this may result in an overall reduction in solute clearance and the risk of underdialysis.

INFECTIOUS COMPLICATIONS OF PERITONEAL DIALYSIS

Peritonitis

Peritonitis has been cited in the literature as the single biggest cause of peritoneal membrane failure (Davis *et al.*, 1993). Although in recent years the incidence of peritonitis amongst patients treated by PD has markedly decreased due to the emergence of disconnect systems for CAPD and the use of APD, it is still a common problem.

In the early days of PD, CAPD patients experienced episodes of peritonitis as frequently as twice a year (Bruun, 1992). CAPD patients using the integrated disconnect system can now expect to experience one episode of peritonitis approximately every 30 patient months (Balteau, 1991; Dratwa, 1992; Lewis, 1992; Stregmayr, 1992; Tielens, 1993). The rate for APD patients is even lower, up to 1 episode in 60 patient months (King *et al.*, 1992), probably due to the reduction in the number of connections made during APD.

Causes of peritonitis

Most episodes of peritonitis are caused by organisms which are normal skin and nasal flora, for example *Staphylococcus epidermis* and *Staphylococcus aureus*. Occasionally, water-borne organisms such as *Pseudomonas* may also cause this infection.

There are five main routes of infection causing peritonitis, each one giving rise to common organisms.

Intraluminal (contamination at the solution bag and transfer set connection site) This contamination occurs most frequently when incorrect techniques have been used to make the connection. Good patient training and education regarding bag exchange procedure techniques and hand washing are essential. It is the nurse's responsibility to provide on-going education and retraining in order to prevent the development of poor exchange technique amongst PD patients. The incidence of this cause of infection has reduced in recent years due to the use of disconnect systems. These systems incorporate a 'flush before fill' into the procedure, which has been shown to remove organisms caused by touch contamination. The design of the Baxter Integrated Disconnect system (Balteau, 1991) is based on research by Verger and Luzar (1986) which reported that 100 ml of dialysis fluid flushed past the patient connection would be effective in removing 100% of *Staphylococcus epidermis*, 60% of *Staphylococcus aureus* and 30% of *Pseudomonas*.

The most common organisms seen when intraluminal contamination has occured are *Staphylococcus epidermis* and *Staphylococcus aureus*.

Periluminal (infection introduced via the catheter tunnel from the exit site)
Bacteria present on the skin surface can enter the peritoneal cavity via the catheter tunnel. This infection can occur if there is infection present at the exit site or in the subcutaneous tunnel, which has migrated into the peritoneal cavity.

The most common organisms seen when periluminal contamination has occurred are *Staphylococcus epidermis*, *Staphylococcus aureus*, *Pseudomonas*, *Proteus* and yeast.

Transmural (infection through the gut wall)   This infection occurs most commonly in patients with diverticular disease or bowel perforation, but can occur in other patients due to bacteria of intestinal origin entering the peritoneal cavity by migrating through the bowel wall.

The most common organism seen during transmural cause of peritonitis is *Escherichia coli*, although multiple contamination with anaerobes and fungi may also be isolated.

Haematogenous (infection via the blood stream)   This is a rare cause of peritonitis and it may be the peritonitis itself which causes septicaemia. The most common organisms associated with this cause of peritonitis are *Streptococcus* and *Mycobacterium*.

Vaginal (ascending through the vagina)   This is thought to be from bacteria entering the peritoneum via the fallopian tubes. The most common causative organisms seen here are *Candida* and *Pseudomonas*.

Diagnosis of peritonitis
Early diagnosis allowing prompt treatment of peritonitis is essential in minimising damage to the peritoneal membrane. Diagnosis is when two or more of the following conditions are present:

- cloudy PD effluent containing > 100 white blood cells μl^{-1} (more than 50% of which are neutrophils);
- abdominal pain and tenderness and pyrexia;
- identification of micro-organisms in the PD effluent by positive Gram stain or culture.

The process of diagnosis of peritonitis is summarised in Fig. 8.25.

Obtaining a PD effluent specimen

CAPD patients   After disconnecting the drainage bag containing the effluent from the patient's transfer set, the bag should be inverted several times to mix the contents. Using strict aseptic technique a sample is taken by sterile needle and syringe from the sample port on the bag (Fig. 8.26). Great care must be taken to avoid contamination of the sample during collection, as this will affect the culture result.

The sample can then be transferred to the appropriate container used in each centre (some laboratories prefer to receive the whole bag of effluent) and sent for microscopy, culture and sensitivity.

APD patients   In APD patients a sample may either be taken from the day time dwell, if the patient utilises a 'wet' day (i.e. dialysate in the peritoneum during the day), by attaching a drainage set and bag to the patient's extension set. The sample is then taken in the same way as for CAPD patient. Alternatively, if the patient is usually 'dry' during the day (i.e. no dialysate in the peritoneum during the day), there are a number of options. Some APD machines have a sample bag which can be attached to the drainage tubing. Alternatively, the patient may be taught how to take a sample from the drainage solution containers themselves. If this is not possible, the patient may be asked to detach the drainage solution container from the machine following treatment and take this into their unit. Many APD patients have a supply of CAPD equipment at home for use when travelling if their APD machine is not a portable version; in this case, the patient may be asked to perform a CAPD exchange at home and then attend the clinic with fluid in the peritoneal cavity which can then be drained and sampled in the usual way.

Calculation of peritonitis rates

When evaluating the quality of any treatment it is important to be able to measure its success. Recording the incidence of peritonitis within a group of patients provides us with one way in which we can appraise the standard of patient care. Measuring peritonitis in terms of patient months giving intervals between episodes of peritonitis is a convenient and reliable way of measuring peritonitis in individual centres on a regular basis. It also allows intercentre comparisons and comparisons at different time points.

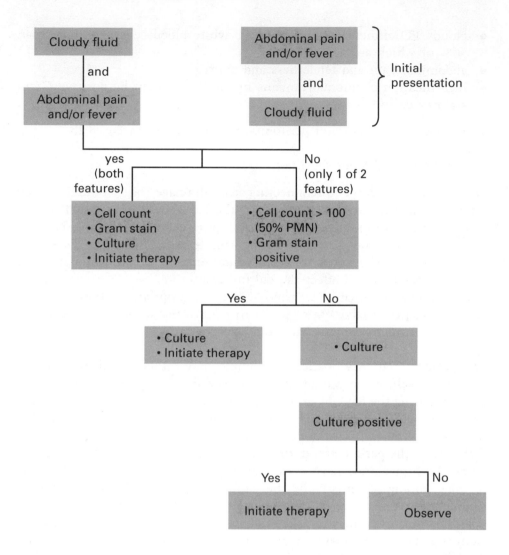

Fig. 8.25 *Initial clinical and laboratory assessment of patient for peritonitis. PMN, polymorphic neutrophils..*

Peritonitis rates are expressed as episodes per patient month and are calculated by dividing the total number of episodes by the total number of patients treated each month. For example, if 100 patients were on PD in January and four had an episode of peritonitis, the rate for January would be 4 in 100 or 1 in 25.

Any patient on PD for 2 weeks is counted as 0.5 of a month. Similarly a patient on for 1 or 3 weeks is counted as 0.25 and 0.75 respectively. Peritonitis rates have a cumulative value as demonstrated in Table 8.6. The most accurate peritonitis rate is one which is cumulative on 12 months. Culture negative or no-growth peritonitis episodes are included in

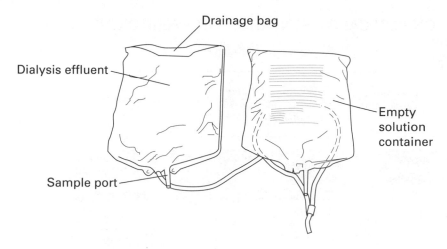

Fig. 8.26 *Sample port on drainage bag.*

peritonitis rates. Recurrence of the same organism within 14 days of completion of treatment is not included in peritonitis rates.

Many peritonitis episodes are mild and can be treated at home. Usually the incubation period from time of contamination for bacterial peritonitis is 24–48 h. Any symptoms should resolve quickly following the initiation of therapy. If the infection shows either a slow response or no response to treatment the choice of antibiotics could be inappropriate.

The PD patient should be taught how to recognise the signs and symptoms of peritonitis during their initial training period and at regular intervals, perhaps at clinic or home visits, whilst they are treated by PD. Each patient should know the importance of prompt treatment for this infection and should therefore be taught to contact the PD clinic for advice at the first sign of infection. Ideally the patient, if on CAPD, should complete the bag exchange at home (the presence of PD fluid in the peritoneum may provide some pain relief from inflammation of the peritoneal membrane), and to bring the bag of cloudy dialysate effluent into the clinic for sampling. Treatment can then be initiated immediately. The *ad hoc* advisory committee on peritonitis management (Keane *et al.*, 1993) produced a document outlining treatment recommendations for PD-related peritonitis (Fig. 8.27).

There is current debate as to the necessity to perform a 'peritoneal lavage' immediately after the diagnosis of peritonitis, as it is thought to reduce the number of phagocytes present in the peritoneum available to fight infection. Peritoneal lavage is therefore thought by some to be of benefit only to patients with purulent effluent and abdominal pain as a pain-relieving exercise. There is no evidence to suggest that a transfer set change performed at this time is of any benefit. On admission to the PD clinic the usual fill volume for the patient is medicated with antibiotics. The

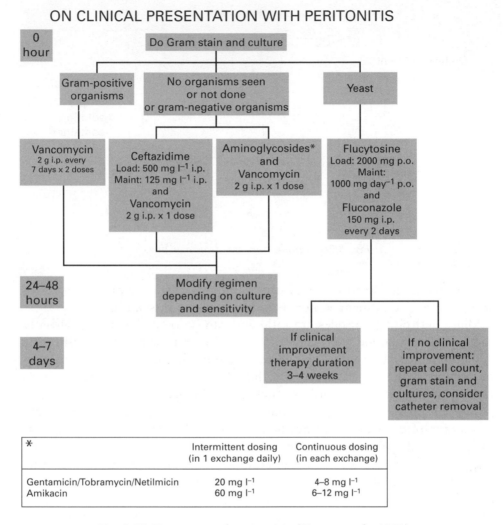

Fig. 8.27 *Treatment of peritonitis (Keane et al., 1993).*
See note added in proof on page 317.

choice is based on the result of the Gram stain (Fig. 8.28 and 8.29; Keane *et al.*, 1993), although it is unusual for any hospital laboratory to perform such a prompt Gram stain that the most appropriate antibiotics be administered immediately. It is more usual for the initial antibiotic therapy to cover a wide range of Gram-negative and Gram-positive organisms (e.g. vancomyocin and aminoglycosides) which can then be changed following identification of the causative organism.

Antibiotics are then added to each subsequent bag of dialysis fluid before each exchange. The patient can be taught how to add the antibiotics to the dialysis fluid to facilitate self-care. Alternatively, the community nursing services can be employed to add the antibiotics to all bags of CAPD

Table 8.6 *Calculation of peritonitis rates.*

Month	Jan	Feb.	March	April	May
Episodes	3	1	2	4	1
Patient month experience	80	86	90	92	94
Monthly peritonitis rate	3/80	1/86	2/90	4/92	1/94
Cumulative	3/80	4/166	6/256	10/348	11/442
Total peritonitis rate	1/26.6	1/41.6	1/42.6	1/34.8	1/40.1
No growth	0	0	1	0	1
Recurrence	0	0	0	1	0

fluid. Heparin (200–500 units l⁻¹) may also be added to the fluid to prevent the formation of fibrin, which is more likely in the presence of infection.

APD patients may receive antibiotics intraperitoneally by adding the antibiotics to the dialysis solution at the start of the therapy. The i.p. antibiotics may be continued during the long daytime dwell period.

Peritonitis is monitored closely and dialysate effluent should be clear within 48 h of commencing treatment. If the peritonitis resolves, antibiotics are discontinued 7–10 days after the start of therapy.

Absorption of antibiotics into the serum through the peritoneum from the dialysate is rapid. Therefore, in most cases, administration of intravenous antibiotics is unnecessary. The outcome of peritonitis treated by either intravenous or intraperitoneal antibiotics is comparable and therefore the choice of route for administration should be tailored to suit the patient's needs. Oral antibiotics have been used occasionally for the treatment of peritonitis (Pérez-Fontan *et al.*, 1991).

Permeability changes during peritonitis

The peritoneal membrane permeability tends to increase during episodes of peritonitis, perhaps due to increased blood flow through the peritoneum. Clearances of both large and small molecules increase, as does the absorption of glucose. This can result in marked increases in protein loss through the peritoneum and poor ultrafiltration. Patients need to be educated as to the need to increase dietary protein intake during episodes of peritonitis and to care for their fluid balance, ensuring that, if they have no residual renal function, fluid intake is kept to a minimum. Rarely, patients are severely ill with peritonitis and need to be treated in hospital.

The use of prophylactic antibiotics

This is not recommended as it encourages the emergence of resistant organisms.

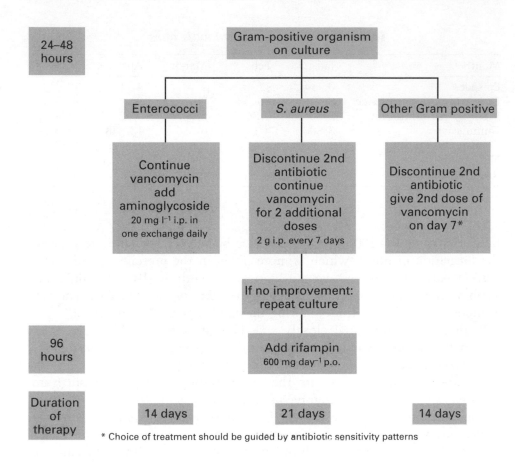

Fig. 8.28 *Treatment of peritonitis – Gram-positive organism on culture (Keane et al., 1993).*

Culture-negative peritonitis

If the dialysate effluent culture results are negative after 24 h the most likely explanation is that although bacterial infection did cause the peritonitis, the organism failed to grow in culture due to a variety of technical reasons.

According to the *ad hoc* advisory committee (Keane *et al.*, 1993), if the patient is clinically improving after 4–5 days and there is no suggestion of Gram-negative organisms on Gram stain, only vancomycin needs to be continued for the normal duration of therapy (i.e. 7–10 days). However, if there is no clinical improvement in the patient, repeat medical evaluation is necessary and the possibility of removing the PD catheter considered.

Fungal peritonitis

Fungal peritonitis, although rare, does occur occasionally, the most common organism being *Candida*. In the past, amphotericin was used to

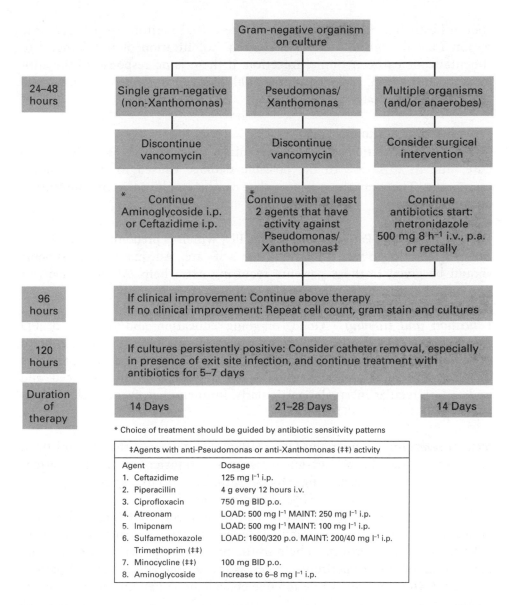

Fig. 8.29 *Treatment of peritonitis – Gram-negative organism on culture (Keane et al., 1993).*

treat these infections; however, its toxicity was seen to be a problem limiting its effectiveness. Keane *et al.* (1993) suggest using imidizoles/triazoles, although catheter removal may be resorted to eventually.

Relapsing peritonitis

Relapsing peritonitis is diagnosed as a reoccurrence of the same organism within 4 weeks of completion of the course of antibiotics. These infections should be treated in the same way as the initial peritonitis; however, the reason may be due to abscess formation, colonisation of the catheter or subcutaneous catheter tunnel infection. If there is no response to the antibiotics within 96 h, consideration should be given to catheter removal and replacement at a later date.

Prevention of peritonitis

As with any infectious disease, prevention of peritonitis is preferable to cure, due in this case to the possible damage caused to the peritoneal membrane. There are three factors that can be employed in the prevention of peritonitis.

Patient selection   Patients selected for PD, which is predominantly a home therapy, should be well motivated for self-care. Adequate home support should be given to those patients requiring extra help. Absence of diverticular disease in the patient is also a major consideration.

Education and training   Good, on-going education and training of PD patients and their families and carers are essential. Education should be in the prevention of peritonitis as well as in its detection and prompt access to treatment. All education should be on-going, being reinforced and updated at regular intervals, particularly following an event such as peritonitis or a break in PD treatment.

System selection   Verger and Luzar (1986) demonstrated that 100-ml flush of dialysate past the connection between the transfer set and the patient was effective in removing 100% *Staphylococcus epidermis*, 60% *Staphylococcus aureus* and 30% *Pseudomonas*.

This flush before fill procedure has been incorporated into the integrated disconnect system originally developed by Baxter Healthcare (Balteau, 1991) and has been proven to help in the prevention of peritonitis by many authors, giving rise to peritonitis rates as low as one episode in 172 patient months (Owen and Fair, 1994) and one episode in 32 patient months (Lewis, 1992).

Exit Site Infection

An exit site infection is defined by the presence of erythema and purulent exudate at the catheter exit site from the skin (Luzar, 1991). The presence of erythema alone may be an early indication of exit site infection. If purulent discharge is present, a swab should be taken and sent to the laboratory for culture, microscopy, Gram stain and sensitivity.

Treatment for exit site infection, usually by oral antibiotics as suggested by Keane *et al.* (1993), is outlined in Fig. 8.30.

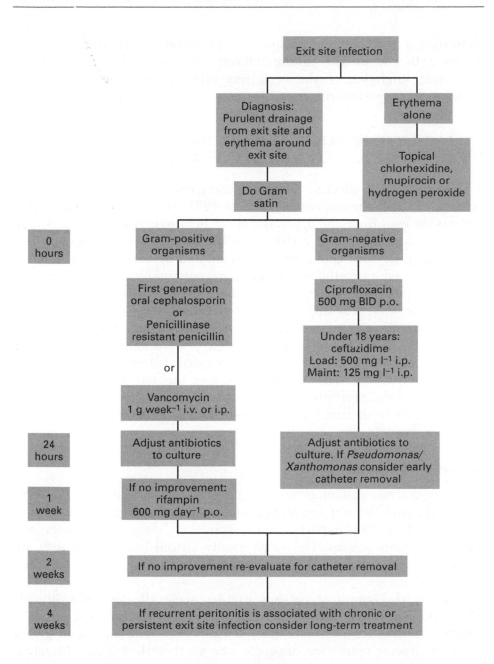

Fig. 8.30 *Treatment for exit site infection (Keane et al., 1993).*

Tunnel Infection

Tunnel infection can present as an extension of the exit site infection into the catheter tunnel and swelling, pain and redness over the subcutaneous tunnel are observed. Tunnel infections do not often respond well to antibiotic treatment and it is usual to remove the PD catheter in these cases, reinserting a new one after about 1 month. Antimicrobial therapy should be given to the patient in the interim time to resolve the infection preventing migration of the organisms into the peritoneum, therefore predisposing to peritonitis.

EDUCATION AND TRAINING IN THE PERITONEAL DIALYSIS PATIENT

It is essential that effective education takes place before patients can be expected to treat themselves at home. In 1983, Wilson-Barnett noted that patients do gain from and appreciate more information and that this may result in less anxiety, more participation and an increased feeling of control over their lives. This comment is substantiated by the earlier findings of Boore (1978), who concluded that giving patients information and a role in their own care will reduce their level of anxiety, reduce postoperative complications and generally enhance recovery.

Many patients who embark on a dialysis training programme are adults and as such, their learning needs are seen to be different from those of children (Tarnow, 1979). Adults are usually motivated to learn and are often learning from choice. They bring a wealth of life experiences with them that influence their learning and response to teaching. However, the extent to which this holds true for patients, including those with chronic renal failure, is questionable.

Barriers to Learning

The new dialysis patient is often frightened – the prospect of dialysing oneself at home may not appeal. Many new patients are uraemic, the symptoms of which can include nausea, vomiting, sleep disturbances and confusion. Many patients feel so physically unwell by the time they are to commence dialysis that they lack motivation to learn, feeling that they will never recover.

Teaching this group of patients can be made all the more difficult when other barriers to learning become apparent. A fundamental barrier is language. In the UK for instance, there is a growing ethnic population, giving rise to a growing proportion of people who speak little English. There are limited resources available for translation and it is frequently the responsibility of a younger member of the family, often a son or daughter, to act as translator during training. It may thus be difficult to assess who is learning, and with no knowledge of the language being translated the trainer finds it difficult to ascertain just who has grasped the concept or answered the question, the patient or the translator. Language may also become a barrier when speaking to patients with no previous medical knowledge. Jargon and clinical terminology can be frightening and confusing.

Many patients who are to learn PD are elderly and having to learn new concepts and procedures on which their life will depend may seem an overwhelming task. This sometimes makes learners feel vulnerable and inadequate, particularly if they are slow to learn. Short-term memory loss is a problem suffered by many elderly patients and is a source of great frustration to both learner and trainer. These patients frequently have added physical barriers to learning, such as poor vision or lack of manual dexterity. Varying levels of deafness may also be a problem – the learner is trying not only to understand what has been said but also straining to hear.

A study conducted some years ago by the UK Department of Education's Adult Literacy and Basic Skills Unit (ALBSU) estimated that between 10 and 13% of the adult population lack the literacy skills needed to function effectively in today's society; that is, they have 'functional literacy difficulties'. This figure does not include those who have numeracy difficulties, who probably account for a further 2 million or 6% of the population. If we consider this problem in relation to the concepts and procedures which need to be taught to dialysis patients, it becomes apparent that the information given must be clear, unambiguous and readily understood, particularly if the patient's literacy difficulty is paired with a second and even third barrier to learning.

Resources

Resources available to staff who are to train dialysis patients are often limited. The learning environment, although important to the learning process, is often not appropriate. Valuable opportunities for teaching patients are often lost in the hospital setting due to clinical duties (Ersser *et al.*, 1984). The nurses who teach patients often have many other responsibilities but training should not take second place (Cohen, 1981). Lack of time, heavy workload and inadequate staffing are often cited as reasons for this (Phol, 1965) and although these reasons may be valid, Winslow (1976) has suggested that it is occasionally due to lack of desire or poor organisation. Winslow also puts some of the blame for inadequate patient education on to the patient who does not 'take the initiative and ask for information'. This again may be the case, but for many patients it is difficult to ask questions on a subject about which they know very little.

Training Materials

It has been well documented that visual, audio and audio-visual materials are an essential part of any training programme (Frantz, 1980; Zappacosta and Lander, 1988). It is important, however, that the material used is appropriate to the learner. Patients have many different learning styles and it is important to accommodate these within the training programme.

The Learning Environment

One of the fundamental needs for effective training to take place is that of a good learning environment. A good training environment is one which is comfortable, non-clinical, free from interruptions and has a welcoming and friendly atmosphere.

Home Training

If patients are ultimately to dialyse at home, the clinical environment of a hospital is not an ideal place in which to learn this therapy. Teaching patients in their own home may be the ideal situation, particularly when teaching patients about CAPD. It will be easier for patients to adapt the therapy to their own lifestyle and if they learn on their own territory some reduction in fear may be achieved. Each patient will almost certainly have uninterrupted one-to-one teaching and the educator will have the opportunity to give practical help and advice about where the dialysis can be performed. Family members may also find it easier to be involved in such education. However, the constraints associated with training patients in their own homes may prevent many renal units from implementing this strategy. One nurse has to be removed from the hospital setting for some days at a time. It may also prove difficult to implement this method of training for patients who were not planned admissions – the patient who needs dialysis very shortly after being diagnosed with renal failure. Having a homely setting within the hospital environment or an off-site training centre may bridge the gap between hospital and home.

Recommendations for Training Within Renal Units

- Set aside an area specifically for teaching purposes. The area should preferably be away from the ward, be non-clinical and quiet. A television and video can be used in this area for teaching.
- Designate a team of nurses for training duties only. Establish some continuity of care by allocationg each patient to a designated nurse.
- Invite family members/partners to participate in the teaching programme.
- Use a wide variety of training materials. Five points to good presentation of these materials:

    (a) teach the smallest amount possible for the job required;
    (b) make the point as vividly as possible;
    (c) review repeatedly;
    (d) have the learner restate and demonstrate material;
    (e) the subject matter should be relevant.

- Any material should be presented in a way that is comprehensible to the learner. There are more than 40 different formulae for assessing the degree of difficulty in reading materials (Doak *et al.*, 1985). However, the most common characteristics on which they focus are:

  (a) difficulty of the vocabulary, particularly the number of syllables in the word;
  (b) average sentence length (McLaughlin, 1969; Seels and Dale, 1971; Fry, 1977).

  Despite the fact that the readability of the material can be measured by the same formula, readers' skills may vary with their interest and background of experience in a particular topic area (Doak *et al.*, 1985).
- Training materials are most effective when presented in an interesting and appropriate manner. Both the language used and the material's degree of complexity need to be taken into account.
- The material should be presented in a memorable fashion. Any visual aids need vivid, simple messages which are easy for patients to remember.

Finally, but perhaps most importantly:

- it is essential that the patients want to learn what is being taught.

The training programme should be designed to prepare patients fully for return to the community. The aim of a training programme is to educate patients to a standard whereby they can confidently care for themselves and perform their CAPD in the community. For some learners this may mean that they learn only how to perform CAPD, troubleshoot and manage their renal diet. For others much more detail may be desired; for example, learning how dialysis works.

Group teaching is an excellent way for patients to learn. This not only enables patients to learn from each other, but also helps the teacher, as many patients can be taught the same subject at the same time. The bulk of the training programme should focus on the patients themselves, relating all they are learning to their disease, treatment and, ultimately, their lifestyle. Sessions should be designed to last for no longer than 20 min and visual aids such as flipcharts, acetates and videos are used to make the material interesting and varied.

What to Teach Patients

It is important that new patients to PD are discharged from the renal unit with enough knowledge to care for themselves safely on dialysis. The amount of information new patients need to know can be overwhelming and provide quite a barrier to learning at the beginning of their treatment.

It is the nurse's responsibility to distinguish just how much information each patient can assimilate at any one time, and give this information in digestible chunks. There are many patients who will have a desire to learn all that there is to know about the therapy, whilst others may only wish to learn the basics. Broadly speaking, when each patient is taught, priority should first be given to what they must know, then to what they should know, and finally to what they could know.

The following topics should be included in a PD training programme:

- *Medication*. The patient's own medication can be used as the central focus for this session. The aim is to ensure that the patient knows how often and why each medicine is taken.
- *Normal functions of the kidney*. This session can be given in groups using a set of overhead projection acetates to explain in a simple way the basic functions of the kidney, relating these to the symptoms they suffer when kidneys fail.
- *CAPD and APD procedures*. These are most easily taught on a one-to-one basis. Demonstration techniques can be used to explain the procedure. A PD simulator (plastic torso with a PD catheter) is an excellent tool on which patients can practise their exchanges.
- *Catheter and catheter exit-site care*. This can be taught to the patient on a one-to-one basis. The PD simulator can be used to practise exit-site dressing technique as can getting the patient to practise the technique in front of a mirror. Photographs are useful to help explain visually the difference between a healthy and an infected exit site.
- *How PD works*. Osmosis and diffusion can be explained using simple 'experiments' or diagrams. A video is also available called 'How does CAPD work?' which explains these simple concepts in more detail.
- *Diet*. Eating is an activity which most people enjoy and therefore takes up a rather large part of their lives. Maybe it is for this reason that many patients focus on diet and want to know all there is to be taught. Plastic models of food can be used in training sessions to make the learning fun. Further discussion of dietary issues for renal patients is presented in Chapter 9.
- *Infections*. It has been well documented that peritonitis is a major complication of PD and can be associated with inadequate self-care and lack of education (Westman *et al.*, 1991). It is therefore important that peritonitis is explained to patients well, using a purpose-printed flipchart.
- *Fluid balance*. Fluid overload can be associated with excessive fluid intake and poor education. It is a common experience that one of the most difficult aspects of treatment to adhere to is the restriction of fluid intake. This subject can also be taught in groups using a purpose-printed flipchart. Weighing a jug of fluid can also be useful to demonstrate the difference between fluid weight and flesh weight.

- *Ordering and delivery of PD supplies.* The practicalities of ordering and delivery of the PD supplies to the patient's home prove a great worry for many patients and their families. It can often be compounded by the problem of where to store this large amount of equipment. A comprehensive video explains in a simple way the ordering and delivery of the dialysis supplies not only to the patient's home but also to other holiday or travel destinations. Patients can be encouraged to talk amongst themselves to gain ideas from each other as well as utilising the experience of nurses.
- *Exercise for PD patients.* The nurse's role is to promote a healthy lifestyle for patients. The training period is an ideal opportunity during which to discuss which type of activities are best suited to that individual patient. A booklet is available which explains the best forms of exercise as well as giving advice and instruction on abdominal and back muscle strengthening exercises for PD patients.

To complement the training programme reading materials should be made available, along with posters and videos. Many training materials have been translated into other languages for use by those patients whose first language is not English.

Assessment of how much information the patient has retained is difficult to make accurately. Testing can be seen as a threatening procedure even though it is essential. Games, therefore, make a valuable contribution to the task of assessing learning and can be used in a variety of forms. Simple, home-made crosswords, wordsearches and quizzes can be fun for patients and relatives to do at the end of their training. 'Renal Bingo' is an excellent way of assessing groups of patients together (Robinson *et al.*, 1988).

SUMMARY

On-going education and support is vital in ensuring the success of patients on PD. Continuing educational support will help to prevent problems such as peritonitis or fluid overload from occurring. As patients gain experience with the therapy, questions may arise which they had not thought of or which were not relevant during the initial training period. It is therefore important to make time available for patients to feel able to ask such questions in an environment where they can be answered fully. Follow-up workshops and home visits by the community nursing team provide an opportunity for patients to discuss the successes and problems they have encountered. Clinical procedure technique can be checked for accuracy by the trainer in a non-threatening environment. Many patients gain an enormous amount from group support sessions (Said, 1995); however, other patients may feel threatened in this environment and one-to-one teaching may be more appropriate.

Above all, teaching and learning should be simple and fun, it should be available in an understandable form to all patients all of the time and ultimately promote the self-care of the patient.

REFERENCES

ARMSTRONG, A. AND CUNNINGHAM, J. (1994) The treatment of metabolic bone disease in patients on peritoneal dialysis. *Kidney International*, **46**(Suppl. 48): S51–7.

BALTEAU, P. (1991) Design and testing of the Baxter Integrated Disconnect System. *Peritoneal Dialysis International*, **11**: 131–6.

BAXTER HEALTHCARE, Caxton Way, Thetford, Norfolk, UK (1992) *UK PET Survey*.

BERGNER, M., BOBBITT, R.A., POLLARD, W.E., MARTIN, D.P. AND GILSON, B.S. (1976) The sickness impact profile: validation of a health status measure. *Medical Care*, **14**: 57–67.

BLAKE, P.G., BALASKAS, E.V., IZALT, S. AND OREOPOULOS, D.G. (1992) Is total creatinine clearance a good predictor of clinical outcomes in continuous ambulatory peritoneal dialysis? *Peritoneal Dialysis International*, **12**: 353–8.

BOORE, J. (1978) *Prescription For Recovery*. London: Royal College of Nursing.

BRUUN, K. (1992) *A Retrospective Study of Peritonitis in CAPD Patients on Different PD Systems*. Syllabus: 12th Annual Conference on Peritoneal Dialysis. Seattle, February.

BURKART, J.M. (1993) Adequacy of peritoneal dialysis. *Dialysis and Transplantation*, **May**: 234–43.

BURTON, H.J., KLINE, S.A., LINDSAY, R.M. AND HEIDEMHEIM, A.P. (1986) The relationship of depression to survival in chronic renal failure. *Psychosomatic Medicine*, **48**: 261–9.

CAMPBELL, A. (1976) *The Quality of American Life*. New York: Russell Sage Foundation.

CHURCHILL, D.N., THORPE, K., TAYLOR, D.W. AND KESHAVIAH, P. (1994) *Adequacy of peritoneal dialysis*. For the Canada–USA Study of Peritoneal Dialysis Adequacy. Abstract 75P. American Society of Nephrology Meeting. Orlando, October 1994.

CHURCHILL, D.N., TAYLOR, D.W., KESHAVIAH, P.R. AND THE CANUSA PERITONEAL DIALYSIS STUDY GROUP (1996) Adequacy of dialysis and nutrition in continuous peritoneal dialysis: association with clinical outcomes. *Journal of American Society of Nephrology*, **7**: 198–207.

COHEN, S.A. (1981) Patient education. A review of the literature. *Journal of Advanced Nursing*, **6**: 11–18.

COLES, G.A., SLINGENEYER, A., FALLER, B. *et al.* (1994) *The effect of intranasal mupirocin on CAPD exit site infection*. Abstract of Presentation. American Society of Nephrology Conference, Orlando, November.

COOPER, A., HENDERSON, I.S. AND JONES, M.C. (1995) Daytime dwell with 7.5% dextrin in automated peritoneal dialysis (APD). *Journal EDTA – ERCA*, **21**(Suppl. 1): 21.

DAVIS, S., BRYAN, J. AND RUSSELL, G.I. (1993) Longitudinal changes in peritoneal kinetics: the influence of dialysis and peritonitis. *Nephrology, Dialysis and Transplantation*, **8**(12): 14–15.

DETSKY, A.S., McLAUGHLIN, J.R. AND BAKER, J.P. (1987) What is subjective global assessment of nutritional status? *Journal of Parental and Entral Nutrition*, **11**: 458–82.

DIAZ-BUXO, J.A. (1984) Intermittent, continuous ambulatory and continuous cycling peritoneal dialysis. In *Clinical Dialysis* (ed. A.R. Nissenson *et al.*). Appleton-Century-Crofts, Norwalk. p. 48.

DOAK, C.C., DOAK, L.G. AND ROOT, J.H. (1985) *Teaching Patients with Low Literacy Skills*. Lippincott, Philadelphia.

DOBBIE, J. (1989) Monitoring peritoneal hystopathology in peritoneal dialysis. The role of the biopsy registry. *Dialysis and Transplantation*, **18**(6): 319–35.

DRATWA, M. (1992) Peritonitis prevention: Twin bag better than Y-set. *Peritoneal Dialysis International. XI Annual CAPD Abstracts*, No. 72.

DUBOIS, D. AND DUBOIS, E.F. (1916) A Formula to Estimate the Approximate Surface Area if Height and Weight is Known. *Arch. Interm. Med.* **17**: 863–71.

ENIA, G., SICUSO, C., ALATI, G. AND ZOCCALI, C. (1993) Subjective global assessment of nutrition in dialysis patients. *Nephrology, Dialysis, Transplantation*, **8**: 1094–8.

ERSSER, S. TAYLOR, S. AND WILKINSON, J. (1984) Healthy and wise. *Nursing Times*, **80**: 54–5.

FALLER, B. AND MARICHAL, J.F. (1984) Loss of ultrafiltration in CAPD: a role for acetate. *Peritoneal Dialysis Bulletin*, **4**: 10–14.

FLEMING, L.W., STEWART, W.U., HALLIDAY, A.A. AND JAMES, N.A. (1985) Treatment of ultrafiltration loss in CAPD. *Nephron*, **39**: 398–9.

FRANTZ, R. (1980) Selecting media for patient education. *Topics in Clinical Nursing/Education for Self Care*, **2**: 77–83.

FRY, E. (1977) Fry's readability graph: clarifications validity and extensions to level 17. *Journal of Reading*, **9**: 242–52.

FUCHS, J., GALLAGHER, M.E. AND JACKSON-BEY, D. (1990). A prospective randomised study of peritoneal catheter exit site care. *Dialysis and Transplantation*, **19**: 81–4.

GOKAL, R., ASH, S.R., HOLFRICH, B.G. *et al.* (1993) Peritoneal catheters and exit site practices. Toward optimum peritoneal access. *Peritoneal Dialysis International*, **13**: 29–39.

GOKAL, R. AND THE MIDAS GROUP (1994) A UK multi-centre study of icodextrin in CAPD. *Peritoneal Dialysis International*, **14**(Suppl. 2): S22–S27.

GOTCH, F.A. AND SARGENT, J.A. (1985) A mechanistic analysis of the National Co-operative Dialysis Study (NCDS). *Kidney International*, **28**: 526–34.

GOTCH, F.A., SARGENT, J.A., PARKER, T.J. *et al.* (1983) National co-operative dialysis study: comparison of the study groups and a description of morbidity, mortality, and patient withdrawal. *Kidney International*, **26**(Suppl. 23): S42–S49.

HOU, S. (1990) Pregnancy in CAPD patients. Editorial. *Peritoneal Dialysis International*, **10**: 201–4.

HUNT, S.M. AND McEWAN, J. (1983) The Nottingham health profile. In *Measuring Health: A Practical Approach* (ed. G. Teeling-Smith). John Wiley, Chichester, pp. 165–9.

HUTCHISON, A. (1992) Peritoneal dialysis solutions for the future. Do we have the solution? *Dialysis and Transplantation*, **21**(2):57–63.

KEANE, W.F., EVERETT, E.D., GOLPER, T.A. *et al.* (1993) Peritoneal dialysis related peritonitis treatment recommendations, 1993 update. *Peritoneal Dialysis International*, **13**: 14–28.

KELMAN, B. (1995) The roles of the peritoneal dialysis nurse. *Peritoneal Dialysis International*, **15**: 114–15.

KESHAVIAH, P.R., NOLPH, K.D. AND VAN TONE, J.C. (1989) The peak concentration hypothesis: a urea kinetic approach to comparing peritoneal and haemodialysis. *Peritoneal Dialysis International*, **9**: 257–60.

KESHAVIAH, P., CHURCHILL, D.N., THORPE, K. AND TAYLOR, D.W. (1996) *Impact of nutrition on CAPD mortality*. For the Canada–USA Study of Peritoneal Dialysis Adequacy. Abstract 9P. American Society of Nephrology Meeting, Orlando. October 1994.

KHANNA, R. AND TWARDOWSKI, Z.J. (1989) Peritoneal dialysis access. In *Peritoneal Dialysis* (ed. K.D. Nolph). Kluwer Academic, Dordrecht, pp. 261–88.

KHANNA, R., BRECKENBRIDGE, C., RONCARI, D., DIGENIS, G. AND OREOPOULOS, D.G. (1983) Lipid abnormalities in patients undergoing CAPD. *Peritoneal Dialysis Bulletin*, **3**(Suppl.): S13–S15.

KHANNA, R., NOLPH, K.D. AND OREOPOULOS, D.G. (eds) (1993). Complications during peritoneal dialysis. In *The Essentials of Peritoneal Dialysis*. Kluwer Academic, Dordrecht, p. 89.

KHANNA, R., WU, G., PROWANT, B. *et al.* (1986) CAPD in diabetics with ESRD: a combined experience of two North American centres. In *Diabetic Renal Retinal Syndrome 3* (eds E. Friedman and F. l'Esperance). Grune and Stratton, New York, pp. 363–81.

KING, L.K., KINGSWOOD, J.C. AND SHARPSTONE, P. (1992) Comparison of the efficacy, cost and complication rate of APD and CAPD as long term treatments for renal failure. *Advances in Peritoneal Dialysis*, **8**: 123–6.

KREDIET, R.T., BOESCHOTEN, E.W., ZUYDERHOUDT, F.M.J. AND ARISZ, L. (1986) Peritoneal transport characteristics of water and low molecular weight solutes on patients during long term peritoneal dialysis. *Peritoneal Dialysis Bulletin*, **6**(2): 61–3.

LAMEIRE, M., DHAENE, M., MATTHYS, E. *et al.* (1993) Experience with CAPD in diabetic patients. In *Prevention and Treatment of Diabetic Nephropathy* (eds H. Keen and M. Legrain). MTP, Lancaster, pp. 289–97.

LEWIS, J. (1992) CAPD disconnect systems: UK peritonitis experience. *Advances in Peritoneal Dialysis*, **8**: 306–12.

LINDBALD, A.S. (ed), NOVAK, J.W., NOLPH, K. *et al.* (1989) *CAPD in the USA*. Kluwer Academic, Dordrecht, pp. 63–74.

LINDHOLM, B., KARLANDER, S.G., NORBECK, H.E. AND BERGSTROM, J. (1983) Hormonal and metabolic adaptation to the glucose load of CAPD in non-diabetic patients. In *Prevention and Treatment of Diabetic Nephropathy* (eds H. Keen and M. Legrain). MTP Press, Boston, pp. 353–9.

LUZAR, M.A. (1991) Exit site infection in CAPD: a review. *Peritoneal Dialysis International*, **11**: 333–40.

MACTIER, R.A. (1991) Investigation and management of ultrafiltration failure. *Advances in Peritoneal Dialysis*, **7**: 57–62.

MAKI, D. (1991) *Improving Catheter Site Care*. Royal Society of Medicine Services, London.

MCLAUGHLIN, G.H. (1969) SMOG grading – a new readability formula. *Journal of Reading*, **12**: 639–46.

MISTRY, C.D., MALLICK, N.P. AND GOKAL, R. (1987) Ultrafiltration with iso-osmotic solution during long peritoneal dialysis exchanges. *Lancet*, **ii**: 178–82.

MONCRIEF, J.W., POPOVICH, R.P., SEARE, W. *et al.* (1996) New microporous (MP) epidermal cuff at the catheter exit site for access in peritoneal dialysis. *Peritoneal Dialysis International*, **16**(Suppl. 2): S53.

NOLPH, K.D., RYAR, L., MOORE, B.S. *et al.* (1984) A survey of ultrafiltration in peritoneal dialysis. *Peritoneal Dialysis Bulletin*, **4**: 137–42.

NORBECK, H.E. AND LINDHOLM, B. (1982) Long term effects of peritoneal versus haemodialysis on serum lipoproteins. Abstract. *European Journal of Clinical Investigation*, **12**: 29.

OWEN, G. AND FAIR, P.A. (1994) Eradicating peritonitis, a six stage approach. Poster Presentation at the British Renal Symposium, Harrogate.

PARK, M.S., LEE, H.B., LIM, A.S. *et al.* (1996) Effect of prolonged subcutaneous implantation of peritoneal catheter on peritonitis rate during CAPD: a prospective randomised study. *Peritoneal Dialysis International*, **16**(Suppl. 2): S54.

PEERS, E.M., SCRIMGEOUR, A.C. AND HAYCOX, A.R. (1995) Cost containment in CAPD patients with ultrafiltration failure. *Clinical Drug Investigations*, **10**(1): 53–8.

PÉREZ-FONTAN, M., ROSALES, M., FERNANDEZ, F. AND MONCALIAN, J. (1991) Ciprofloxacin in the treatment of Gram positive bacterial peritonitis in patients undergoing CAPD. *Peritoneal Dialysis International*, **11**: 233–6.

PHOL, M.L. (1965) Teaching activities of the nursing practitioner. *Nursing Research*, **14**: 4–11.

PIRAINO, B., BERNARDINI, J. AND SORKIN, M. (1986) The influence of peritoneal dialysis catheter exit site infections on peritonitis, tunnel infections and catheter loss in patients on CAPD. *American Journal of Kidney Disease*, **8**: 436–40.

PROWANT, B.F., SCHMIDT, L.M., TWARDOWSKI, Z.J. *et al.* (1988) Peritoneal dialysis catheter exit site care. *American Nephrology Nurses Association Journal*, **15**: 219–22.

RAMOS, J.M., HEATON, A., MCGURK, J.G., WARD, H.K. AND KERR, D.N.S. (1983) Sequential changes in serum lipids and their subfractions in patients receiving CAPD. *Nephron*, **35**: 20–3.

RANDERSON, D.H., CHAPMAN, G.V. AND FARRELL, P.C. (1989) Amino-acids and dietary status in CAPD patients. In *Peritoneal Dialysis* (eds R.C. Atkins, N.M. Thompson and P.C. Farrel). Edinburgh, Churchill Livingstone, pp. 179–91.

ROBINSON, J.A., ROBINSON, K.J. AND LEWIS, D.J. (1988) Games: a motivational education strategy. *American Nephrology Nurses Association Journal*, **15**: 277–9.

ROUTTEMBOURG, J. (1988) Peritoneal dialysis in diabetics. In *Peritoneal Dialysis* (ed. K.D. Nolph). Kluwer Academic, Dordrecht, pp. 365–79.

ROUTTEMBOURG, J., ISSAD, B. AND LANGOLIS, P. (1985) Loss of ultrafiltration and sclerosing encapsulating peritonitis during CAPD: evaluation of potential risk factors. *Proceedings of the National Conference on CAPD*, pp. 109–17.

SAID, V. (1995) Beyond adventure. *Lifeline – the CAPD Newsletter*, **12**: 2.

SHAMBYE, H. *et al.* (1993) The cytotoxicity of CAPD solutions with different bicarbonate/lactate ratios. *Peritoneal Dialysis International*, **13**: S116–S118.

SEELS, B. AND DALE, E. (1971) *Readability and Reading. An Annotated Bibliography*. Newark: International Reading Association.

STARZOMSKI, R.C. (1984) Three techniques for peritoneal catheter exit site dressings. *American Nephrology Nurses Association Journal*, **11**: 9–16.

STREGMAYR, B. (1992) Lower incidence of peritonitis in CAPD with integrated disconnect system than with an UV flash system. *Peritoneal Dialysis International*, **12**, Abstract 272.

TARNOW, K. (1979) *Special Programmes in Continuing Education for Nursing in Working with Adult Learners*. Nurse Educator, Texas Woman's University, College of Nursing.

TEEHAN, U.P., SCHLEIFER, C.R., BROWN, J.M., SIGLER, M.H. AND RAIMONDO, J. (1990) Urea kinetic analysis and clinical outcome in CAPD: a five year longitudinal study. *Advances in Peritoneal Dialysis*, **6**: 181–5.

TIELENS, E. (1993) Major reduction in CAPD peritonitis after introduction of the twin bag system. *Nephrology, Dialysis and Transplantation*, **8**: 1237–43.

TWARDOWSKI, Z.J. (1989) Clinical value of standardised equilibration test in CAPD patients. *Blood Purification*, **7**: 95–108.

TWARDOWSKI, Z.J. (1990) Tidal peritoneal dialysis. *EDTNA Journal*, **XV**: 4–9.

TWARDOWSKI, Z.J., NOLPH, K.D., KHANNA, R. *et al.* (1987) Peritoneal equilibration test. *Peritoneal Dialysis Bulletin*, 7(3): 138–47.

UTTLEY, L. AND GOKAL, R. (ed.). (1986) Organisation of a CAPD programme – the nurse's role. In *Continuous Ambulatory Peritoneal Dialysis*. Churchill Livingstone, pp. 162–5.

VAS, S. (1996) Randomised clinical trial with silver coated PD catheter. *Peritoneal Dialysis International*, **16**(Suppl. 2): S56.

VERGER, C. (1986) Clinical significance of ultrafiltration alterations on CAPD. In *Proceedings of 2nd International Course in Peritoneal Dialysis* (eds G. La Greca and C. Ronco). Witching Editor, Milan, pp. 91–4.

VERGER, C. (1989) Anatomy and physiology of the peritoneum in continuous peritoneal dialysis. Evaluation and methods of surveillance. *Nephrologie*, **10**(Suppl.): 22–9.

VERGER, C. AND CELICONT, B. (1985) Peritoneal permeability and encapsulating peritonitis. *Lancet*, **1**: 986–7.

VERGER, C. AND LUZAR, M.A. (1986) In vitro study of CAPD Y-line systems. *Advances in Peritoneal Dialysis*, **2**: 160–4.

WARE, J.E. AND SHELBOURNE, C.D. (1992) The MOS 36 item short-form health survey (SF-36): I. Conceptual framework and item selection. *Medical Care*, **30**: 473–83.

WELCH, G. (1994) Assessment of quality of life following renal failure. In *Quality of Life Following Renal Failure* (eds H. McGee and C. Bradley). Harwood Academic, Switzerland, pp. 55–98.

WESTMAN, J., GEORGE, S., PAVELKA, C. AND SWEENEY, J. (1991) Psychosocial issues on dialysis management. *Peritoneal Dialysis International*, **11**(Suppl. 1): 290.

WILSON-BARNETT, J. (1983) Patient teaching. *Recent Advances in Nursing Series*. Churchill Livingstone, Edinburgh.

WINSLOW, E.H. (1976) The role of the nurse in patient education. *Nursing Clinics of North America*, **11**: 213–22.

WOLFISH, N.M. (1983) Loss of ultrafiltration capacity in infants. *Nephron*, **38**, 277–8.

YOUNG, G., KOPPLE, J.D., LINDHAN, B. *et al.* (1991) Nutritional assessment of continuous ambulatory peritoneal dialysis patients: an international study. *American Journal of Kidney Disease*, **17**(4): 462–71.

YOUNG, M.A., NOLPH, K., DUTTON, S. AND PROWANT, B. (1984) Anti-hypertensive drug requirement in CAPD. *Peritoneal Dialysis Bulletin*, **5**: 85–8.

ZAPPACOSTA, A.R. AND LANDER, S.M. (1988) Components of a successful CAPD education programme. *American Nephrology Nurses Association Journal*, **15**: 243–7.

Note added in proof:

Since the submission of this chapter there have been some reported incidences of Vancomycin resistant enterococci (VRE). The *ad hoc* advisory committee on peritonitis management therefore made further recommendations at the end of 1996. These can be found in *Peritoneal Dialysis International*, **16**(6): 557–73.

CHAPTER 9

DIETARY MANAGEMENT OF CHRONIC RENAL FAILURE

A HISTORICAL REVIEW OF DIETARY MANAGEMENT, WITH AND WITHOUT HAEMODIALYSIS

1965–1970

Dietary treatment was considered to be a very important component of the treatment of patients with end-stage renal failure (ESRF) before haemodialysis was accepted as a regular form of renal replacement therapy (RRT) during the 1960s and 1970s.

Professors Sergio Giovanetti and Camello Giordano from Italy developed during this period a very low protein diet for patients approaching ESRF, with gastrointestinal symptoms (Berlyne, 1968). This diet was prescribed to selected patients with a serum creatinine clearance of 3 ml min^{-1} or a urea level of 200 mg 100 ml^{-1} (33 mmol l^{-1}).

Dr Geoffrey Berlyne modified this Giovanetti/Giordano diet for British patients, as the original was based on Italian eating habits (Berlyne, 1968). This modified diet contained 20 g protein, mostly high biological value (HBV) protein, to cover essential amino acid requirements. To prevent loss of muscle weight and maintain nitrogen balance, at least 50 kcal per kilogram ideal body weight (kg^{-1} ibw) were prescribed.

Therefore, the daily HBV protein intake consisted of 1 egg, 180 ml milk and 150 g potatoes. There was no limit on vegetables and fruit. Low protein (LP) foods replaced cereal products such as bread, biscuits, flour and pasta. The majority of energy was supplied by sugar, glucose polymers like Hycal (Beecham) and similar liquid glucose/glucose syrup solids, cream, butter, margarine and oil for food preparation. This was a difficult diet to follow and required total dedication from the patient, their family and carers.

Blood chemistry (urea, serum creatine and phosphate levels) improved to such an extent that the patient's appetite returned to normal and was able to return to work. For many patients this was the only alternative to reaching a vicious circle of uraemic vomiting and salt depletion, leading to death some weeks or months later.

Regular haemodialysis (HD) became an alternative RRT for selected patients during the latter part of the 1960s – early 1970s. These patients were usually young and without other complicating organic disease. They received two or three dialysis treatments per week. Although the HD diet was not as strict as the Giovanetti–Giordano diet, an intake of 50 g protein, mainly HBV, low salt (approximately 20–25 mmol Na), low potassium (50 mmol K) and 3500 kcal were still necessary to control the patient's blood chemistry.

1970–1980

There have been periods when predialysis dietary protein restriction was in and out of fashion. A badly managed low protein diet resulted in severe protein and energy malnutrition, prolonging the rehabilitation of patients who were initially 'selected' for HD. The energy content of protein-restricted diets did not receive sufficient attention and the selection of commercial low protein, prescribable foods was very limited in palatability and supply.

The quote 'The patient reduces to the size of his kidneys' is well remembered by the older generation of nephrology health care workers.

During this decade dialysis technology enabled more patients to receive treatment and predialysis dietary treatment relaxed somewhat to a protein restriction of $0.5–0.75$ g kg^{-1} and a $30–40$ kcal kg^{-1} body weight energy intake.

As treatment became more efficient and frequent the HD diet also relaxed to 60 g protein, Na 60 mmol, K 60 mmol and $2500–3000$ kcal day^{-1}.

1980–1990

In the early 1980s, Dr Barry Brenner introduced the hyperfiltration, hyper-perfusion hypophesis, induced by dietary protein, diabetes and nephron destruction. His results, and those of others, showed that progression of renal failure could be delayed by early protein restriction in partially nephrectomised rats (Brenner 1983).

Many retro- and prospective randomised trials were initiated to study this effect in humans. This hypophesis has been difficult to prove in humans, and patient's compliance on a 0.6 g kg^{-1} low protein diet was also a problem as this diet was initiated during the early stage of chronic renal disease, before the patient became symptomatic.

In 1985 the National Institute of Health (NIH) in the USA launched the three-phased study on the modification of diet of renal disease (MDRD) using four different types of diet:

- usual protein intake;
- moderate protein restriction (1.3 g kg^{-1} and $16–20$ mg kg^{-1} phosphorus restriction);
- a low protein diet, 0.6 g kg^{-1} and $5–10$ mg phosphorus kg^{-1};
- very low protein diet, 0.3 g kg^{-1} with a phosphorus restriction of $5–10$ mg kg^{-1} and supplemented with keto acids.

(The preliminary results were published in 1994 and are discussed below.)
Several questions needed to be answered:

- Will the low protein/low phosphorus diet with adequate counselling delay the rate of progression?

- Will the diet cause malnutrition?
- Will the diet be acceptable to patients for a long period of time (Snetselaar, 1990)?

During this decade, peritoneal dialysis (PD) became widely recognised as an alternative treatment for HD, and dietary recommendations were introduced, recognising peritoneal losses of protein. Diabetic and elderly patients were now also accepted for RRT and this provided a challenge for dietary treatment, to accommodate special requirements for the diabetic and elderly patients.

The quality of a dialysis patient's life changed with the development of recombinant human erythropoietin (RHu EPO), resulting in an improved feeling of well being and improvement in appetite.

Other advances in dietary management developed as a result of long-term aspects of treatment of chronic renal failure (CRF):

- prevention of renal bone disease, emphasising early phosphorus restriction;
- prevention of cardiovascular disease (CVD) by including 'healthy eating' guidelines.

The development of sophisticated dialysis machines for continuous haemofiltration (CHF) changed the dietary management of acute renal failure with or without nutritional support.

CURRENT CONCEPTS ON DIETARY INTERVENTION

Attitudes towards dietary protein restriction varies in European countries. The EDTA Registry Report published in 1992 provided information on the overall pattern for greater protein restriction as renal function declines (Raine et al., 1992).

Forty-five per cent of centres advised a degree of protein restriction even when creatinine clearance (cr/cl) was over 60 ml min^{-1} and 89% of centres did so when cr/cl was less than 10 ml min^{-1}.

In Italy, 13% of centres restricted protein intake to 0.8 g kg^{-1} with a cr/cl of > 60 ml min^{-1} and 63% centres reduced protein to 0.6 g kg^{-1} when cr/cl was < 10 ml min^{-1}. In the UK, very few centres restricted protein with cr/cl of > 60 ml min^{-1} and only 16% restricted protein when cr/cl was < 10 ml min^{-1}.

The NIH completed their three-phase study on MDRD launched in 1985, using the four different types of diets and different levels of blood pressure control. The preliminary results were published in 1994 and showed initially a slower decline in progression of renal disease in the absence of

...

severe proteinuria and hypertension. There appeared no further advantage in using a very low protein (VLP) diet supplemented with essential amino acids or keto acids (Klahr *et al.*, 1994).

Amongst other findings the following implications were included:

- that patients with proteinuria and polycystic kidney disease had a faster rate of progression;
- patients with chronic renal disease and proteinuria should lower blood pressure below the level recommended for the prevention of CVD;
- that patients with a renal function of < 20% of normal should reduce their protein intake;
- those with a renal function of 20–40% of normal may only slightly benefit from a low protein diet.

The report cautioned that while lowering blood pressure and protein intake appear to be safe, both must be carefully monitored.

Additional secondary results are in the process of being published. A meta-analysis which includes the MDRD study indicates that a low protein diet reduces the risk of renal failure or death in patients with non-diabetic renal disease (Levey *et al.*, 1995).

Besides strict control of blood pressure, treatment includes dietary phosphorus restriction to prevent renal bone disease and a modest degree of protein restriction, but not as severe as previously. However, this needs close dietetic supervision to prevent malnutrition and enhance dietary compliance.

Malnutrition must be detected and treated early. Severe weight loss and a steady decline in serum albumin (S-Ab) levels in non-nephrotic patients are obvious clinical signs.

The provision of good-quality treatment at optimal efficiency at the lowest cost possible has become essential to accommodate this growth in the dialysis population. Starting dialysis early preserves residual renal function for a longer period. It also promotes rehabilitation, and this approach is now accepted as the way forward to reduce the cost of treatment whereby expensive hospitalisation is kept to a minimum. Quality of dialysis should not be compromised by inadequate treatment in an aim to reduce cost that could lead to underdialysis, a return of unrecognised uraemia, loss of appetite and malnutrition, leading to an increase in morbidity and mortality.

In 1993, the NIH stated that the nutritional health of a patient prior to dialysis is an important indicator of outcome (NIH, 1993) and that all patients are entitled to receive a nutritional assessment by a trained renal dietitian. In the absence of obvious malnutrition, a moderate low protein diet of up to 0.7–0.8 g protein kg^{-1} ibw day^{-1} should be prescribed. When malnutrition is present, the amount of energy is increased and the amount of protein is raised to 1.0–1.2 g kg^{-1}, to allow for nutritional repletion or to counter the catabolic effects of stress. Dietary prescriptions should include guidelines for energy, fat and carbohydrate, fluid, sodium, phosphate and potassium, as well as other nutrients and micronutrients (personal communication).

Although modification of the diet to minimise lipid abnormalities is reasonable, such modifications should not be so rigid that they limit energy intake below daily requirements. Lipid abnormalities, particularly hypertriglyceridaemia and reduced high density lipoprotein (HDL) cholesterol along with elevated levels of lipoprotein (a), are common in ESRF, but there are limited data to support the efficacy of diet or drug therapy.

THE AIMS OF CONSERVATIVE DIETARY MANAGEMENT

The nutritional content of a protein-restricted diet should be specifically adapted to each patient's individual needs and personal circumstances. This should result in the reduction of accumulated metabolic waste products which can be controlled as chronic renal disease progresses.

Regular dietary follow-up should provide maintenance of optimal nutritional status by ensuring that sufficient protein and energy (expressed as kcal or kJ) continues to be taken by the patient and that other important nutrients such as vitamins and minerals are prescribed as supplements.

The diet should help prevent long-term effects of renal disease such as CVD by manipulating the intake and type of fat as a source of energy, but not compromise adequate energy intake. The diet should provide sufficient dietary freedom and enable the patient to lead a near normal life. This means that dietary flexibility must be incorporated and relatives or friends should be involved while educating the patient to promote maximum dietary compliance.

The following are important in the dietary therapy of conservative management:

- protein
- energy (carbohydrate and fat)
- sodium and fluid
- potassium
- phosphorus
- other minerals, such as calcium, iron and zinc
- vitamins.

Table 9.1 *Protein restriction and energy requirements versus degree of renal function*

Glomerular filtration rate (GFR) (ml min^{-1})	*Protein (g kg^{-1})	Energy (kcal kg^{-1})
> 30	Free	RDA
20–30	0.8–1.0	30–35
5–20	0.8	35
<5 Dialysis indicated		

* 60–70% high biological value (HBV).
* 40–30% low biological value (LBV).
RDA, recommended daily allowance.

Protein

Protein is an important nutrient for repair and maintenance of tissue and for growth. There are two important aspects to consider when prescribing a protein-restricted diet:

- the quantity of protein
- the quality of protein.

Quantity

The level of dietary protein in a retricted diet should maintain nitrogen balance and nutritional status as previously discussed. The calculation should be based on the ideal or acceptable body weight and not on actual body weight, taking the patient's residual renal function into consideration (see Table 9.1). For instance, if a patient consumes a high protein diet a reduction to 1.0 g kg^{-1} ibw day^{-1} may initially be sufficient and can be reduced to 0.8 g kg^{-1} ibw if renal function deteriorates at a later stage. This is an acceptable degree of protein restriction for long-term use and is well within the limit advised by the World Health Organisation, assuming the energy content of the consumed diet is sufficient (see Table 9.2).

Quality

It is equally important that the correct type of protein is prescribed for similar reasons, especially when protein restriction is < 0.8 g kg^{-1} ibw.

The majority of protein should be obtained from animal sources, such as meat, fish, eggs and some milk. These foods contain a higher percentage of essential amino acids. Ideally 60–70% should be of HBV protein (type of protein that contains a high percentage of essential amino acids) and the remainder from low biological value (LBV). This may not always be an achievable goal as many patients, such as Asian women, follow a vegetarian diet.

Table 9.2 *Dietary aspects of conservative management of chronic renal failure (CRF)*

Protein	0.8–1.0 g kg^{-1} ibw
	60–70 HBV%
	40–30 LBV%
Energy	35–30 kcal kg^{-1} ibw
	↓ malnutrition
	↑ obesity
Fat	40% of energy
	↑ SFA (animal fat)
	↓ PUFA & MUFA
Carbohydrate	50% of energy
	↓ monosaccharides
	↑ polysaccharides
	↑ fibre
Phosphorus	800–1000 mg
Sodium	↑ Na with depletion
	↓ with fluid retention
Potassium	approx. 1.0 mmol kg^{-1} ibw
Minerals	Ca (CaCO$_3$ containing PO$_4$ binders)
	Fe and folate with RHuEPO
Vitamins	'Renal' formula

HBV, high biological value; LBV, low biological value; SFA, saturated fatty acid; PUFA, polyunsaturated fatty acid; MUFA, monounsaturated fatty acid; RHuEPO, recombinant human erythropoietin; ibw, ideal body weight.

Dietary advice must be excellent to prevent malnutrition and to alleviate boredom leading to non-compliance. This can be achieved by using the expertise of an experienced renal dietitian with frequent follow-up sessions either at clinic or by telephone.

The effect of protein restriction

An improvement in well-being is first noticed with often a corresponding decrease in serum urea and creatinine levels. Some patients notice that mild symptoms like 'morning sickness' and a 'metallic taste' in the mouth disappear. The initial fall in creatinine is due to a reduction in the consumption of muscle protein (i.e. meat or fish).

If urea levels do not show an improvement, the following should be investigated:

- Urinary urea excretion should be measured, indicating the amount of dietary protein intake (Maroni, 1994).
- The protein content of the diet may be too high.
- The intake of energy (carbohydrate and fat) is too low and protein is used to supplement energy requirements.

- Other extrarenal catabolic factors can lead to excess breakdown of protein due to lack of energy. This may occur as a result of a serious infection or major surgery.
- Steroid therapy, to treat inflammatory disease or to prevent and treat rejection after transplantation. Steroids increase catabolism and this in turn releases nitrogen from tissue, with a corresponding increase of urea. Elevated urea levels need then to be considered as acceptable.

In most cases treatment can continue, after correcting any of the dietary and/or metabolic aspects.

Energy

The amount of energy required for maintenance is just as important as the quantity and quality of the protein itself. Insufficient energy will lead to protein catabolism, a negative nitrogen balance, to protein and protein-energy malnutrition and weight loss.

Too much energy leading to obesity is equally undesirable, especially with replacement therapy in mind. The formation of a fistula becomes difficult and the possibility of further weight gain with PD is preventable. A low energy diet should then be considered at an early stage to achieve weight loss in preparation for RRT later on. The minimum requirement is not less than 30 kcal (126 kJ) for the 0.8–0.9 g kg^{-1} ibw diet for patients with a normal body mass index (BMI) range.

> Example: to calculate energy requirements for a 70-kg person (ideal weight):
> 70 × 35–30 kcal (150–126 kJ) = 2450–2100 kcal (14.7–8.8 mJ).

Carbohydrate (1 g equals 4 kcal (18 kJ))

Ideally, 50% of the dietary energy should be obtained from carbohydrate, the majority from starch and fibre-containing foods (i.e. wholemeal bread, whole grain cereals, biscuits, potatoes, brown rice and pasta and small amounts in vegetables and fruit). These foods contain some protein and some are high in potassium and need to be avoided in the case of hyperkalaemia.

Fat (1 g = 9 kcal (38 kJ)

Fat is a concentrated form of energy and makes food palatable, providing a feeling of satiety.

The recommended dietary guideline on the intake of fat is about 30–35% of the total energy intake. To achieve a satisfactory energy intake this figure needs to be increased for patients on a protein-restricted diet (1 g protein = 4 kcal (18 kJ); see Table 9.2).

Table 9.3 *Management of nephrotic syndrome*

- Treatment of hypertension
- Moderate protein restriction:
  - 0.8–1.0 g kg^{-1} ideal body weight (ibw)
  - adequate energy
- Treatment of hyperlipidaemia
  - manipulate fat intake
  - lipid lowering drugs

The nephrotic syndrome   The nephrotic syndrome is associated with proteinuria. The majority of the protein loss is albumin, but other proteins with an intermediate molecular weight are also secreted. These proteins bind nutrients, such as the iron, vitamin D, copper and zinc (Kaysen, 1992).

Hypoalbuminaemia can lead to severe fluid retention, which is difficult to treat by diuretic therapy and dietary sodium and/or fluid restriction alone.

Current practice is to optimise blood pressure control with angiotensin-converting enzyme (ACE) inhibitors and to normalise the dietary protein to 0.8–1.0 g kg^{-1} ibw and to modify the intake of energy to 35 kcal kg^{-1} ibw if the patient consumes a high protein diet and/or has a high or low energy intake (see Table 9.3).

The nephrotic syndrome is associated with hyperlipidaemia due to lipoprotein abnormalities. Hyperlipidaemia and proteinuria disappear when the nephrotic syndrome is successfully controlled.

General advice regarding weight loss would be to increase exercise, eliminate smoking and commence a low animal fat, low cholesterol diet which is high in polyunsaturates. This, together with lipid-lowering drugs, may help to reduce the long-term risk of CVD with a morbidity and mortality rate of > 50% in patients with CRF (Harris, 1994).

Sodium and Fluid

Mild to moderate sodium (Na) and fluid retention occurs in most types of renal disease and contributes to high blood pressure. Diuretic drug treatment controls fluid retention by increasing Na and fluid excretion (urine).

A moderate salt-restricted diet (about 80–100 mmol Na) will help to prevent excessive accumulation of Na. In practice this means very simple advice:

- Use a little salt in meal preparation.
- Avoid adding salt to food after preparation.
- Avoid excessive amounts of salty foods such as cured foods and convenience meals (see Appendix 9.1).

- Avoid monosodium glutamate. This is added liberally to enhance the taste of Chinese, Asian and other Far Eastern meals.

Patients diagnosed as 'salt losers' need to add salt to their meals and/or use salt supplements, such as Slow Sodium. One Slow Sodium tablet equals 10 mmol Na and can be replaced by 1 OXO cube, containing 26 mmol Na.

Potassium

Body stores

The total amount of potassium (K) found in a healthy individual is about 50 mmol kg^{-1}. About 98% (140 mmol l^{-1}) is found in the intracellular and the remaining 2% in the extracellular fluid (4–5 mmol l^{-1}).

Intake

Depending on the dietary intake, approximately 100 mmol K is absorbed from the food and about 90% is excreted by the kidneys. The remainder is excreted via the gastrointestinal route. The intracellular potassium uptake is mediated by insulin.

Hyperkalaemia

Progressive renal failure is often complicated by hyperkalaemia, a potassium level of > 6.0–6.5 mmol l^{-1}, and may occur when renal function has declined to a glomerular filtration rate (GFR) of 5 ml min^{-1} with normal urine output. Severe hyperkalaemia can also occur at an earlier stage when patients receive ACE inhibitors for blood pressure control combined with a high intake of potassium-rich foods.

This is potentially life threatening, is not associated with physical warning signs and requires immediate treatment. Dietary and non-dietary causes for hyperkalaemia should both be investigated at the same time (Bansal, 1992).

A dietary intake of no more than 60–70 mmol day^{-1} (1 mmol kg^{-1} ibw) is sufficient to prevent or treat hyperkalaemia by dietary means in the presence of an adequate urine output or dialysis treatment. However, serum K levels in anuric non-dialysed patients would rise by 1 mmol day^{-1} despite gastrointestinal adaption to eliminate dietary K in CRF.

Examples of non-dietary hyperkalaemia are:

- metabolic acidosis;
- increased catabolism;
- endocrine abnormalities;
- drugs such as potassium supplements (i.e. Slow K), potassium-sparing diuretics (i.e. Frumil K), ACE inhibitors, non-steroidal anti-inflammatory drugs (NSAIDS) and cyclosporin;
- excessive exercise, heat stroke and rhabdomyelosis cause hyperkalaemia due to tissue cell destruction (Bansal, 1992);

- blood used for transfusions can contain up to 30 mmol l^{-1} potassium, if stored for too long.

Potassium exchange resins

Potassium binders such as calcium or sodium ion exchange resin (i.e. calcium- or sodium resonium) may be used to control hyperkalaemia. Calcium ions are exchanged for K ions in the gut and the potassium salt is then eliminated.

Calcium resonium is a gritty textured powder, to be taken in measures of 15 g once, twice or three times daily. The resin is best taken with a low K, sweet soft drink to mask its taste. The long-term use of calcium resonium should be reconsidered in order to prevent severe constipation, unless appropriate laxatives are prescribed (check K content of laxatives and bulking agents). Calcium resonium may be administered rectally in cases of oral intolerance. The dose is doubled to achieve the same effect as oral administration.

Most foods contain K, but the majority is found in vegetables and fruits, some varieties containing more than others. Staple foods such as potatoes, yam, sweet potatoes, green bananas and plantain contain a lot of K, but can be included in a K-restricted diet. Potassium is also found in salt substitutes whereby the sodium component is replaced by K. Potassium-containing salts, such as dipotassium phosphate, are used as food additives but in small quantities. Dietary K restriction may be initiated either to prevent or to treat hyperkalaemia alongside correcting other reasons for hyperkalaemia.

Patients should receive dietary advice regarding the K content of specific foods, avoiding high K foods and including fruit and vegetable portion exchanges, depending on their low, medium or high K content (see Appendix 9.2).

Some K can be removed by the process of leaching. The most effective procedure for removing K from potatoes (a high K staple food) is the double cooking technique, whereby the water is exchanged for fresh half way during boiling. Cooking until 'ready' is sufficient and retains the quality of boiled potatoes. This method removes 72% of K but nutrient losses, such as that of vitamin C, are likely (Bower, 1989).

Potassium and high-fibre foods

Constipation is a problem for sedentary and continuous ambulatory peritoneal dialysis (CAPD) patients especially. High-fibre cereal products are recommended to control constipation and hyperlipidaemia. High-fibre foods are also high in K and some is absorbed, although it is unclear what percentage is available for absorption in the gut (Pagenkemper et al., 1994). The overall effect of a high-fibre diet on serum K levels is not significant, about 0.3 mmol l^{-1} (McKenzie and Henderson, 1986).

In considering the benefits and possible side-effects, one should remember that high-fibre cereal products improve bowel habits, contributing to the medical and general well-being of patients on dialysis treatment.

Phosphorus

Renal osteodystrophy

The balance between calcium (Ca) and phosphorus (P) is carefully maintained in health. Ca and P are the main substances of bone tissue. The formation of growth and the maintenance of healthy bone tissue is mediated by the active vitamin D3 metabolite 1,25-$(OH)_2$ D3 called calcitriol, by increasing the absorption of Ca from food.

Ca and P are obtained from foods with a high protein content. Examples are milk and its products, hard cheese being especially rich in Ca and P. P also appears in fibre-rich cereal foods and fish with edible bones.

Vitamin D3 is obtained from food (i.e. added to margarine and butter) and exposure to sunlight. Vitamin D3 is converted by the kidneys to its active metabolite.

Renal osteodystrophy (ROD) is a major long-term problem of CRF and undetected chronic hyperphosphataemia is one of several causes. There are two types of ROD:

- high-turnover osteodystrophy associated with hyperparathyroidism;
- low-turnover osteodystrophy as seen with a dynamic bone disease in CAPD patients.

In CRF, the balance between calcitriol, Ca and P is disrupted as vital functions fail:

- the conversion of vitamin D3 to its active form calcitriol;
- impairment in the Ca and P balance caused by a reduced phosphate excretion as renal function declines. Hyperparathyroidism further contributes to hyperphosphataemia as P is released from high bone turnover.
- A high Ca to P ratio (Ca × P product > 5.0 mmol l^{-1}) may eventually lead to secondary soft tissue and vascular calcification.

Management of hyperphosphataemia

Hyperphosphataemia starts to occur when renal function is reduced to 25% or less. This equals a serum creatinine level of 250 µmol l^{-1} (Coburn and Salusky, 1989). Abnormalities in bone histology can already be demonstrated when GFR falls to 50% or less of normal, although patients are clinically asymptomatic.

Hypocalcaemia develops progressively alongside and is due to a reduction in gastrointestinal Ca absorption from food due to calcitriol deficiency.

Therefore, hypocalcaemia can be treated by controlling hyperphosphataemia, maintaining normal Ca levels with calcitriol administration.

Hyperparathyroidism is a result of hyperphosphataemia and insufficient circulating 1,25 vitamin.

The overproduction of parathyroid hormone causes excess calcium release from bone tissue leading to 'brittle bones'.

ROD develops over many years but can be prevented by starting dietary P restriction and Ca CO_3-based phosphate binders to prevent hyperphosphataemia early in addition to calcitriol drug therapy, normalising serum levels of 1,25 D3.

Treatment with calcitriol is only successful when serum phosphate levels remain within acceptable levels (Slatopolsky and Delmez, 1996).

Dietary Management

Hypocalcaemia   The recommended Ca intake for predialysis patients is 1000–1500 mg daily. A protein- and/or phosphate-restricted diet tends to be Ca deficient as foods with a high P content are rich in Ca. Ca supplements (i.e. calcium carbonate) should be taken away from food, preferably at bedtime to maximise Ca absorption in addition to calcitriol drug therapy.

Hyperphosphataemia   Hyperphosphataemia is difficult to control by dietary manipulation alone and needs to be combined with phosphate binders.

Dialysis helps to eliminate P, but as dietary protein requirements increase, so the intake of P will rise proportionally. Dietary P restriction reduces the intake of protein when prescribed during the predialysis phase of CRF.

Avoid foods with a high phosphorus content in addition to a moderate protein restriction. Foods with a high P content like some types of hard cheese, excessive amounts of milk, yoghurt and foods containing milk or milk powder should either be eliminated or form part of the dietary P intake and phosphate binders prescription (see Appendix 9.3).

Phosphate binders   Calcium carbonate is an effective phosphate-binding agent. It produces a beneficial rise in serum Ca and bicarbonate levels in predialysis patients (Williams et al., 1989). Phosphate binding occurs in the gut. P from food forms with Ca (or aluminium (Al)) from the binders an insoluble salt and this product is eliminated via the gastrointestinal route.

Phosphate binders should be taken with food, main meals in particular and with snacks containing P, such as nutritional supplements containing milk.

Al-containing phosphate binders are not routinely prescribed and may cause aluminum bone disease if incorrectly prescribed and taken by the patient. However, $Al(OH)_3$ is a very potent binder and can be used for a short period to lower serum phosphate levels, which can then be maintained with calcium carbonate.

To minimise the risk of hyperphosphataemia the following principles should be observed (Vennegoor and Nunan, 1990):

- Restrict the dietary intake of P to 0.5 mmol (15 mg) kg^{-1} ibw.
- Individualise the prescription for phosphate binders. Phosphate binders should supplement a P-restricted diet, to minimise the dose required and not become the sole form of treatment. Ideally, the renal dietitian plays an important role to adapt the dose of phosphate binders to the P content of the diet and help promote diet and drug compliance.
- Change partly to $Al(OH)_3$ combined with $CaCO_3$ or consider calcium acetate as an alternative phosphate binder, which appears more effective than $CaCO_3$. Monitor progress and return to $CaCO_3$ once the patient's P levels have improved.
- Monitor Al levels at regular intervals if Al-containing binders are used for a longer period.
- Avoid prescribing iron (Fe) supplements with phosphate-binding agents as it impairs Fe absorption.
- Avoid calcium citrate as Al absorption from food containing some Al is enhanced. Al toxicity can still develop over a long period of time.
- The treatment of hyperphosphataemia should be approached at a multi-disciplinary level.

Foods with a high fibre content It has been suggested earlier that increasing the dietary intake of fibre improves bowel habits and the general well-being of patients. Serum phosphate levels may slightly rise by 0.25 mmol l^{-1} (Pender, 1989); however, the benefits of a high fibre intake outweigh the risk of hyperphosphataemia, which can be treated by increasing phosphate-binding agents.

Magnesium Magnesium (Mg) is retained with impaired kidney function. Mg-containing antacids to relieve gastrointestinal problems are potent phosphate binders, but may cause diarrhoea.

Other Important Nutrients

Iron

A low protein intake may cause iron (Fe) deficiency. Fe supplements are essential to correct anaemia in patients on RHuEPO.

Abnormal ferritin levels will indicate Fe deficiency. As a guide, some patients may need an oral supplement of 200–300 mg Fe day^{-1} to restore Fe status when on HD or PD with a serum ferritin level of < 100 ng ml^{-1}

or a relative Fe deficiency with a transferrin saturation of < 20% (Makoff, 1992).

Avoid prescribing Fe supplement with phosphate binders; these should be taken separately (i.e. bedtime).

Fe should be taken in combination with folate, pyridoxine (B6), B12 and vitamin C (see below).

Lastly, hyperparathyroidism may blunt the response to RHuEPO.

Zinc

Meat, fish, pulses and wheat products are rich in zinc (Zn). Zn deficiency may occur in patients taking insufficient protein before or during dialysis. This could be treated with supplements if Zn deficiency has been established.

Vitamins

CRF causes abnormalities in the effective levels of water-soluble vitamins. This is due to abnormal patterns of vitamin absorption and excretion, interaction of metabolites and toxins, and the protein binding of certain vitamins may be abnormal (Makoff, 1991).

The ideal supplement should contain all vitamins of the B group, including folic acid and vitamin C in a moderate dose. The intake of vitamin C will be reduced once hyperkalaemia prevents the intake of sufficient fresh vegetables and fruit.

Too much vitamin C can eventually lead to oxalosis. Vitamin C provides 30–50% of the daily endogenous production of oxalic acid and the excess is excreted by the kidneys. Renal patients retain oxalic acid as calcium oxalate. An increased amount of this product is found in soft tissue, such as muscle tissue, and vital organs, such as the heart and kidneys.

Vitamin supplements containing vitamin A and D are contraindicated in patients with CRF. The vitamin A metabolites are less well excreted and accumulate over time. The 1,25 D3 vitamin is the only form of any use to this group of patients. These must be used under close medical supervision only. Table 9.4 lists the recommended vitamin requirements in conservative and dialysis treatment (Kopple, 1981).

DIETARY MANAGEMENT OF RENAL REPLACEMENT THERAPY

During the predialysis period, patients with ESRF will receive information on HD, PD and transplantation (TLN). Changing these modes of treatment will be necessary when one of these therapies fails and any specific dietary requirements need then to be adjusted.

Table 9.4 *Recommended daily supplement (Kopple, 1981)*

Water-soluble vitamins	
Thiamine (B1)	1.5 mg
Ribiflavin (B2)	1.8 mg
Pantothenic acid	5.0 mg
Niacin	20.0 mg
Pyridoxine	5.0 mg
Vitamin B12	3.0 μg
Ascorbic acid (vitamin C)	70–100 mg
Folic acid	1.0 mg
Fat-soluble vitamins	
Vitamin A	None
Vitamin D	Calcitriol as required
Vitamin E	?
Vitamin K	None

Table 9.5 *Dietary recommendations for patients on renal replacement therapy*

	Haemodialysis (HD)	Continuous ambulatory peritoneal dialysis (CAPD)	Transplantation (TLN)
Protein (g kg^{-1} ibw)	1.0–1.2	1.1–1.3	1.0
Energy (kcal kg^{-1} ibw)	RDA	RDA-400	RDA
Carbohydrate (%)	50	35	50
Fat (%)	35	30	35
Na (mmol kg^{-1} ibw)	1.0	1.5	1.0–1.5
K (mmol kg^{-1} ibw)	1.0	1.2	Free
P (mg)	1000	1200	Free/supplement
Vitamins (H$_2$O soluble)	Renal	Renal	NA
PO$_4$ binders	Yes	Yes	NA

NA, not applicable; ibw, ideal body weight.

Current recommendations for dietary requirements for HD, PD, and TLN are shown in Table 9.5.

Protein Requirements

During dialysis all water-soluble products, such as urea, creatinine, K, Na and fluid, phosphates and other waste are removed. Nutrients such as amino acids and vitamins of the B complex and C are also water soluble.

During HD approximately 8–12 g amino acids are lost per treatment. The normal recommended intake of protein is 1.0 g protein kg⁻¹ ibw. A supplement of 0.1–0.2 g kg⁻¹ is needed to cover these losses. Therefore, the recommended intake of protein for HD patients totals 1.2 g kg⁻¹ ibw.

During PD, a mean of 9 g albumin (Ab) is lost daily in addition to 5 g amino acids. About two-thirds of this protein is Ab. There may be a 10-fold difference in protein losses between patients and this is dependent on the molecular weight of the protein, the permeability of the peritoneal membrane, the composition of the dialysate, and serum protein concentration, as well as clinical status (Kopple and Blumenkrantz, 1983).

During peritonitis, protein losses increase due to changes in the permeability of the membrane. This should correct once the peritonitis has been treated.

Nephrotic and diabetic patients suffer the greatest losses, as proteinuria continues to exist until renal function ceases.

The protein requirement for a patient with a good functioning transplant returns to normal: 1.0 g kg⁻¹ ibw to be reduced once again in the case of TLN failure (Pagenkemper and Foulks, 1991).

Energy Requirements

The energy requirement for HD and TLN can be adapted to recommended values for age and activity. Patients on dialysis need 20–25 kcal kg⁻¹ to lose weight and 45–50 kcal kg⁻¹ to gain weight.

The energy intake for PD may need to be adapted as dialysate glucose could provide 700 kcal of the total energy intake, depending on the strength of the solution. The recommended energy intake for a non-obese, non-malnourished CAPD patient is therefore 35 kcal kg⁻¹ ibw to maintain ideal body weight and this includes energy obtained from dialysate (Lindholm and Bergstrom, 1989).

Potential energy uptake from peritoneal dialysate
Up to 70% of glucose may be absorbed from the dialysate (Kopple and Blumenkrantz, 1983).

  2 l isotonic (1.36% dextrose) dialysate contains 27 g glucose.
  2 l medium strength (2.27% dextrose) dialysate contains 45 g glucose.
  2 l strong (3.86% dextrose) dialysate contains 67 g glucose.

Assuming that 70% of glucose is absorbed, the non-dietary energy supply may be as follows: 76 kcal for isotonic, 182 kcal for medium strength and 308 kcal for the strong 2-l bag of dialysate.

A patient receiving the following dialysis prescription may receive:

- 4×2 l isotonic dialysate = 4×76 kcal = 302 kcal or
- 3×2 l isotonic plus ⎤ 410 kcal or
  1×2 l medium strong ⎦
- 3×2 l isotonic plus ⎤ 536 kcal or
  1×2 l strong   ⎦
- 4×2 l isotonic plus ⎤ 612 kcal
  1×2 l strong   ⎦

Sodium

The intake of sodium (Na) may need to be reduced to control thirst with a fluid-restricted diet. Patients with a good urine output do not need to drastically reduce their salt intake.

A restriction of 80–100 mmol day^{-1} is usually sufficient to control thirst and helps the patient to manage their fluid restriction.

Foods with a very high salt content are to be avoided. Very little salt should be added to food during the cooking process and it should be avoided after preparation (see Appendix 9.1).

Fluid

The intake of fluid needs to be restricted as the patient's urine output reduces.

Until recently, an interdialytic weight gain (IDWG) in excess of 1.5–2.0 kg was considered unacceptable. Studies in recent years have found little or no relationship between IDWG and predialysis or interdialytic blood pressure. Sherman found that IDGW affected predialysis blood pressure in less than 25% of patients (Sherman et al., 1993). Excessive weight gain complicates dialysis with symptomatic hypotension and cramps. An IDGW of 2.5–3.0 kg could be acceptable for the larger patient.

A daily fluid allowance of 500 ml plus the volume of urine from the previous day is usually sufficient to prevent severe fluid overload.

The restriction of fluid is one of the most difficult parts of the dialysis diet for the patient to adhere to. Up to 86% of patients may exceed the fluid weight guideline of 1.5 kg and diabetics do not differ from non-diabetic patients (Halverson et al., 1993). A multidisciplinary approach to this aspect of general management is essential, as patients are often confused between flesh and fluid weight.

$$\text{Flesh weight} + \text{Fluid weight} = \text{Total weight.}$$

Some hints for fluid control

- Avoid salt and highly salted foods.
- Avoid meals prepared with monosodium glutamate (i.e. Chinese, Asian and other Far Eastern meals).

- Measure the fluid allowance in a water jug.
- Divide the fluid allowance during the whole day, using small cups (150 ml each) instead of mugs (250 ml each). Drink only ½ cup each time.
- Ice cubes may be more thirst quenching, but each cube equals 30 ml fluid (two tablespoons).
- Rinse the mouth with water, gargle, but do not swallow.
- Stimulate saliva production by sucking slices of lemon, sherbets or chewing gum.
- Take medicines with the main meals unless contraindicated.
- When going out, save the allowance of fluid. This allows for an extra drink(s) when socialising.
- A patient may be preoccupied by the desire for fluid. It is important to keep occupied.
- A daily weight check will reveal the rate of fluid accumulation in between HD treatments and fluid status of PD.

Potassium

The risk of hyperkalaemia is higher in anuric patients. The dietary intake of K should be reduced to 1.0 mmol kg^{-1} ibw for intermittent HD and to 1.2 mmol kg^{-1} ibw daily for CAPD patients.

Most patients starting dialysis continue to produce good quantities of urine and this helps with the excretion of Na and K. At this time, it may be possible to relax the intake of Na, fluid and K but urine output must be monitored regularly. Dietary K, salt and fluid restrictions should then be adapted as the urine output diminishes.

Hyperkalaemia is a frequent problem, especially with HD, and dietary indiscretion is partly to blame. The amount of K removed during dialysis can vary as much as 71%.

Inadequate dialysis and non-selective beta-blockers (e.g. propanolol) also contribute to hyperkalaemia.

Some HD patients consume foods with a high K content during the first or second hour of dialysis. The transit of food and fluid through the gastro-intestinal tract may take 9–12 h before any of the nutrients and fluid are absorbed in the blood stream (Gardner, 1979). This means that the K in food consumed during the early part of dialysis will not be removed during dialysis.

Foods with a high K content should be avoided when dietary intake of K needs to be adjusted (see Appendix 9.2).

Phosphorus

The recommended intake is approximately 1000 mg (33 mmol day^{-1}) for HD and 1200 mg (40 mmol day^{-1}) for CAPD, to prevent hyperphosphataemia.

Table 9.6 *Dietary phosphorus intake versus treatment*

Treatment	Protein (g)	Phosphorus (mg)	Clearance
Conservative	0.8–1.0	800	Poor
Haemodialysis (HD)	1.0–1.2	1000	24 mmol protein week^{-1}
Continuous ambulatory peritoneal dialysis (CAPD)	1.1–1.3	1200	70 mmol protein week^{-1}
Transplantation (TLN)	1.0	Free	Sufficient

Dietary P restriction combined with phosphate binders and dialysis helps to prevent severe hyperphosphataemia (see Appendix 9.3).

Table 9.6 shows the dietary P intake versus modes of treatment. P depends on protein intake and the removal of P depends on mode of dialysis.

With a daily dietary intake of 1000 mg (32 mmol) P, only 3×240 mg (8 mmol) P is removed by HD three times per week (= 24 mmol). This is a net gain of 200 mmol week^{-1}.

With PD, the dietary intake is 1200 mg (39 mmol) daily, while only 300 mg (10 mmol) is removed daily by CAPD (= 70 mmol). This is a net gain of 203 mmol week^{-1}. Thus, the net gain of P can only be controlled by using appropriate phosphate binders.

Vitamins

It is recommended that dialysis patients should supplement their water-soluble vitamin intake. Table 9.4 lists the recommended intake of vitamins for dialysis patients (Makoff, 1992).

Erythropoietin (EPO)

Patients on RHuEPO treatment experience an improved feeling of well-being and an improvement in nutritional status (Bennett *et al.*, 1991).

In addition to haemoglobin measurements, ferritin levels should also be monitored to detect possible Fe depletion causing failure to respond to RhuEPO. Ferritin levels can be raised by providing Fe supplements together with folic acid, vitamin C and vitamin B12 (Makoff, 1992) (see Chapter 6).

PRESCRIPTION DIALYSIS

Urea Kinetic Modelling in HD and PD

Urea Kinetic Modelling (UKM) is used to prescribe dialysis treatment, using noted formulas. UKM includes the calculation of protein catabolic rate

(PCR). Malnourished patients can be easily identified, alerting dietitians to spend time on those that are at risk (Goldstein and Frederico, 1987).

Urea Reduction Rate (URR)

This is an alternative method of calculating dialysis adequacy.

Method

$$URR = \frac{predialysis\ urea - postdialysis\ urea}{divided\ by\ the\ predialysis\ urea.}$$

A urea reduction ratio of 50% = Kt/V of 0.8 and each additional 5% reduction equals an increase of the Kt/V by 0.2.

Ideally, the percentage should be 70–75% per HD treatment. This equals a Kt/V of 1.4 (Lowrie and Lew, 1991).

There are pros and cons to both methods of assessing the quality of dialysis. Table 9.7 shows the relationship between the two types of assessments compared to mortality rates.

Table 9.7 *Relationship between urea reduction rate (URR),* Kt/V *and mortality.*

(URR) (%)	Kt/V	Mortality (%)
50	0.82	25
60	1.05	22
70	1.40	17

These figures are derived from several databases in the USA (Boag, 1994).

MALNUTRITION

Malnutrition is recognised as a common and important problem amongst dialysis patients and contributes to morbidity and mortality. It is a preventable condition. In dialysis patients malnutrition is linked to inadequate dialysis but also with the loss of renal function and failure to adjust the dialysis prescription.

Approximately 47% of HD patients and 44% of PD patients are clinically malnourished (Marckman, 1988). This must be corrected to avoid preventable morbidity and mortality related to malnutrition and inadequate dialysis. For instance, each $10\,\mathrm{g\,l^{-1}}$ decrease in serum albumin levels increases the likelihood for hospitalisation and in diabetics, this is 10-fold (Spiegel *et al.*, 1993).

Consequences of Malnutrition

Malnutrition is associated with:

- delayed wound healing;
- decreased resistance to infection;
- electrolyte imbalance;
- prolonged hospitalisation increasing the cost of treatment.

There are several reasons for malnutrition in dialysis patients and these are multifactorial, leading to protein and/or protein-energy malnutrition.

Reasons for Malnutrition

Reduced dietary intake

- Existing malnutrition at the start of dialysis due to uraemia and unsupervised predialysis dietary restriction.
- Inadequate dietary nutrient intake. Most patients consume less protein than is recommended. This may not always lead to a negative nitrogen balance in stable patients, and some patients achieve this on a protein intake of $0.7\,g\,kg^{-1}$ ibw day^{-1} with a high energy consumption of 35–$38\,kcal\,kg^{-1}$ ibw day^{-1} (Bergstrom, 1993).
- Conflicting dietary recommendations: increase in protein, while reducing dietary phosphorus.
- Financial constraints.

Reduced appetite

- Inadequate dialysis, leading to uraemic symptoms.
- Suppression of appetite due to glucose absorption with PD, intra-abdominal compression and constipation.
- Chronic depression.
- Coexisting gastrointestinal disease and comorbidity such as cardiac failure and cancer.
- Prolonged hospitalisation contributing to an inadequate nutritional intake.

Increased nutritional losses

- Water-soluble nutrient losses such as albumin, amino acid and vitamin losses during dialysis.
- Persistent proteinuria.

Altered metabolism

- Protein degradation as a result of the dialysis process (HD).
- Untreated acidosis contributes to protein catabolism.

Assessing the Nutritional Status of Dialysis Patients Using Subjective Global Assessment

It is important to identify malnutrition early to rehabilitate the patient early and to improve the clinical outcome.

Subjective global assessment (SGA) classifies patients in three groups: well nourished, mildly malnourished or suspected of malnutrition, and severely malnourished.

Treatment of Malnutrition

Intervention should start as soon as malnutrition is identified. This consists of dietary review and counselling by an experienced renal dietitian who will:

- increase the existing dietary prescription as required;
- modify its consistency if chewing and/or swallowing are a problem;
- gradually motivate the patient to improve their appetite if active depression is an underlying cause of inadequate intake;
- introduce nutritional support at an early stage;
- monitor progress frequently.

NUTRITIONAL SUPPORT

Methods of Nutritional Support

- Oral or sip feeding for patients who are able to eat and drink normally.
- Nasogastric or gastrostomy feeding for patients who are unable or unwilling to eat or drink normally. Oral and tube feeding can be combined, for instance tube feeding overnight, while the patient sleeps, and normal eating/drinking during the day.
- Intraperitoneal nutrition on PD (IPN).
- Interdialysis parenteral nutrition during HD (IDPN).
- Total parenteral nutrition (TPN) for patients who are unable to receive oral/sip or enteral methods of nutritional support.

Nasogastric and sip feeding
Concentrated oral supplements could be used once malnutrition is diagnosed and these should be prescribed as a medicine.

Table 9.8 Commercial nutritional products for sip or tube feeding

Product per unit	Energy (kcal)	Protein (g)	K (mmol)	P (mg)
[1]Nepro (237 ml)	475	17	6	171
[1]Suplena (237 ml)	475	7	7	173
[1]Ensure Plus (200 ml)	300	13	9	212
[2]Entera (200 ml)	300	11	9	103
[3]Fortisip (200 ml)	300	10	8	100
[2]Protein Forte (200 ml)	200	20	8	200
[4]Maxijul (200 ml)	400	—	—	—

[1]Ross/Abbott Ltd;
[2]Fresenius Ltd;
[3]Cow and Gate Nutricia Ltd;
[4]Scientific Hospital Supplies Ltd.

The insertion of a percutaneous enteral gastrostomy feeding tube enables long-term tube feeding without the discomfort of a nasogastric feeding tube.

The manufacturers of nutritional support products have improved their range for oral consumption and enteral tube-feeding products. The high protein and energy-dense products are best for the anuric patient requiring additional support, while patients on PD would benefit from high protein formulas. Low volume enteral tube feeding regimes can be made to the patient's individual needs. These are highly viscous and need the assistance of a special feeding pump for tube feeding. Some formulas available are shown in Table 9.8.

Nutritional peritoneal dialysis

Recent studies indicate that using dialysate with a 1.1% amino acid concentration, providing a net gain of 18 g amino acids in 2 l dialysate, improves the nutritional status of PD patients (see Chapter 8).

Interdialysis parenteral nutrition (IDPN)

Parenteral formulas containing approximately 65–70 g protein and 1000 kcal (mainly glucose) can be delivered during HD treatment. Glucose monitoring during treatment is essential to prevent hyperglycaemia. The fluid balance can be adjusted accordingly. It is a useful mode of nutritional support for patients for whom other forms of nutritional support have failed or are contraindicated (Seeley, 1993).

Monitoring Nutritional Support

Biochemistry

Serum albumin   Patients with a chronic illness or underlying liver disease are not expected to show an improvement in serum albumin (S-Ab) levels until recovery takes place.

    S-Ab levels depend on fluid status and will be lower in fluid overloaded patients.

Serum C-reactive protein   Until recent S-Ab levels were considered to be a marker of nutritional status and an indicator for survival. Serum C-reactive protein (CRP) levels rise with inflammation infection and tissue damage. When S-Ab levels are corrected for CRP, S-Ab loses its significance as a nutritional marker (Bergstrom et al., 1995).

Anthropometric measurements

Weight loss of more than 10% in less than 3 months is a nutritional risk factor. If available, anthropometric measurements are useful to assess lean body mass. The patient will be their own control but fluid status can flaw the results. It is therefore necessary to perform these measurements *after* dialysis. Fistula arms should not be used to perform these measurements.

    There are limitations to anthropometry, due to observer error, instrument error and recording techniques. Other considerations are errors related to patients' status and interpretation of measurements. Anthropometry should therefore only be measured by well-trained personnel (Nelson, 1991).

QUALITY STANDARDS FOR DIALYSIS PATIENTS

Table 9.9 shows recommended nutritional standards for dialysis patients. These are based on the publications of the The Health Care Finance Administration in the USA (Medford, 1992). The British Renal Association and Royal College of Physicians (1995) issued standards and audit measures to guarantee adequate treatment. The second revised edition is due for publication during 1997. The Nutritional Standards produced by the Renal Nutrition Group of the British Dietetic Association will also be issued during 1997.

TRANSPLANTATION

Some nutritional problems occurring after transplantation are specific to immune suppressive therapy. Side-effects include protein hypercatabolism, obesity, hyperlipidaemia, glucose intolerance (steroid-induced diabetes),

Table 9.9 *Nutritional standards for patients on renal replacement therapy*

	Haemodialysis (HD)	Continuous ambulatory peritoneal dialysis (CAPD)
Albumin $(g\,l^{-1})$	>35	>35
Urea $(mmol\,l^{-1})$	20–30	20–30
K $(mmol\,l^{-1})$	>3.5–6.5	>3.5–6.5
P $(mmol\,l^{-1})$	1.1–2.0	1.1–2.0
Ca $(mmol\,l^{-1})$	2.12–2.60	2.12–2.60
Urea kinetic modelling (UKM) (Kt/V)	>1.2–1.4 per treatment	1.7 per week
Urea reduction rate (URR)	70–75%	

hyperkalaemia and interference with the action of vitamin D. Post-transplantation dietary treatment should be taken into consideration.

Protein

The immediate post-transplant recommended intake of protein ranges between 1.3 and 1.5 g kg^{-1} ibw, to a maintenance protein intake of 1.0 g kg^{-1} ibw. The protein intake may need to be reduced with transplant failure (Pagenkemper and Foulks, 1991).

Energy

Obesity is common with a successful transplant and is multifactorial:

- the patient's appetite increases due to an increased feeling of well-being;
- steroids stimulate the patient's appetite;
- lack of exercise.

Obesity contributes to hypertension, hyperlipidaemia and these in turn to CVD.

Maintenance of ideal body weight for height can be achieved with an energy intake of 28–30 kcal kg^{-1} ibw. The patient should be made aware of the risk of obesity at an early stage.

Hyperlipidaemia Post-Transplantation

The majority of transplant patients show signs of hyperlipidaemia with elevated serum triglyceride and cholesterol levels. This is due to steroid and cyclosporin drug therapy causing glucose intolerance (insulin resistance) and hyperlipidaemia.

Table 9.10 *Recommendations for healthy eating*

Sources of energy:	
Carbohydrate:	50% of energy
	↑ Polysaccharides
	↓ Monosaccharides
	↑ Fibre
Fat:	30–35% of energy
	↓ Saturated fatty acids
	↑ monounsaturated fatty acids
	↑ polyunsaturated fatty acids

The effect of changing from saturated to unsaturated fat may not result in a change of serum lipid levels (Lawrence *et al.*, 1995).

Dietary treatment of hyperlipidaemia

Hyperlipidaemia is a common feature of the nephrotic syndrome and of PD. The latter is linked to continuous glucose absorption from the dialysate. It is obvious that patients with a long history of hypertension, hyperlipidaemia and diabetes are prone to CVD.

It is important that guidelines for healthy eating and regular excercise are incorporated whenever a renal patient is counselled for dietary advice (Table 9.10).

DIABETIC PATIENTS

One of the major complications of insulin-dependent diabetes mellitus (IDDM) is diabetic nephropathy (DN). It takes 10–20 years to develop and occurs in 30–40% of patients who will eventually require RRT.

DN is initially diagnosed when small quantities of protein are found in the urine (microproteinuria). Progression to macroproteinuria and ESRF can be delayed by early intervention, normalising hypertensive blood pressure and hyperglycaemia. Genetic predisposition, dietary protein intake, serum lipid levels and smoking may also influence the rate of progression. The higher rate of mortality compared to non-diabetic patients is mainly due to CVD.

Non-insulin dependent diabetes patients also develop DN. Most patients suffer from diabetic retinopathy. This further adds to the limitations of the diabetic patient and severely affects their quality of life.

Studies have shown that a moderate protein restriction (0.8 g kg^{-1} ibw) implemented early (Viberti *et al.*, 1993), together with optimal glucose and blood pressure control using ACE inhibitors, will reduce the decline in GFR (Stenvinkel, 1993).

Hyperlipidaemia is more common in IDDM and any dietary guidelines will include modification of fat intake. Also important is to reduce energy if the patient is overweight and to provide general advice on healthy eating and living (stop smoking and taking exercise).

Drugs to control hyperglycaemia will need to be adjusted regularly, as requirements diminish as renal function declines.

A renal diet combined with that of diabetes, hyperlipidaemia and possibly energy restriction to treat or prevent obesity is highly complex, needs dedication from the patient, family and carers, especially when started early when the patient feels relatively well.

Renal Replacement Therapy in Diabetic Patients

Diabetic renal patients can be treated as successfully as non-diabetics by HD, PD and TLN.

The dietary requirements are not different from non-diabetics (Nunan and Vennegoor, 1986). As with non-diabetic renal patients, dialysis is started early and the production of urine is an advantage. The disadvantage is that existing proteinuria will continue, resulting in an additional loss of protein and lower than acceptable S-Ab levels. These patients will benefit from protein-enriched nutritional supplements.

Glycaemic Control on Dialysis

Drugs used to lower blood sugar levels need to be adjusted to the patient's dietary intake on HD. The peritoneal dialysate prescription will also change the need for hypoglycaemic agents, depending on the dextrose content of the dialysate.

DIETARY MANAGEMENT IN PAEDIATRICS

CRF may present shortly after birth or later in life and can proceed into ESRF during childhood (Watson, 1991). The profound effects CRF can place upon growth (Hokken-Koelega, 1995) and development, particularly during infancy, necessitate nutritional management on a long-term basis. Fluctuating clinical and biochemical disturbances with changes in treatment require constant readjustment of the nutritional prescription by an experienced dietitian (Coleman, 1994). Infants may present with particular problems such as anorexia and vomiting, and an understanding of the psychosocial effects often proves to be as important as the dietary advice (Norman *et al.*, 1995).

Nutritional assessment should include the regular monitoring of growth and dietary analysis by means of food diaries. Biochemical assessment with frequent review of fluid balance and prescribed medication such as phosphate binders is recommended. The maintenance of normal serum calcium and phosphate levels is crucial to achieve normal bone development, and nutritional measures have a large part to play, particularly in controlling phosphate levels. The dietary aims in managing children with CRF are dependent upon age, stage of management and nutritional assessment.

Nutritional supplements, unlike specialist low protein products, are frequently used and should be encouraged orally. However, experience has shown that attempting to achieve adequate nutrition this way can be stressful for families.

A proactive approach to maintaining good nutrition and growth without the use of growth hormone has resulted in a programme of early dialysis in combination with nutritional support in our unit. Although nasogastric tubes are used successfully, supplementary feeding with use of a gastrostomy button device, particularly in children under 5 years of age, may be more suitable in the long term (Coleman and Watson, 1992). The button also provides a convenient route for the administration of medication, which has undoubted benefits for the child and family.

PD is the preferred dialysis treatment for children in most centres. It generally allows a more liberal diet when compared to HD. Performed overnight by an automatic cycling machine (continuous cyclic peritoneal dialysis – CCPD), often in combination with overnight feeding, it enables the child to be managed at home, attend school and be encouraged to participate in family meals.

Dialysis is seen only as a holding measure before TLN. It may be of benefit for those children who required nutritional support on dialysis to avoid using the existing tube route following TLN. Appetite is usually restored with good renal function and high dose corticosteroids. Post-TLN, energy intake may need to be restricted in some children to prevent rapid weight gain and a healthy eating diet should be encouraged with on-going dietetic advice.

Maintaining good nutrition in this group of children requires support from all members of the multidisciplinary team (Collier and Watson, 1994). Dietetic time to regularly attend ward rounds, outpatient clinics and psychosocial meetings is essential. Home and school visits with frequent telephone contact are invaluable supportive measures.

CONCLUSION

Advances in nephrology and dialysis technology have brought about an increase in the number of patients treated by RRT. These changes have created new challenges and opportunities for everyone involved in the care of renal patients.

In conservative management, prevention or a delay in progression to ESRF is important. Dietary treatment is important for several reasons:

- normalising protein intake or a moderate reduction in diabetic patients may help to reduce the decline in renal function;
- controlling the accumulation of urea, potassium and phosphates including the correction of metabolic acidosis;
- to prevent malnutrition prior to RRT.

The dietary requirements of RRT depend on the mode of treatment. Individualised dietary treatment is just as important as individual dialysis prescriptions in patients of all ages and cultural backgrounds.

Dietary manipulation to help prevent malnutrition, renal osteodystrophy and CVD is an important component of the general management of patients with ESRF.

REFERENCES

BANSAL, V.K. (1992) Potassium metabolism in renal failure: nondietary rationale for hyperkalemia. *Journal of Renal Nutrition*, **2**(3): 8–12.

BENNETT, S.E., EDMUNDS, M.E., FEEHALLY, J. AND WALLS, J. (1991) Nutritional status of hemodialysis patients receiving recombinant human erythropoietin therapy. *Journal of Renal Nutrition*, **1**(3): 125–9.

BERGSTROM, J., HEIMBURGER, O., LINDHOLM, B. AND QURESHI, A.R. (1995) Elevated serum C-reactive protein is a strong predictor of increased mortality and low serum albumin in haemodialysis (HD) patients. *JASN*, **6**(3): 573 (abstract).

BERGSTROM, J. (1993) Nutritional requirements of hemodialysis patients. In *Nutrition and the Kidney*. (W.E. Mitch and S. Klahi, eds). Boston: Little, Brown and Co. pp. 263–89.

BERLYNE, G.M. (1968) *A Course in Renal Disease*, 2nd edn. Blackwell Scientific Publications, Oxford.

BOAG, J.T. (1994) Basic truths in optimal hemodialysis. *Dialysis and Transplantation*, **23**(11): 636–42.

BOWER, J.A. (1989) Cooking for restricted potassium diets in dietary treatment of renal patients. *Journal of Human Nutrition and Dietetics*, **2**: 31–8.

BRENNER, B. (1983) Hemodynamically mediated glomerular injury and the progressive nature of kidney disease. *Kidney International*, **23**: 647–55.

BRITISH RENAL ASSOCIATION AND ROYAL COLLEGE OF PHYSICIANS (1995) *Treatment of adult patients with renal failure: Recommended standards and audit measures*. The Renal Association and the Royal College of Physicians of London, Royal College of Physicians Publication Unit, London.

COBURN, J.W. AND SALUSKY, I.B. (1989) Control of serum phosphorus in uremia (editorial). *New England Journal of Medicine*, **320**(17): 1140–1.

COLEMAN, J.E. (1994) The kidney. In *Clinical Paediatric Dietetics*, (eds V. Shaw and M. Lawson). Blackwell Scientific Publications, Oxford, pp. 125–43.

COLEMAN, J.E. AND WATSON, A.R. (1992) Gastrostomy buttons: The optimal route for nutritional support in children with chronic renal failure. *Journal of Renal Nutrition*, **2**(Suppl.): 21–6.

COLLIER, J. AND WATSON, A.R. (1994) Renal failure in children: specific consideration in management. In *Quality of Life Following Renal Failure* (eds H. McGee and C. Bradley). Harwood Academic Publishers, Chur, pp. 225–45.

GARDNER, J.L. (1979) The G.I. lag and its significance to the dialysis patient. *Dialysis and Transplantation*, **8**(2): 132–3.

GOLDSTEIN, D.J. AND FREDERICO, C.B. (1987) The effect of urea kinetic modeling on the nutrition management of hemodialysis patients. *Journal of the American Dietetic Association*, **87**(4): 474–9.

HALVERSON, N.A., WILKENS, K.G. AND WORTHINGTON-ROBERTS, B. (1993) Interdialytic fluid gains in diabetic patients receiving hemodialysis treatment. *Journal of Renal Nutrition*, **3**(1): 23–9.

HARRIS, K.P.G. (1994) Hyperlipidaemia of renal disease: a treatment dilemma? *EDTNA–ERCA Journal*, **XX**(3): 26–9.

HOKKEN-KOELEGA, A.C.S. (1995) Growth and growth promotion in children with renal disease. *Paediatrics*, **8**(2): 31–7.

KAYSEN, G.A. (1992) Nutritional management of nephrotic syndrome. *Journal of Renal Nutrition*, **2**(2): 50–8.

KLAHR, S., LEVEY, A.S., BECK, G.J. *et al.* (1994) The effects of dietary protein restriction and blood-pressure control on the progression of chronic renal disease. *New England Journal of Medicine*, **330**(13): 878–84.

KOPPLE, J.D. (1981) Nutritional therapy in kidney failure. *Nutrition Review* **39**(5): 193–206.

KOPPLE, J.D. AND BLUMENKRANTZ, M.J. (1983) Nutritional requirements for patients undergoing continuous ambulatory peritoneal dialysis. *Kidney International*, **24**(Suppl. 16): S295–302.

LAWRENCE, I.R., THOMSON, A., HARTLEY, G.H. *et al.* (1995) The effect of dietary intervention on the management of hyperlipidaemia in British renal transplant patients. *Journal of Renal Nutrition*, **5**(2): 73–7.

LEVEY, A.S., PEDRINI, M.T., LAU, J., CHALMERS, T.C. AND WANG, P.H. (1995) Effect of dietary protein restriction on the progression of non-diabetic renal disease: meta-analysis. *Nephrology Dialysis Transplantation*, **10**(6) Abstracts: 985.

LEVEY, A.S., BECK, G.J., CAGGIULA, A.W. *et al.* (1995) Trends towards a beneficial effect of a low protein diet during additional follow-up in the modification of diet in renal disease study. *EDTA–ERA* Abstracts: 985.

LINDHOLM, B. AND BERGSTROM, J. (1992) Nutritional aspects of peritoneal dialysis. *Kidney International*, **42**(Suppl. 38): 165–71.

LINDHOLM, B. AND BERGSTROM, J. (1989) Nutritional management of patients undergoing peritoneal dialysis. In *Peritoneal Dialysis* (ed. K.D. Nolph). Boston: Kluwer Academic, pp. 230–260.

LOWRIE, E.G. AND LEW, N. (1991) The urea reduction ratio (URR): a simple method for evaluating hemodialysis treatment. *Contemporary Dialysis and Nephrology*, **February**: 11–20.

MAKOFF, R. (1991) Water-soluble vitamin status in patients with renal disease treated with hemodialysis or peritoneal dialysis. *Journal of Renal Nutrition*, **1**(2): 56–73.

MAKOFF, R. (1992) The importance and use of iron supplementation in uremia. *Nephrology News & Issues*, **June**: 14–19.

MARCKMAN, P. (1988) Nutritional status of patients on hemodialysis and peritoneal dialysis. *Clinical Nephrology*, **29**(2): 75–8.

MARONI, B.J. (1994) Nutrition in the predialysis patient. *Dialysis and Transplantation*, **23**(2): 76–94.

MCKENZIE, S.I. AND HENDERSON, I.S. (1986) The effect of increased dietary fibre intake on regular haemodialysis patients. In *Aspects of Renal Care* Baillière Tindall, London, pp. 172–78.

MEDFORD, S. (1992) Medical review criteria – HCFA. *Journal of Renal Nutrition*, **2**(2): 77–8.

NATIONAL INSTITUTE OF HEALTH (1993) Morbidity and Mortality of Dialysis. *NIH Consens Statement* Nov 1–3, **11**(2): 1–33. National Library of Medicine, Office of Medical Applications of Research, National Institutes of Health, Bethesda, MD.

NELSON, E.E. (1991) Anthropomometry in the nutritional assessment of adults with end-stage renal disease. *Journal of Renal Nutrition*, **1**(4): 162–72.

NORMAN, L.J., COLEMAN, J.E. AND WATSON, A.R. (1995) Nutritional management in a child on chronic peritoneal dialysis; a team approach. *Journal of Human Nutrition*, **8**: 209–13.

NUNAN, T.O. AND VENNEGOOR, M.A.A. (1986) Dietary guidelines for the management of diabetic patients with chronic renal failure. *Diabetic Medicine*, **3**: 75–9.

PAGENKEMPER, J.J., BURKE, K.I., RODERICK, S.L., MARTIN, D.M. AND SHAVLIK, G.W. (1994) Potassium availability in selected bran products: implications for the renal patient. *Journal of Renal Nutrition*, **4**(1): 27–31.

PAGENKEMPER, J.J. AND FOULKS, C.J. (1991) Nutritional management of the adult renal transplant patient. *Journal for Renal Nutrition*, **1**(3): 119–24.

PENDER, F.T. (1989) The effect of increasing the dietary fibre content of diets of patients with chronic renal failure treated by haemodialysis at home. *Journal of Human Nutrition and Dietetics*, **2**: 423–7.

RAINE, A.E.G., MARGREITER, R., BRUNNER F.P. *et al.* (1992) Report on management of renal failure in Europe (xii, 1991) In *Nephrology, Dialysis, Transplantation*. Vol 7, Suppl 2. Oxford: Oxford University Press. pp. 13–19.

SEELEY, L. (1993) Intradialytic parenteral nutrition. In *Renal Handbook of Nutrition*. National Kidney Foundation/Council of Renal Nutrition of New England, USA. pp. 86–98.

SHERMAN, R.A., DANIEL, A. AND CODY, R.P. (1993) The effect of interdialytic weight gain on predialysis bloodpressure. *Journal of Artificial Organs*, **17**: 770–4.

SLATOPOLSKY, E. AND DELMEZ, J.A. (1996) Pathogenesis of secondary hyperparathyroidism. *Nephrology, Dialysis and Transplantation*, **11**(Suppl. 3): 130–5.

SNETSELAAR, L. (1990) MDRD study enters clinical phases. *Nephrology News and Issues*, **March**: 14–15.

SPIEGEL, D.M., ANDERSON, M., CAMPBELL, U. *et al.* (1993) Serum albumin: a marker for morbidity in peritoneal dialysis patients. *American Journal of Kidney Diseases*, **21**(1): 26–30.

STENVINKEL, P. (1993) Factors influencing the development and progression of diabetic nephropathy. *EDTNA–ERCA Journal*, **XIX**(4): 2–4.

VENNEGOOR, M.A.A.A. AND NUNAN, T.O. (1990) Recommendations to improve phosphate control in patients with chronic renal failure. *ERCA–EDTNA Journal*, **13**(March): 10–12.

VIBERTI, G.C., DODDS, R., EARLE, K. AND MATTOCK, M. (1993) Reduction of proteinuria and diminished glomerular filtration rate fall by low protein intake: long term effects. *XIIth International Congress of Nephrology*: p. 419 (abstract).

WATSON, A.R. (1991) Disorders of the urinary tract. In *Jolly's Diseases of Childhood*, 6 edn (ed. M.I. Levine). Blackwell Scientific Publication, Oxford, pp. 226–68.

WILLIAMS, B., VENNEGOOR, M.A.A.A., NUNAN, T.O. AND WALLS, J. (1989) The use of calcium carbonate to treat the hyperphosphataemia of chronic renal failure. *Nephrology Dialysis Transplantation*, **4**: 725–9.

APPENDIX 1

FOODS WITH A HIGH SODIUM (SALT) CONTENT

These foods should be taken in moderation with a sodium restricted diet.

Dairy Products

- Salted butter, margarine, low fat spreads. Use unsalted or salt reduced alternatives instead.
- All types of hard or soft cheeses (also high in phosphorus).

Meat and Meat Products

- Smoked and cured meats such as bacon, gammon, salt beef, corned beef, ham, tongue, black pudding, all types of sausages, pâtés.
- Meat pies, quiches and sausage rolls.
- Ready-to-cook meals or meals for reheating: frozen or purchased from supermarkets and take-away shops, e.g. as beefburgers, fish and (salted) chips, curries, and other meals.

Fish and Shell Fish

- All types of *smoked* fish or *dried* fish such as cod, haddock, kippers, bloaters, salmon, trout, mackerel.
- Canned fish in tomato sauce, oil or brine: salmon, sardines, herrings, tuna, anchovy.
- Shell fish: crab, lobster, crayfish, prawns, scampi, shrimps, cockles.
- Fish products: fish fingers, cakes, fish paste, fish roes.

Vegetables

- All canned vegetables (unless preserved without salt).
- Sauerkraut, instant potato powder, salted potato crisps.

Nuts

- Roasted and salted nuts, peanut butter.

Miscellaneous

- Salt, mayonnaise, salad dressings (unless home made).
- Bottled sauces, pickles.
- Canned, packet soups or ready made soups for reheating.
- Pasta sauce, curry paste, soya sauce.
- Meat or yeast extracts and bouillon cubes, packet gravy, gravy cubes or powders.
- All meals containing monosodium glutamate.
- Salted savoury snacks.

Asian Foods

- Papadums, samosas, savoury snacks, chutneys, pickles, chevra, Chana.

Greek Foods

- Taramasalata, canned vine leaves, houmous.

Chinese Foods:

- Dried fish, salted fish, dried shell fish or squid.
- Peking duck and similar products

(these foods may form part of Chinese-style diets).

It may not be possible to eliminate all above foods or meals, unless a low sodium alternative is available. A compromise may be reached by allowing some salty foods for sandwiches or main meals, but preparing the rest of the meals at home without salt. Adding herbs and spices during meal preparation or thereafter compensates for the loss of salt.

APPENDIX 2

FOODS WITH A HIGH POTASSIUM CONTENT

Snacks

- Bombay mix, curu snacks, peanuts and raisins, potato crisps, potato hoops, tortilla chips, Twiglets, vegetable samosas.

Sweets

- Chocolate, plain, milk or white, and all sweets containing chocolate or cocoa.
- Liquorice Allsorts, toffees, fudge and other sweets containing nuts, chocolate and dried fruit.

Beverages

- Herb teas brewed for a long period of time.
- Coffee in excess of one cup per day (either instant or fresh).
- Milk powder and drinks containing milk powder such as Ovaltine, Horlicks, Complan, Build up, drinking chocolate, milk shakes, Nutrament, cocoa powder.
- Fruit juices unless exchanged for fruit, tomato juice, carrot juice, vegetable juice, cane sugar juice, pomegranate juice, guava, mango and lychee juice.
- Strong ale (e.g. Guinness).

Fruit (See also Fruit Exchange List)

- Avocado pear, banana, fresh black or redcurrants.
- Dried fruit such as dried apples, dried apricots, dried banana chips, currants, dates, dried figs, prunes, raisins, sultanas and other dried fruits.

Nuts

- All types of nuts, including peanut butter and marzipan.
- All types of seeds such as sesame seeds. Chocolate and nut spread.

Vegetables

- Ackee, Jerusalem artichokes, beetroot (only as part of a salad), mushrooms in excess, spinach, celeriac, squash, grilled or fried tomatoes, fried onions in excess, potato waffles.
- Plantain and green bananas in small portions only to replace potatoes.
- Sun-dried tomatoes.
- Dried pulses such as dried beans, red kidney beans, broad beans, butter beans, black eyed beans, dried peas, chick peas, lentils.

Vegetables which can be taken instead of potatoes
- Yam, sweet potato and pulse vegetables and parsnips.
- Green banana and plantain in small amounts (half the amount of the potato allowance).

Cereals

- All bran, branflakes, oatbran flakes, Fruit and Fibre, oat and wheat bran, Raisin Splitz, Shredded Sultana Bran.

Cakes and Biscuits

- Fruit cake, mince pies, Christmas cake, ginger nuts.
- Oat cakes, Rye crispbread.
- All biscuits and cakes containing dried fruit, nuts or chocolate.

Pudding and Desserts

- Bread pudding and Christmas pudding.
- Desserts containing chocolate.

Meat Substitutes

- Fresh soya bean products, vegetarian meat substitutes, bean milk.

Condiments and Miscellaneous

- Sauces such as tomato ketchup, tomato chutney, tomato purée, tomato sauce (in small quantities).

- Meat and yeast extracts (dried or paste). Salt substitutes containing potassium chloride (i.e. Low Salt products).

FOODS WITH A LOW POTASSIUM CONTENT

These can be given as alternatives to high potassium foods.

Sweets

- Sugar, jam, marmalade, honey, lemon curd, Golden Syrup.
- Boiled sweets, barley sugars, peppermints, plain fudge, butterscotch toffee and Turkish Delight, fondant sweets, Jelly Babies, fruit pastilles, fruit gums, sherbets, marshmallows, lollipops, ice lollies, chewing gum.

Drinks

- Tea, black or with a little milk or Coffeemate.
- Fizzy drinks: tonic, Seven-Up, Coca Cola, Pepsi Cola, lemonade, Lucozade (bottled only), soda water, mineral water, dry ginger ale, ginger beer, American ginger ale, bitter lemon, sparkling orange and other soft drinks with a low juice content.
- Fruit squash or barley water with a low natural juice content.
- Whisky, gin, vodka, brandy, rum and liqueurs in small quantities. These can be mixed with water, soda, lemonade, tonic and any of the above soft drinks.

Fruit

- Crystallised or glacé fruit.
- Olives.

Cereal

- Rice, wild rice noodles, pasta.
- Bread, pitta bread, croissant, puri, chapati.
- Cream crackers, water biscuits.
- Corn Flakes, Rice Krispies.
- Plain cake, pastry and biscuits.
- Flour, barley, sago, semolina, tapioca.
- Gelatin and yeast for baking.

Fat (See Advice on The Use of These Products).

- Margarine, butter, low-fat spreads, oil, olive oil.
- French dressing, mayonnaise, salad cream.
- Double cream, crème fraîche, cream cheese.

Condiments

- Spices such as allspice, cinnamon, ginger powder, mustard powder, nutmeg, pepper.
- Vinegar, Worcester sauce, mustard, chili sauce.

Dried Herbs or Spices in Moderation

- Basil, bayleaf, caraway seeds, chili powder, cloves, coriander, curry powder, dill, mint, oregano, paprika, parsley, sage, tarragon, thyme, tumeric, etc.
- Garlic, lemon juice, Tabasco.
- Piccalilli, horseradish, chutney and sweet pickles.

Fresh Herbs in Moderation

- Basil, bayleaf, coriander, dill, oregano, mint, tarragon, thyme, etc.

LEACHING

Potassium can be removed from vegetables and fruit by the process of leaching (boiling in plenty of water). For example, the potassium content of potatoes can be reduced effectively by the double cooking method and slicing the potatoes. This results in a loss of approximately 70% of potassium.

Potatoes should be peeled, thinly sliced and brought to the boil in twice the volume of water, then drained, fresh water added, and brought to the boil again for 20 min or until 'ready'. There is no need for presoaking.

Sweet potatoes and yams can be treated similarly.

Vegetables

1. Peel and cut in small pieces.
2. Boil in plenty of water to remove potassium.
3. Drain the vegetables well, then measure the portion.
4. Do not use a microwave oven or pressure cooker to cook vegetables; potassium does not leach sufficiently. Avoid stir frying vegetables unless preboiled.

5. A microwave oven may be used to reheat food.
6. Canned vegetables contain more salt.

POTASSIUM EXCHANGES

Potassium exchanges can be used to encourage variety. Most fruits and vegetables contain potassium in varying quantities. Each portion contains approximately 5 mmol (200 mg) potassium. Quantities are based on fresh or boiled vegetables or on fresh, stewed or canned fruit.

Potatoes (One Portion Contains 10 mmol Potassium)

150 g Boiled potatoes may be replaced by:

- 150 g new potatoes, peeled
- 75 g baked potato in skin
- 75 g new potatoes, boiled in skin
- 75 g roast potato
- 50 g chips (2 tablespoons): or 6 oven chips
- 25 g = 1 small packet potato crisps (no salt)
- 2 potato croquettes
- 150 g boiled parsnips
- 150 g risotto
- 150 g ravioli or spaghetti in tomato sauce
- 150 g yam, sweet potato, dasheen, eddoes, coco, boiled bread fruit
- 150 g rice and peas (without coconut)
- 75 g boiled green banana or plantain.

Pulses, Boiled Weight, to be Used Instead of Potatoes (For Dialysis Patients Only)

- 150 g soaked and boiled butter beans, haricot beans, black eyed beans, baked beans in tomato sauce, dried peas, split peas, chick peas
- 100 g lentils, boiled
- 75 g red kidney beans, boiled

Vegetables (One Portion is Approximately 5 mmol (200 mg) Potassium)

Low potassium content
The following vegetables are low in potassium. As a guide one unit is 150 g boiled and drained vegetables such as:

- Asparagus (six medium spears)
- Runner beans

- Beansprouts
- Bamboo shoots
- Cauliflower
- Carrots
- Globe artichoke
- Red, white or savoy cabbage
- Chinese leaves
- Marrow
- Pumpkin
- Peas (processed, canned, frozen, mushy peas)
- Onions boiled, pickled or silverskin
- Spring greens.

Medium high potassium content

The following vegetables have a medium high potassium content. As a guide one unit is 100 g of boiled, drained vegetables such as:

- Aubergine
- French beans
- Broccoli
- Celery
- Courgettes
- Curly kale
- Mange tout
- Leeks
- Capsicum (red or green)
- Turnip
- Sweetcorn kernels, on the cob or baby sweetcorn, fresh or canned
- Turnip.

Fairly high potassium content

The following vegetables have a fairly high potassium content. As a guide one unit is 75 g of boiled, drained vegetables such as:

- Brussels sprouts (six)
- Okra (six pods)
- Fennel
- Kohlrabi
- Mushrooms (boiled in water first)
- Tomatoes (canned).

Raw Vegetables

One unit is 75 g of salad vegetables (use a mixture of the following):

- Beetroot
- Red cabbage
- Carrots
- Celery
- Chicory
- Coleslaw
- Corn kernels
- Cucumber
- Lettuce
- Mustard and cress
- Peppers (red, green, yellow or orange)
- Radish
- Spring onions
- Tomato
- Watercress.

Fruit

Canned, bottled, stewed or baked fruit in water contains less potassium than raw fruit. Drain fruit before measuring a portion, as the juice also contains potassium and should be discarded.

Low potassium content
The following fruits have a low potassium content. As a guide, one unit of fruit is 150 g of the following (canned):

- Apples
- Blackberries
- Cranberries
- Cherries
- Fruit cocktail
- Gooseberries
- Grapefruit
- Guava
- Loganberries
- Lychees
- Mandarins
- Mango
- Paw paw
- Peaches
- Pears
- Pineapple
- Plums
- Raspberries

- Strawberries

or 150 g fresh:

- Apple
- Clementine
- Grapefruit
- Mango
- Melon (cantaloupe, galia, honeydew, water)
- Orange
- Passion fruit
- Peach
- Pear
- Satsuma
- Tangerine

Medium high potassium content

The following fruits have a medium high potassium content. As a guide, one unit is 100 g (canned or fresh):

- Apricots (in syrup or juice only)
- Blackberries (fresh or stewed)
- Blackcurrants (stewed only)
- Cherries
- Gooseberries (stewed)
- Kumquats
- Lemon or lime
- Loganberries (fresh)
- Lychees (fresh)
- Nectarines
- Paw paw (papaya)
- Peaches (fresh or in natural juice)
- Pineapple
- Pomegranate
- Plums (stewed only)
- Raspberries (fresh)
- Rhubarb (stewed or canned)
- Sharon fruit
- Strawberries

Fairly high potassium content

The following fruits have a fairly high potassium content. As a guide, one unit is 75 g of canned or fresh:

- Damsons
- Dates (fresh or dried)

- Figs (fresh)
- Greengages (fresh)
- Kiwi fruit
- Prunes (6)

APPENDIX 3

FOODS WITH A HIGH PHOSPHATE CONTENT

All foods with a high protein content also contain a fair amount of phosphorus. However, some of these foods are an essential part of the diet and cannot be eliminated.

The following foods can be excluded without altering the nutritional quality of the diet:

- Most types of hard cheese.
- Milk powder, cocao powder, chocolate (also high in potassium).

The following foods should be restricted to a minimum as part of the diet:

- Milk and milk puddings, yoghurt, buttermilk
- Eggs (no more than one daily).

However, these quantities may need to be adapted for vegetarian diets.

High-fibre foods with a high phosphorus content include:

- Bran, All-Bran, Fruit and Fibre, Raisin Splits.
- Crispbread containing rye, oatcakes, scones.
- Pulses such as dried peas, dried beans and all dishes containing these foods. Pulses can be exchanged for potatoes, but for dialysis patients only.
- Nuts and seeds and all types and foods containing these, peanut butter, marzipan.

TO BE AVOIDED

- Offal: liver and kidneys.
- Fish with edible bones: whitebait, kippers, anchovies (remove bones from canned fish such as herrings, tuna and salmon).
- Fish paste, fish roe.

CHAPTER 10

CHILDREN WITH RENAL PROBLEMS

INTRODUCTION

The aim of this chapter is to reflect the special nursing needs of a child with a renal deficit, including the need for family-centred care. Paediatric nephrology is a small speciality and renal disease is uncommon in childhood. Consequently, there are only 13 paediatric renal units in the UK. With more centres, patient numbers would be too low to maintain expertise in the care of these children (Report of a Working Party of the BAPN. March 1995).

As a result of this, many families travel long distances for treatment, adding to the stress of having a sick child in the family. Paediatric renal units must provide good facilities such as parent and sibling accommodation. Nurses and doctors must have expertise in paediatrics and renal disease, and a multidisciplinary team with the skills of a dietitian, psychologist, social worker, pharmacist and school teacher is essential. Good links with the community are important to provide support for the families at home. Many centres provide their own community staff to visit the family and liaise with local services.

This chapter concentrates on four main areas: acute renal failure, nephrotic syndrome, chronic renal failure and transplantation. The intention is to highlight the differences between care of the child and care of the adult. Most of the information in the adult chapters of the book is broadly relevant and should be read in conjunction with the appropriate section of this chapter.

ACUTE RENAL FAILURE

Acute renal failure (ARF) is a sudden potentially reversible reduction in renal function, although severe disease or late presentation may result in permanent renal damage. The cause may be acute renal disease or secondary to other serious illness. Acute renal failure is seen less often in children than in adults (Arbus *et al.*, 1994).

The causes of ARF in childhood are similar to those of adulthood but in different proportions. Neonates are susceptible to ARF following complications such as birth asphyxia or haemorrhage. Haemolytic uraemic syndrome is the most common cause of ARF in childhood and is described in more detail later in the chapter.

Most children with ARF will be transferred from a local hospital to a specialist renal or intensive care unit. This in itself is traumatic for the child and family, who are often too shocked to take in information on arrival. It is important to give information simply, clearly and often.

On admission, it is important to assess the child's condition quickly with observations of:

- blood pressure
- pulse
- respirations
- central and peripheral temperature gap
- weight
- oedema
- jugular venous pressure (JVP)

It is also important to assess the child's fluid state. Blood urea, electrolytes and creatinine should be checked to determine the level of renal function and assess the need for dialysis.

Choice of Dialysis Treatment

Peritoneal dialysis (PD) is often the dialysis treatment of choice for children with ARF, unless contraindicated. If the underlying cause of renal failure requires treatment with plasma exchange, haemodialysis (HD) may be chosen, as the vascular access would be suitable for both. Haemofiltration is an alternative to HD, chosen in the intensive care setting. Technical problems often occur with dialysis, so it is important, therefore, that specialist centres offer more than one approach. Today, HD is a well-accepted short-term treatment in all age groups starting from the full-term neonate.

Contraindications to PD include severe burns to the abdomen, recent intraperitoneal surgery, scarring and adhesions following previous major surgery or peritonitis. In children with severe spina bifida or prune belly syndrome, PD may not be possible. In cases of severe poisoning, such as iron overdose, haemodialysis removes the poison more efficiently. A small number of children congenitally have a small hole in the diaphragm, and on starting PD the child shows signs of respiratory difficulty as dialysate leaks into the chest. A chest X-ray may be confused with pulmonary oedema. PD in this case must be discontinued immediately.

Dialysis is discussed in more detail in the section on chronic renal failure (CRF).

Care of the Child

Explanations should be given to the child at a level appropriate to the age. A good play specialist can reinforce information through play. Depth of understanding of the information given should be checked.

One child with renal failure became upset at the prospect of a blood test. On questioning the refusal was because 'the doctor is stupid, he is taking blood from my arm, when everyone else knows it is my kidneys that are not working'. A quick, simple physiology lesson allowed venepuncture to continue without further problem.

The child in ARF requires some dietary manipulation. The parents lose confidence when they realise they no longer understand what to feed their child. A compromise between a renal failure diet (which is discussed in more detail in the section on CRF) and a diet which causes as little distress to the child and family as possible will be initiated.

A high calorie, low electrolyte, low fluid diet is necessary. In a small child it is often kinder to pass a nasogastric tube and feed overnight to avoid battles at each mealtime. Children in renal failure are anorexic and cannot be expected to eat well. The parent and child should be encouraged to see a nasogastric tube as part of the treatment and not a failure on their part. Older children can usually be persuaded to take calorie supplements, and a variety of flavours and types are commercially available. Dietary restriction should be kept to a minimum, as a child who is restricted and anorexic will eat nothing at all. Once the child is on dialysis usually most foods, except an excessive amount of salt, are allowed. If a child craves a food such as crisps, it is better to allow a small portion than ban the food and make an issue out of it.

In ARF, fluid restriction causes distress to most children. A typical restriction for an anuric child is 500 ml per 24 h. Teaching a child to measure and record their fluid intake with parental supervision can help understanding. Tiny cups, ice cubes and ice lollies help to make the fluid last longer. Despite this, most renal wards ring with the words 'I want a drink now!'.

Haemolytic Uraemic Syndrome

The most common cause of ARF is haemolytic uraemic syndrome (HUS) (Rizzoni, 1988). At the height of the summer the larger centres may have up to six children suffering from various stages of the disease at any one time.

The most common form of HUS is typically preceded by an *Escherichia coli* gastroenteritis with several days of bloody diarrhoea. Often other members of the same family will have the same diarrhoeal illness which does not progress to renal failure, though it is not uncommon for siblings to present with HUS together. HUS is less common in adults; it is most common in the 1–5 year age group, who also have the best prognosis.

Often the parents of a child with HUS will have taken the child to the GP or casualty department with the diarrhoeal illness one or more times before the renal failure presents or before a diagnosis is made. By the time the child reaches a specialist paediatric renal unit they are extremely ill, often near death. The parents are anxious and often blame themselves, because instinctively they have known the child was ill. The parents may also be tired after several sleepless nights. Introducing the parents to other parents of children in the recovery phase, or fully recovered children visiting outpatients, or failing that showing a photo of a recovered child, can be reassuring.

A typical child presenting with HUS will be pale and anaemic, will have lost weight from several days of diarrhoea and be irritable and lethargic. They may be either dehydrated from the diarrhoeal illness or fluid over-loaded as a result of oliguria or anuria, depending on the stage of illness. Any urine is usually blood stained. Blood chemistry will reveal renal failure, raised creatinine uraemia and deranged electrolytes. Haematology will show a low haemoglobin, fragmented cells and a low platelet count. The low platelet count causes impaired clotting.

Dialysis and blood transfusion is often a medical emergency. Occasionally, a child whose parents are Jehovah's Witnesses will present with HUS. The anaemia of HUS is so severe, often dropping daily despite blood transfusion, and for children presenting with haemoglobin as low as $4 \, g \, dl^{-1}$ transfusion is a life-saving procedure. If the parents will not agree to transfusion, and the child is not able to show competence to make the decision, current paediatric practice is to obtain a court order. Although this is the subject of enormous ethical debate, sensitive handling often enables good relationships with the parents to continue.

The main treatment for HUS is supportive:

- blood transfusions to correct the anaemia;
- dialysis;
- tube feeding until the renal function recovers;
- whilst the haematology is altered, some units transfuse daily with fresh frozen plasma to treat the disease. The benefits of this have not been conclusively proven.

The most severe cases of HUS may require plasma exchange.

Most children given good nursing and medical care will make a rapid recovery. Usually, the first sign of recovery is the child looking better, then the haematology improves and finally renal function recovers. Typically, this takes 2–3 weeks.

Many children who are admitted seriously ill with HUS are discharged home 3 weeks later. Nevertheless, HUS is a serious disease with a significant mortality (10%). Cerebral involvement can occur, in which case prognosis is poor. It is important not to understimate the seriousness of the disease when talking to parents. HUS is a seasonal illness with epidemics in the summer months. Some children will have residual renal damage; all children with HUS should be followed up throughout childhood with a yearly check of blood pressure and renal function.

Familial HUS is a rare form of HUS with a much higher mortality rate.

Although the child may recover from the disease quickly, it takes the family much longer to recover from the stress. Links with the community and maintained links with the hospital must be available to provide continuing support.

Many parents feel a sense of panic the first time their child has a minor ailment following HUS and need to be able to ask for help and reassurance until they have regained their confidence.

NEPHROTIC SYNDROME

The nephrotic syndrome is defined as heavy proteinuria, hypoproteinaemia and oedema. There are several different diseases causing nephrotic syndrome, the most common of which in children is minimal change nephrotic syndrome. Minimal change commonly presents in the preschool child.

Whilst medical treatment and prognosis may vary according to the underlying disease, the nursing care is related to the severity of symptoms. For discussion of the disease process and medical management, see Haycock (1994) and Trompeter (1994). This section concentrates on the nursing care of the child with nephrotic syndrome.

The priority upon admitting a child with nephrotic syndrome is to assess the child's fluid status (see ARF section above). The low plasma albumin can cause hypovolaemia. Because nephrotic children are oedematous, fluid status is more difficult to assess. Skin turgor is less helpful, weight merely reflects the level of oedema and the oedema often masks the low JVP. On recording the blood pressure, the oedema must be taken into account when choosing the appropriate cuff. Central peripheral temperature gap in association with blood pressure are the most reliable indicators of fluid state. If a child has normal blood pressure for age and a temperature gap of less than 2°C, they are not hypovolaemic. A urinary sodium of less than 10 mmol l^{-1} is an indicator of hypovolaemia; however, this investigation is only useful in the absence of frusemide. Children often complain of abdominal pain when hypovolaemic.

Severe, prolonged hypovolaemia can result in clotting of major blood vessels, so must be regarded as an emergency. If normal saline is given as in conventional treatment of hypovolaemia, the saline will quickly leak out of the circulation to become oedema. The circulation will therefore not be increased.

In severe hypovolaemia the child should be rehydrated with 4.5% plasma albumin which temporarily replaces both albumin and fluid into the circulation. If hypovolaemia is less severe, 20% plasma albumin is given slowly over at least 4 h. The dose is 1 g of protein per kilogram body weight. This delivers concentrated albumin into the circulation, temporarily increasing the plasma albumin; this increases the oncotic pressure in the circulation, resulting in oedema fluid returning from the tissues to circulation.

It is important, therefore, to nurse nephrotic children in the sitting position during plasma infusions to minimise the risk of pulmonary oedema. The child should be nursed where they can be easily seen, and blood pressure, pulse and respiratory rate recorded quarter- to half-hourly, even if the child appears well and stable. If the child shows signs of fluid overload, oxygen saturation should be checked, the infusion discontinued and intravenous frusemide given.

Children with nephrotic syndrome are often extremely oedematous. Altered body image can be difficult for both child and parents. Children are self-conscious and may be teased by their peers. Parents make remarks like 'I have forgotten what my child really looks like'.

The oedema causes physical as well as psychological problems. If oedema is incapacitating, then albumin and frusemide can be given to reduce the oedema. Unfortunately, this is very short acting. Oedema can cause difficulty in movement; walking becomes difficult with a swollen vulva or scrotum. The child should be encouraged to move as much as possible, to prevent deep vein thrombosis and chest infection. Blood is hypercoagulable in the nephrotic child and gross ascites can splint the diaphragm. A good play specialist is invaluable to occupy and distract the child in whom movement is difficult, and relieve the parents' anxiety.

The parents should be encouraged to continue the child's care, but may need help. A nephrotic child is often heavy and difficult to lift. Oedematous skin should be kept clean and dry; skin folds are susceptible to thrush. Oedematous skin is prone to pressure sores so frequent repositioning is important. If oedematous skin is broken, oedema fluid leaks from the wound and often will not heal until the oedema is no longer present.

All types of nephrotic syndrome are treated with immunosuppression. This adds to the changed appearance and perception of body image. Whilst many side-effects of immunosuppression are well recognised by health care professionals, including change of appearance, poor growth and susceptibility to infection, many parents describe the mood swings and behavioural changes associated with steroids as extremely distressing. Acknowledgement and discussion of the problems, together with advice from a psychologist on management of behaviour, may be helpful. The effect of steroids on behaviour is often underestimated by doctors and nurses.

Conventionally, the advice to nephrotic children has been to eat a high protein diet. The proteinuria is usually too great to replace the protein by dietary intake, therefore it is kinder to let the child eat their normal diet. A salt restriction can help minimise oedema; a salt-free diet is unpalatable, so a low-salt diet is recommended during relapse. Fluid restriction is dangerous, adding to the risk of hypovolaemia. Unless the child has impaired renal function as a consequence of nephrotic syndrome, free access to fluids is essential.

Fluid intake and output are recorded to help assess fluid state. In a severely nephrotic child, urine output may be low. Urine is tested daily to assess response to treatment. The child or parents are encouraged to measure proteinuria in preparation for discharge, as home urine testing is necessary.

Some fortunate children have only one episode of nephrotic syndrome, some relapse rarely. At its worst, children relapse frequently and eventually require dialysis and transplantation. Some nephrotic syndromes recur in the transplanted kidney.

The severity of nephrotic syndrome inevitably interferes with the child's life. Frequent hospital visits, changed appearance, altered behaviour, together with an uncertain future, affect the whole family. Good information, good medical care and good nursing care preventing complications can help to minimise the problems.

On discharge, liaison with the community is important. Discussion with the school can promote understanding of changed behaviour and alert the school staff to the risk of chickenpox in an immunosuppressed child. Some schools are extremely supportive. The parents need to know what to do when the child relapses, and who to telephone for advice.

As well as susceptibility to infection due to immunosuppression, nephrotic children often relapse in association with a mild infection, such as a cold or sore throat. It is difficult to avoid unnecessary infection from interfering with the child's social life. Often parents need help and encouragement to allow the child to be normal.

CHRONIC RENAL FAILURE

Chronic renal failure (CRF) is an insidious disease. It often does not present till late in its progression. It is irreversible and, fortunately, rare. The incidence in the UK is about 5.2 children per million child population. As CRF is not often detected early in a child, it may present as ARF, where the child may be hyperkalaemic, fluid overloaded, hypertensive and requiring dialysis.

There are many causes of CRF. Many large studies have shown that glomerulonephritis and pyelonephritis appear to be the main causes of renal failure in children, followed by urinary tract anomalies and hypoplasia. Routine antenatal screening has greatly helped in detecting renal tract anomalies in the foetus. This means that with close liaison between the obstetrician and paediatrician, the newborn baby can be referred to the specialist unit for the care it needs. CRF is usually defined as when glomerular filtration rate (GFR) falls to below 50 ml min^{-1} 1.73 m^2 Body surface area (BSA). At this level, growth begins to be impaired, and metabolic abnormalities occur. CRF progresses relentlessly into end-stage renal failure (ESRF), but many children can now be managed meticulously for a long period of time before renal replacement therapy (RRT) is needed.

Signs and Symptoms of CRF

- *Failure to thrive, poor growth.* The majority of children in CRF present with failure to thrive. In the young infant there is a failure to gain weight, and in the older child a marked loss in height velocity. These children are nauseated and vomit frequently so adequate intake of nutrition is impaired. There is also a degree of anorexia in the older child, where they 'go off their food'.
- *Lethargy and pallor.* Children in CRF are anaemic. This may be due to the reduction in production of erythropoietin together with a depletion of iron and folate stores. The resulting anaemia causes listlessness and lethargy.
- *Hypertension.* Owing to fluid overload as the kidney continues to deteriorate or owing to the underlying cause of the CRF, for example polycystic disease.
- *Frequent urinary tract infections (UTIs).* Many children present with a long history of frequent UTIs and possibly bed-wetting. On investigation the underlying cause may be due to reflux nephropathy.
- *Congestive cardiac failure (CCF).* Children in CRF may present with CCF due to fluid overload.

Electrolyte abnormalities are detected when serum is analysed. Hyperkalaemia, high urea and creatinine, acidosis and high phosphate levels are demonstrated. Serum albumin may be low due to heavy protein loss and inadequate protein intake. This applies particularly in nephrotic syndrome.

The pale, thin child who is constantly tired, complaining of headaches, does not eat or want to go to school, must never be ignored. Many children on the end-stage programme have presented with this history. There are also parents, who when faced with the diagnosis of CRF, feel angry, bitter and guilty that they have not insisted on a second medical opinion. Despite specialist referral and outreach clinics, paediatric units in the UK still see children presenting in CRF when dialysis is needed.

Investigating CRF

When CRF is suspected, investigations need to be carried out to confirm diagnosis and establish the cause.

Meticulous preparation of the child and family is essential to ensure successful results. Those investigations may be invasive and unpleasant or non-invasive. Play therapists and specialist nurses using dolls, pictures, videos and clear simple explanations are involved in the preparation and carrying out of these tests:

- *Urinalysis.* The most basic non-invasive test carried out to detect protein, blood, ketones and pH.
- *Height and weight.* Both these growth parameters have to be measured accurately and plotted on a growth chart.
- *Ultrasound.* Detects renal tract anomalies and any abdominal mass. 'Jelly on the tum' does not hurt and even younger children can be persuaded to lie still while this procedure is carried out.
- *Abdominal X-ray.* To detect renal calculi and spina bifida.
- *Serum.* As mentioned before for electrolytes and a full blood count to detect anaemia.
- *Micturating cysto-urethrogram (MCUG).* An MCUG is unpleasant and many children dislike having this procedure carried out. Used widely to detect the presence of posterior urethral values and reflux.
- *Radio-isotope scans.* Used in children to detect size, function and perfusion of the kidneys. Young children may need to be sedated as they are frightened of the camera and are unable to lie still for a period of time.
- *Intravenous pyelogram.* Used when upper renal tract abnormalities are suspected.
- *Wrist X-ray.* Every child with suspected CRF has the left hand and wrist X-rayed to detect any renal osteodystrophy and to calculate actual bone age. Children in CRF often have a bone age younger than chronological age.

• *Renal biopsy*. The best method of ascertaining underlying pathology. The biopsy is carried out under a general anaesthetic (in the young infant) or heavy sedation and local anaesthetic in the older child.

There are many more tests, such as Mag 3, which are too numerous to list in this chapter.

Management of CRF

Diet, medication and psychosocial support are *essential* in the management of a child who will progress to ESRF. In paediatrics, a multidisciplinary approach is vital. Paediatricians, paediatric renal dietitians, paediatric renal pharmacists, social workers, psychologists and paediatric renal nurses form the specialist team who are all involved in the child and the family's care.

Medications

Medicines, unfortunately in the form of pills or solutions, are needed to maintain management of CRF. This is when the problems of compliance begin. These children will have to take:

• phosphate binders – to correct high phosphate levels;
• sodium bicarbonate – to correct acidosis;
• vitamin D – to correct, prevent and alleviate bone disease;
• sodium supplements – to help normal growth;
• erythropoietin – recombinant human erythropoietin – is given as a subcutaneus injection to correct anaemia;
• antihypertensive agents – used if there is an underlying cause of hypertension;
• antibiotics – if the diagnosis of CRF is reflux, and so prevent the child getting more UTIs;
• folic acid – to replenish depleted folate stores;
• iron supplements – as in above to replenish iron stores;
• multivitamins;
• growth hormone injection daily.

Any or all of these drugs are used to maintain normal homeostasis. At a glance it is easy to see why the older child can express a degree of non-compliance. Support for the family and child along with respected education is the only way of ensuring compliance.

Diet

The diet of a child in CRF can be a challenge. As mentioned above, protein restriction is variable from unit to unit. Allowing a child to have their sausages or beefburgers is important to alleviate the unnecessary misery of the chronic disease.

Calories are very important and there are many calorie supplements available on the market. Many children find these sickly sweet and, despite all the various flavours available, soon tire of them. Double cream, and drinks such as Lucozade or Coca-Cola can be used to increase dietary intake. It is not uncommon in our unit for a child to be *prescribed* a litre of one of these drinks per day. Care must be taken of the amount of phosphate in some drinks.

Dairy products usually have to be restricted due to their high phosphate content. This means that the amount of milk on cereal or taken in drinks will need to be adjusted.

Depending on potassium levels, fresh fruit which is high in potassium will also need to be restricted. It is interesting to note that as soon as restriction is applied, the surge in interest in eating oranges or strawberries arises. The diet of children in CRF need not be misery-making. The child must be allowed to eat the normal family meals, and not made to feel different. Sibling animosity and financial burdens may arise with the diet over such expensive items as cream and drinks. These needs must be met by the psychosocial members of the team.

In the young infant and toddler, an adequate protein and calorie intake is usually met by either feeding the child by overnight nasogastric tube (Plate 7c), or gastrostomy feeding. Both these methods have excellent results but have advantages and disadvantages. The crucial point to consider is that both methods achieve good nutrition and excellent growth. It is worth the extra effort to obtain a good calorie and protein intake and see the results in an acceleration of height velocity. With good control of secondary hyperparathyroidism, renal osteodystrophy need never happen. The challenge lies in getting the child to take the prescribed phosphate binders daily and correctly.

Dialysis

Both HD and PD are useful for treating ESRF in children. As mentioned before, the aim of most paediatric units is to transplant the child before they require dialysis.

Haemodialysis

HD as a long-term prospect is extremely difficult in the very young infant because of the difficulty in maintaining vascular access (Plate 7b). HD is viable in the older child as access is easier.

When haemodialysing children, calculation of extracorporeal volume is important, in order not to render the child hypovolaemic. Extracorporeal volume is calculated by using a simple equation:

80 ml kg^{-1} 8–10% of this volume is then used to dialyse the child
e.g. 10-kg child = 10 × 80 = 800 ml
    10% of this volume is 80 ml.

A suitable dialyser and paediatric lines will then be used, ensuring that only 80 ml is outside the child's body at any time. Small fistula needles have also been a boon. Bicarbonate dialysis has been a great asset in dialysing these children. Lactate and acetate as buffers have often made these children unwell, and bicarbonate dialysis not only corrects any acidosis, but also enables the child to have symptom-free dialysis treatment.

Access   This still remains the biggest problem for children who require HD. Who are these children? They are those who cannot have PD perhaps because of major abdominal surgery, severe non-compliance on PD, or in families where home PD is not feasible due to social circumstances. There are many forms of access for HD. They are:

- *Shunt*. Temporary access and rarely used in the chronic HD patient.
- *Fistula*. Excellent when constructed successfully. Children are taught to cannulate themselves and this is indeed the best form of HD access.
- *Gortex and vein grafts*. When a child 'runs out of access' a synthetic or autologous vein graft may be needed. These have the disadvantage of clotting and infection.
- *Haemocatheters/permanent catheters*. Used quite frequently. An excellent method of accessing the circulation, but carries the risks of clotting and infection.

Children who are on long-term HD have to come into a unit three times weekly for HD. This involves several factors:

- Travelling long distances – owing to the distribution of paediatric dialysis units.
- Missing school to attend the dialysis sessions, though this problem has been successfully met by providing on-going education in the unit, by using the hospital school and teachers. Children on HD may even sit GCSEs or any other exam, with liaison between the school and the hospital.

Dietary and fluid restrictions are quite severe. The fluid restriction of children on dialysis, if they are anuric, is usually between 300 and 500 ml of fluid per day. Can you imagine what it is like to have someone tell you as a child that you can only drink approximately two mugs of fluid per day, especially if you were previously allowed to drink 1 l of Lucozade every day?

Dietary restrictions include low phosphate and low potassium meals. The bonus on HD is that when the child is connected to the HD machine, they can be given a huge cooked breakfast of everything possible. They can have crisps, chocolate, a large drink and fresh fruit. Many children love this treat, and accept HD as a way of life. Home HD was accepted practice in the 1970s, but severe family stress, cost, and the advent of continuous ambulatory peritoneal dialysis (CAPD) in the late 1970s stopped this practice in the majority of units.

Financial difficulties have to be met by close liaison with the social worker. The cost of travelling to a unit, very often from long distances, and loss of earnings for a parent have to be met. Care of any other siblings whilst a parent is with one child must also be considered. Financial help may also be needed for any special dietary requirements. Despite this gloomy picture, nurses caring for children in an HD unit have an extremely close relationship with their patients and there is always a noisy, busy and happy atmosphere on the unit, alas lacking in many adult units.

Peritoneal dialysis

PD has been available to children in the UK since the early 1980s. It is a safe, relatively simple procedure that the child and parents can be taught to carry out. All paediatric units advocate the use of home PD. PD is carried out via a Tenckhoff catheter inserted into the peritoneal space. The insertion procedure is always surgically carried out under a general anaesthetic. In this sense it differs from adult practice where catheters are sometimes inserted under local anaesthetic.

Automated PD by way of overnight cycling as opposed to CAPD is the preferred method of treatment. Lack of central government funding has resulted in many units not being able to offer overnight PD, as no money is made available to buy the cycler machines needed for this treatment. Many of these cyclers are bought by charity funding. CAPD is not feasible in the very young, because very small volume dialysate bags are not made. The smallest commercially available bags are 500 ml.

Very small infants can be successfully dialysed at home on PD using a cycler, as it is possible to programme the cycler for small fill volumes (i.e. 50 ml) (Plates 7a and d). Paediatric units in the UK use a variety of Tenckhoff catheters. They can be:

- straight adult size
- short curly
- swan-neck.

All have success and to date there has not been a multicentre study to determine the best position or type of catheter to use in the paediatric units in the UK.

Dialysate is infused at between 30 and 40 ml kg^{-1} into the peritoneal cavity. Aseptic techniques when carrying out the dialysis connectology are largely similar to the adult units. Young children can be safely taught to carry out PD, though many have difficulty in pulling off protective caps and seals. This appears to require the strength of an ox!

Exit site infection and peritonitis remain the biggest problem in children. Many children pick their noses and generally fiddle with their body, including the tube exit site, despite a covering dressing. Poor compliance with bathing/showering and carrying out a dressing procedure (especially in the teenager) lead to severe exit site infections. *Staphylococcus aureus* is the most common bacterium isolated.

Peritonitis occurs with poor technique, usually associated with boredom, which inevitably goes hand in hand with the monotony of carrying out four exchanges per day. It is sometimes a sign or symptom of a cry for help. Teenagers, in particular, feel depressed and different from their peers. Whether it is the body image of a bit of plastic in their abdomen, their fluid restrictions or the restrictive nature of carrying out four exchanges every day, has not been ascertained. CAPD, in particular, can disrupt normal family life and many a child who has been transplanted or put on to an overnight cycler feels that life has been 'transformed'. Fluid restrictions in the anuric child on PD remain the same as the child on HD. Anuria can be a problem on PD where poor ultrafiltration occurs. Recommended dietary protein intake of children on PD is higher than for children on HD due to high protein losses in dialysate. High calorie diets including supplements, either commercially made or otherwise, are a must in both sets of children.

Schooling is not severely affected in children on PD, as they usually can go home or carry out an exchange in a room designated for their use (Plate 5). Close liaison by the community nurse, hospital and school are so important. School visits by the PD nurse to educate staff and children in the class plays a significant role in helping to rehabilitate the child back in the normal environment.

Good psychosocial support is *the key* to enable the child and family to cope with the severe stress of having a child on dialysis at home. It is interesting that many adult units now recognize that psychosocial support is as important as nursing and medical care in delivery of an holistic approach to the patient and family.

Dialysis is a poor quality of life in comparison to transplantation for children in ESRF, but due to the decrease in availability of donor kidneys and an increase in the ability to treat very small children, more and more children are now on dialysis. It is only with education and greater public awareness that this trend can be reversed.

TRANSPLANTATION

Despite improvements in both dialysis equipment and technique, a successful renal transplant remains the only prospect for a near normal quality of life for the child with ESRF. In an ideal world most children would be transplanted before dialysis was necessary. Not only would this be easier for the child and family but cheaper for the National Health Service (NHS).

Pre-emptive transplantation (transplantation before dialysis) is not always possible because:

- ESRF may occur without prior diagnosis.
- Progression from chronic to ESRF may be faster than anticipated.
- The cause of renal failure may be acute. In some diseases, such as vasculitis or Goodpasture's syndrome, transplantation must wait until disease is no longer active so as to avoid the disease reoccurring in the transplanted kidney.
- There may not be a suitable organ available.

Kidneys for transplantation come from two different sources: cadaver or live related donor. In the UK, all cadaver kidneys from donors under the age of 18 years are offered to paediatric units first.

Mothers of children in intensive care approached about organ donation often consider the recipient's mother, typically remarking, 'If I can stop some other mother suffering as I am now, I will'. Parents of recipients often express grief and gratitude for the generosity of the donor family.

Live related donor transplants are most commonly parent to child, though on occasion grandparents, aunts or uncles have donated kidneys. A sibling would offer the best chance of a well-matched graft; however, in the UK this would only be considered if the sibling was over the age of 18 years.

The advantages of live donor transplants are:

- The kidney is available when needed, allowing transplantation to be planned.
- The kidney is often well matched.
- The time between removal of the organ from the donor and transplantation is negligible.
- Long-term results from live related transplantation are excellent.

The donor undergoes painful major surgery, which is not without risk. Live donor transplantation can be of huge benefit to the recipient and psychologically to the donor. Although extremely rare, death of the donor could occur.

It is important that the donor is well informed and makes the decision themselves to donate. The donor should have a separate medical team to ensure their physical and psychological well-being is fully met. This happens naturally in paediatrics with adult and paediatric teams.

The psychology of living related donation is complicated. At its best, to see a sick child on dialysis become a healthy child with a working graft is a positive experience for the donor – anecdotally described by mothers as 'giving birth again'.

The recipient may have mixed feelings about receiving a parent's kidney: not wanting the parent to suffer, worries concerning death of the donor or indeed fear of obligation to the donor. The donor may be angry if the child does not look after 'their' kidney. Most teenagers are non-compliant in some ways; rebellion is a normal part of growing up. If that rebellion takes the form of missing immunosuppression, it is hard for any parent to understand, let alone one who has provided the kidney. If the transplant does not work there are feelings of anger, disappointment and guilt from both donor and recipient. It is important that these issues are discussed before the transplantation with the family.

Despite the potential problems associated with live related donor transplantation, it is probably medically the best option for the child and, given the shortage of cadaver kidneys, sometimes the only option.

The size of the kidney does not have to be well matched to the size of the donor. Cadaver kidneys under the age of 2 years are usually avoided in the UK because results have been universally disappointing. Donor kidneys from tall male adult donors may be too large for the smallest recipients (8–10 kg).

When a young child receives a large kidney it is important to remember the kidney is used to a higher blood pressure than the recipient's. The child may need a blood transfusion to perfuse the kidney and to be maintained at a higher blood pressure than normal to achieve urine output. This is usually only necessary for 2–3 days, after which blood pressure can be allowed to drift back to normal for age.

Preoperative Care

Preparation for transplantation is important. The child and family must receive honest information concerning transplantation, discussing success and failure. It is important to meet other transplant patients and all the multidisciplinary team. A transplant preparation day with professionals giving talks and plenty of discussion time is a useful and popular way of giving information.

The child must be fully vaccinated, as live vaccines cannot be given once immunosuppression is started.

The bladder must be investigated to determine whether reconstructive surgery is necessary. The kidney can be transplanted with a ureterostomy, by-passing an inadequate bladder.

The inferior vena cava is ultrasounded to ensure the child has an adequate blood supply for the transplant operation. Blood groups and tissue typing are undertaken to enable cross-matching of either cadaver or live donor organs (Ward, 1994).

Nursing a child through a renal transplant is exciting. It is one of the few times as a nurse that one cares for a child requiring intensive care who is thrilled to be there. It is important to remember that although parents and children are usually excited about the transplant, they are also apprehensive about the surgery and results. One must be calm, positive and encouraging, whilst making it clear the kidney may not work.

Immunosuppression is started preoperatively; the regime varies from centre to centre. The child is examined to ensure they are well and infection free. Typically, the child is off the ward for 2–3 h, giving plenty of time to prepare the bed space, familiarise the parents with the postoperative surroundings and give them chance to take a meal.

Postoperative Care

Postoperatively, it is important to ensure the kidney is well perfused quickly to minimise graft loss for technical reasons.

On return from theatre, the child will have a central line for central venous pressure (CVP) recordings, and a saline infusion to replace urine output, which can be massive. Dextrose saline is used to replace insensible loss. A dopamine infusion to increase renal perfusion, and the use of a patient- or nurse-controlled analgesia infusion is commenced. Blood and plasma are given according to observations and blood results. A ureteric stent and urethral catheter ensure drainage of urine and protect the ureteric anastomosis.

Ideally, for the first half hour postoperatively two nurses are needed, one to attach and monitor fluids the other to record observations. It is most important to ensure parents feel welcome and necessary at this busy time and not in the way.

The aim of the postoperative care is to:

- achieve a normal blood pressure for age;
- achieve a CVP of around 5–10 cm of water;
- achieve a central peripheral temperature gap of less than 2 °C when the toes are covered with a space blanket.

To achieve this, the children are often slightly fluid overloaded for the first 24 h. Because of this and the long anaesthetic, it is important to nurse the child in the sitting position.

Children can eat and drink postoperatively as soon as bowel sounds return. In most older children this is almost immediately. In the baby and toddler age group, it may be as long as 2–4 days.

By 24–48 h postoperatively the child will usually look well, be out of bed and have *in situ* only a peripheral intravenous line for drugs, the urethral catheter and ureteric stent. It is unnecessary and cruel to isolate children post-renal transplantation but avoiding obvious infection is sensible.

Follow-up Care

The first signs of rejection typically occur at 7–10 days post-transplant. Signs of rejection are:

- creatinine raised by 10% or more or a previously falling creatinine becomes static;
- tender, painful graft;
- hypertension;
- weight gain;
- decreased urine output;
- flu-like aches and pains;
- diarrhoea (this is more common in younger children).

As all these symptoms can be attributed to other diagnoses, a renal biopsy is indicated. Renal biopsies on children are usually performed under heavy sedation. Treatment of rejection is an urgency and consists of an increase in immunosuppression. No matter how well prepared a family is, the first rejection episode is frightening as the prospect of losing the kidney is considered. It is important to be honest when talking to both child and family; children become aware of their condition and the implications at a young age.

Infection can be a problem in the immunosuppressed child. The child treated with increased immunosuppression to treat rejection becomes susceptible to opportunist infections such as cytomegalovirus and pneumocystis. Rarely, a child will die of infection post-transplantation. Occasionally, a decision has to be made to abandon the kidney, rather than risk the child's life with more immunosuppression.

If a transplant fails, the child and family are often bitter and angry. The child has suffered major surgery, immunosuppression and a stay in hospital, all disrupting family life. It may be some time before they can face another transplant, physically or emotionally. A period on dialysis may be indicated.

The drug regime post-transplant causes changes in the children, cushingoid appearance and hirsutism and acne being the most distressing to children. Steroids cause mood swings, high-dose steroids in toddlers often result in serious temper tantrums, an important area of concern to parents; advice from a psychologist can be helpful. The importance of altered body image to the children cannot be underestimated. However, the effects of immunosuppression on appearance do decrease in time.

Once successfully transplanted, children achieve a more normal quality of life. Appetite and growth increase, catch-up growth often occurs. The children report an increase in well-being. An 8-year-old boy post-transplant said 'I didn't know you could feel this well. I didn't know anyone could play football for so long without getting tired'.

Transplanted children have grown up and entered careers as diverse as nursing, law, photography and working on a deep sea oil rig. Many have gone on to be parents themselves.

Younger and younger children are now receiving kidney transplants. Babies as small as 6–10 kg have been transplanted. Transplanting small children is difficult and opens up an ethical debate concerning the issues of balancing suffering against potential gain in children too small to express their opinion. Transplants do not last forever, though some kidneys have now been transplanted for over 20 years. However, young children receiving kidney transplants will inevitably need retransplanting at some stage (Plate 7e).

A transplant recipient will need hospital follow-up for the rest of their life. This may be as infrequently as 3 monthly. They also need immunosuppression for the rest of their life. Good discharge information is essential to both child and family to minimise graft loss. Unfortunately, teenagers do rebel by omitting medicines. Teenage non-compliance is a well-recognised cause of graft loss (Meyers *et al.*, 1995).

CONCLUSION

In this chapter an attempt has been made to point out differences in treating children in renal failure from treating the adult counterparts. The specialist team is essential. In 1976, the European Dialysis and Transplant Association (EDTA) registry proposed a rigorous definition of a paediatric centre. The team included a paediatrician, dietitian, social worker, child psychologist, school facilities, a children's ward and a dialysis and transplant programme. In 1989, 77% of all children in Europe were treated in specialist centres. It is interesting that children who were treated in specialist centres fared better.

The problems of diet, loss of 'normal' freedom due to dialysis, medications, and all its problems of non-compliance, poor school attendance and altered family dynamics, not to mention financial constraints, can only be met by a multidisciplinary team. Weekly psychosocial meetings to discuss problems are invaluable in caring for the child and family with CRF. Paediatric units have always emphasised the psychosocial role, and it is interesting to note that many adult units are beginning to do the same. This support can also have a lighter side. For instance, adolescent groups (teenagers) may be encouraged to meet monthly, to talk about things, swim, eat or go out. It helps with the ghastly sense of isolation, to meet with others experiencing the same problem. 'I'm not the only short one around here' is the sort of remark that can be heard. Dialysis holidays where children are taken away to a resort by nurses and other members of the team give families a much needed break. Home respite care and home liaison nurses help to support and relieve the stress of caring for a child with CRF.

The advent of erythropoietin and growth hormone have given hope to these children. Anaemia is now a problem of the past and participation in normal school activity has improved.

More and more children are now being treated in specialist centres. In December 1992, 570 children were receiving RRT (British Association for Paediatric Nephrology, 1993). A functioning transplant remains the best outcome for growth and normal school attendance, which in turn leads to better rehabilitation into adult life. Unfortunately, until we see a reverse in the current trend, where there is a shortage of donors, we will continue to see children on dialysis for longer periods of time. The aim of the specialist team is to make life for these families bearable.

REFERENCES

ARBUS, G.S., FARINE, M. AND GUIGNARD, J.P. (1994) Acute renal failure. In *Clinical Paediatric Nephrology*, 2nd edn (ed. R.J. Postlethwaite). Butterworth Heinmann, Oxford, p. 248.

HAYCOCK, G.B. (1991) Steroid responsive nephrotic syndrome. In *Clinical Paediatric Nephrology*, 2nd edn (ed. R.J. Postlethwaite). Butterworth Heinmann, Oxford, pp. 210–225.

MEYERS, K.E.C., WEILAND, H. AND THOMSON, P.D. (1995) Paediatric renal transplantation – non-compliance. *Paediatric Nephrology*, **9**: 189–92.

Report of a working Party of the British Association for Paediatric Nephrology. March 1995.

RIZZONI, G. (1988) Plasma infusion for HUS in children – results of a multi-centre controlled trial. *Journal of Paediatrics*, **112**: 284–90.

TROMPETER, R.S. (1994) Steroid resistant nephrotic syndromes. In *Clinical Paediatric Nephrology*, 2nd edn (ed. R.J. Postlethwaite). Butterworth Heinmann, Oxford, pp. 226–34.

WARD, G. (1994) Chronic renal failure in childhood. Guy's Hospital, London, unpublished.

FURTHER READING

Short stature and chronic renal failure – what concerns children and parents? J M Reynolds, A J Wood, D M Eminson, R J Postlethwaite

Archives of disease in childhood. 73. 36–42–1995

Handbook of Renal Investigations in Children C M Taylor, S Chapman Wright – 1989

CHAPTER 11

RENAL TRANSPLANTATION

INTRODUCTION

Renal transplantation is now widely acknowledged as the treatment of choice for patients in end-stage renal failure (ESRF). Since the time of the first transplants in the 1950s, advances in antirejection therapies, surgical techniques and tissue matching have enabled kidney transplantation to evolve from an experimental procedure to the treatment that can offer the best quality of life and the most cost-effective care for kidney patients.

Many patients view a kidney transplant as the gateway to 'personal liberation' and as the opportunity to restore 'control over one's life' (Galpin, 1992). A successful transplant offers freedom from the practical and psychological difficulties and restrictions of long-term dialysis; freedom from dependence upon a machine, fluid bag or partner; freedom from fluid and dietary restrictions; a return of sexual functioning and fertility with the possibility of parenthood; and a return to an almost normal lifestyle.

Medical advances, such as the availability of synthetic erythropoietin (EPO), have dramatically improved the lifestyle of some dialysis patients. However, research studies clearly show that kidney transplantation has the greater rehabilitation potential (Blogg *et al.*, 1973; Petrie, 1989) and that the quality of life for patients with functioning grafts is superior to that which is usually achieved on dialysis (Churchill *et al.*, 1984; Simmons *et al.*, 1984; Evans *et al.*, 1985; Morris and Jones, 1988).

Quality of Life

Quality of life research has received much criticism. Individual perception and assessment of 'quality of life' is known to be affected by a wide range of independent and personal variables. Studies have been discredited because important variables have been excluded or ignored. It is difficult to have a truly comprehensive appreciation of an individual's 'quality of life' and, despite nearly two decades of research, a consensus has still not emerged as how best to conceptualise 'quality of life' (Evans, 1990).

The most extensive data available for comparing dialysis and transplant quality of life come from a large collaborative study led by Roger Evans of the Battelle Human Affairs Research Centre at Seattle (USA). This study, involving more than 800 patients in 11 American centres, is widely accepted as it used both objective and subjective 'quality of life' indicators, investigated all treatment modalities and included new medical advances such as treatment with EPO and new immunosuppression regimens. Evans concludes that 'Transplant recipients generally have a higher level of functional ability, are more likely to return to work, are in better health, and have higher levels of well being, life satisfaction, psychological affect, and happiness than do patients on any form of dialysis' (Evans, 1990).

Therefore, for many kidney patients transplantation offers an improved 'quality of life'. The quality of life issue may be the most significant factor for patients when considering transplantation. Dialysis can offer long-term support, therefore the decision to proceed to transplant does not have to be based on the issue of survival and may be based on life satisfaction needs.

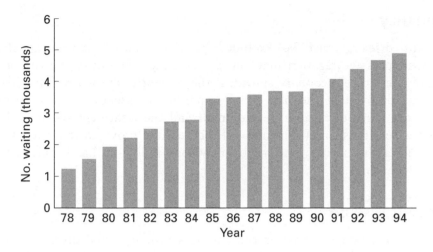

Fig. 11.1 *Kidney waiting list reported to United Kingdom Transplant Support Services Authority (UKTSSA), 31 December 1978 to 1994.*

Cost-Effective Care

Transplantation is the most cost-effective treatment option for end-stage renal disease. The cost of 1 year of haemodialysis or peritoneal dialysis is similar to that of a renal transplant in the first year. However, thereafter, the cost of continuing care for the transplant patient is one-fifth of the cost of dialysis per year.

National Waiting List Figures for Kidney Transplant

The improvement in quality of life and cost effectiveness of this treatment support the suggestion that renal transplantation is the treatment of choice for the majority of patients. Unfortunately, such a goal is not possible at present because of the limited supply of cadaveric organs. The current UK waiting list for kidney transplantation stands at more than 5000 patients (Fig. 11.1). On average, 1700 renal transplants are performed each year.

We therefore need to explore ways of increasing donor numbers in order to offer all suitable patients the chance of a transplant.

CONTRAINDICATIONS TO RENAL TRANSPLANTATION

Although the majority of patients may request a transplant, this treatment may not be suitable for all ESRF patients on medical grounds.

Malignancy

Malignant disease must be excluded prior to transplantation as the immunosuppressive regimen may cause accelerated growth of the tumour and may encourage secondary spread. If the patient is known to have had a tumour removed in the past, it is important to ascertain the type of tumour, the stage of tumour development and the treatment received. In selected cases transplantation may still be possible provided that curative treatment has been given and sufficiently long follow-up has occurred to exclude recurrence.

Recurrent Disease

It is also important to consider the patient's primary renal disease as in some cases the disease may recur and destroy the new kidney. Renal disorders with very high recurrence rate include focal segmental glomerulosclerosis (FSGS) (causing massive proteinuria and scarring of the glomeruli) and mesangio capillary glomerulonephritis (an immunological disorder of the glomeruli). Transplantation would still be considered but only after counselling and explanation of the risks to the patient. Most centres would advise against living related donation in this setting.

Other conditions such as Goodpasture's syndrome (in which an antibody in the blood attacks the kidney), and the other vasculitic illnesses need to have been fully treated before going ahead with transplantation because of the risk of damage in the new kidney in the presence of active disease. Twelve months is normally considered the earliest that transplantation would be considered, to allow antibody levels to fall.

Several other diseases, such as diabetes and immunoglobulin A (IgA) nephropathy, can cause microscopic changes in the kidney after many years but rarely lead to graft loss.

Hepatitis Virus and HIV

Patients who are hepatitis B or hepatitis C positive may be at risk of progressive liver disease after transplantation due to the impact of the immunosuppressive therapy. Similarly, the immunosuppression would have an adverse effect in the presence of human immunodeficiency virus (HIV) accelerating the disease. In most centres, infection with HIV is classed as an absolute contraindication to transplantation. Opinions differ with regard to transplantation in the presence of hepatitis B and hepatitis C. Decisions are taken on an individual basis with regard to level, type of infection and the extent of liver damage.

Diabetes Mellitus: Cardiovascular Disease

Many diabetic patients receive renal transplantation, but it is important to remember that they are likely to have many other complications from their diabetes. Cardiovascular disease is seen primarily in older non-insulin-dependent diabetics, and may contribute to higher levels of morbidity and death. Also it is important to assess vessel patency as severe atherosclerosis of the iliac vessels may at worst preclude transplantation and at best complicate the transplant surgery.

EVALUATION FOR TRANSPLANTATION

Age

Morbidity and mortality after kidney transplantation tend to increase with age and therefore the age of the recipient must be classed as a risk factor. Age must also be considered within the context of other risk factors such as advanced cardiovascular disease. In the past, centres have operated an age barrier to transplant, with cut off ages of 55, 60 and 65 years. However, most centres do not have age barriers today. Health is assessed on an individual basis, and physiological rather than chronological age and the existence of other risk factors are seen as the important assessment issues. Many units have patients of 70 years and over who have progressed well following a kidney transplant. With demand far exceeding supply, some may question the use of such a precious and scarce resource in older patients; should the young receive in preference to elderly recipients? This debate continues with some centres now attempting to match kidneys from older cadaveric donors with the older recipients; however, tissue match is always the major deciding factor.

Polycystic Kidney Disease

This inherited kidney disease can result in several members of a family receiving ESRF treatments. In our own centre we have a father and son with functioning transplants, a daughter on dialysis awaiting a transplant and a younger brother in the predialysis phase.

The native cystic kidneys may be very large, thus leaving little space for the transplant, and there may also be an increased risk of bleeding and infection. Occasionally, it may be necessary to perform a unilateral, or in severe cases a bilateral, nephrectomy prior to transplantation. In the past, nephrectomy led to severe anaemia due to lack of production of EPO; however, synthetic EPO is now available and is usually given following such surgery.

Urinary Tract

It is important to assess that there are no problems with the bladder and urethra and that there will be no difficulties following transplantation; if it is felt that the bladder capacity is unacceptably low, surgical enlargement may be possible. In the presence of a history of repeated urinary tract infections with bilateral reflux, it may be necessary to undertake a bilateral nephrectomy prior to transplantation to reduce the risk of post-transplant infection.

Cardiac Disease

Routine investigations such as an electrocardiogram (ECG) and cardiac history are essential for all patients. Those patients who are in the high-risk groups for cardiovascular disease (e.g. older patients, diabetics and those who have a history of ischaemic heart disease) should be reviewed by a cardiologist. Patients who have a history of myocardial infarction should be symptom-free for 1 year prior to transplant.

Gastric Ulceration

A history of indigestion and/or gastric ulceration most be noted and endoscopy undertaken if active ulceration is a possibility. Patients with active ulceration risk bleeding after transplantation due to the action of the steroid therapy. Treatment with H_2 receptor blocking agents (such as ranitidine) should be given prior to transplantation if active disease is present. Many centres also use ranitidine prophylaxis in all recipients during the first 6 postoperative months.

Respiratory Disease

Routine chest X-ray is essential for all patients, and any infection must be treated. Pulmonary tuberculosis will require treatment before transplantation. Patients with a history of tuberculosis and those who have visited or lived in high-risk areas will require prophylactic treatment with isoniazid and pyridoxine for at least 1 year following transplantation.

   Patients should also be strongly advised to stop smoking and should be offered information regarding antismoking strategies and support systems.

Obesity

Obesity may make the transplant surgery difficult and increase the risk of postoperative complications. Therefore, it is advisable to ask patients to reduce their weight if possible; however, patients treated with continuous ambulatory peritoneal dialysis (CAPD) may find weight loss very difficult due to the absorption of glucose contained in the dialysis fluid.

Oral Hygiene

Dental hygiene and assessment of dental state is essential. Any gum infection or dental problems should be dealt with prior to transplantation. Cyclosporin can cause gum hypertrophy, which is made much worse in the presence of poor hygiene.

Acute Infections

Acute infections should be treated as and when they occur so that the patient is infection free at the time of transplantation. This is particularly relevant for haemodialysis patients with temporary access and CAPD patients prone to peritonitis and exit site infections.

PRETRANSPLANTATION PREPARATION

Psychological Adjustment Stage

Patients may be referred for transplantation during different phases of the disease process; some may be in the predialysis stage, others may already be established on dialysis therapy.

Disease and Dialysis Adjustment (Initial–Early Response)

The diagnosis of ESRF and the subsequent need for treatment will result in shock and fear for both the patient and their family. Emotional adjustments must be negotiated to manage the physical, psychological, marital and dialysis-related changes imposed by the disease. Such adjustments can produce profound stress, adjustment anxiety and depression (Salter, 1988; Petrie, 1989; Surman, 1989).

Various psychological coping strategies may be utilised during this time and, in the early phase, denial and suppression are the most frequently used avoidance techniques (Miller, 1983). Denial as a psychological defence has been shown to be prominent in the haemodialysis population (Surman, 1989).

For patients referred during the predialysis or early phase of the disease process such psychological denial may make communications between patient and staff difficult and may result in unrealistic expectations for post-transplant rehabilitation. Unrealistic expectations may predispose the patient to depression if major complications occur after the transplant

(Dubovsky and Penn, 1980). Early transplantation is often welcomed from a clinical perspective but may prove difficult psychologically if emotional adjustments have not been successfully negotiated and the patient and family are still reeling from the impact of the disease.

Disease: Dialysis Adjustment (Later Response)

Gradually, as the patient adjusts to the dialysis treatment more positive coping strategies may develop with problem solving, seeking of information, enhancement of spiritual life and hope of a transplant among those strategies most commonly utilised (Voepal-Lewis *et al.*, 1990; White *et al.*, 1990). Peretz (1970) defined hope as the capacity to anticipate that even though one feels uncomfortable now, one may feel better in the future. Once a transplant is suggested, many patients make an immediate decision to proceed, whereas others may agonise over the decision. Patients who are doing well on dialysis may express doubt as to whether or not a transplant will improve their quality of life (Weems and Patterson, 1989) and may have heard negative accounts from fellow patients who have experienced problems or a failed graft. Conversely, patients may have been given falsely positive information. Therefore, it is essential that in-depth, realistic and honest information is given and that staff are aware of individual needs so that informed consent is achieved and individual support planned.

Pretransplant Meeting: Assessment and Support

Some patients may receive the initial information about transplantation at a predialysis meeting. Other patients may be given information by the nephrologist or dialysis nursing staff. Written information is essential as verbal information given during a stressful time is often forgotten. Booklets and videos must be expressed in terms that patients can understand and should be offered so that they can be viewed at home in a familiar and safe environment.

Most transplant centres will invite the patient and family to the unit for a discussion meeting. The aim of this visit is to provide a forum to explore transplantation and its suitability for them. This is also an opportunity to meet with all members of the multidisciplinary team to initiate supportive relationships. The patient and family are given the opportunity to meet with the transplant surgeon to discuss the advantages and disadvantages of transplantation. Issues such as patient suitability, risk factors, waiting list procedures, post-transplant medication and lifestyle are explored, with special attention given to the benefits and the side-effects of the immuno-suppression regimens. Questions are answered with complete honesty.

Following this discussion the patient will undergo the necessary pretransplant clinical tests as outlined in Table 11.1. Later, a tour of the transplant

Table 11.1 *Evaluation for transplantation for all potential renal*
transplant recipients

- *Full history*
    Renal disease and disease progression
    Previous medical history — noting previous blood transfusions/
    pregnancies and previous transplants
    Previous surgery
    Current status
    Social history, family status
    Medications, allergies
    Smoking, alcohol and drug abuse

- *Physical examination*
    Assessment of blood pressure
    Cardiac assessment
    Respiratory assessment
    Urological assessment
    Assessment of vascular system with pulses
    Abdominal assessment — previous surgery, Tenckhoff site

- *Routine investigations*
    Urea and electolytes
    Full blood count
    Blood group
    Tissue typing
    Liver function tests and uric acid
    Lipid levels
    Virology screen — human immunodeficiency virus (HIV)
                     hepatitis B & C
                     cytomegalovirus (CMV)
                     Epstein—Barr virus (EBV)
                     varicella zoster virus (VZV)
    Weight
    Chest X-ray
    MSU (mid-stream urine)
    ECG (electrocardiogram)

centre will enable them to meet the unit staff and familiarise themselves with the facilities. Meetings with patients who have received a transplant may be arranged if appropriate and the opportunity to view a video outlining pre- and post-transplant care is offered. Further meetings with the named transplant nurse practitioner to explore individual fears, anxieties and special needs may be arranged. Individual anxieties discussed during such meetings include fear of changes in body image due to the effects of immunosuppression, fear of loss of identity when accepting a 'foreign organ' and fear of surgery, particularly for older patients.

Body Image Changes

Immunosuppression and its side-effects may present a major hurdle for patients following transplantation (Hudson and Hion, 1966; Galpin, 1992). Cyclosporin therapy may induce hirsutism (excessive hair growth, particularly facial hair), gingival hyperplasia (excessive growth of gums) and shaking, and steroid therapy may cause acne and a cushingoid (facial swelling) appearance.

Body image is an individual subject and what is a problem for one person may be insignificant to another (Price, 1990). However, studies show that many renal transplant patients report body image problems, often leading to lower self-esteem and depression. In extreme cases patients may be tempted to stop the immunosuppression and therefore careful preoperative information and counselling concerning expected side-effects is crucial. Patients should be reassured that such side-effects are dose related and will lessen as the drug doses are reduced. Also, practical advice in coping with specific problems may reduce anxiety and fears. A trained skin and beauty therapist may be available to offer extensive advice and free electrolysis treatment to help reduce psychological trauma and aid adjustment.

Psychological Acceptance of the Transplant

Some patients report the anxiety that there may be difficulty accepting the transplant as part of 'self', others fear that they may be accepting the 'persona' of the donor with the kidney. There may also be fears that a kidney from a female donor may feminise a male patient or conversely, a kidney from a male may masculinise a female patient. Such anxieties can be resolved by empathetic discussion and additional information.

Guilt: Benefiting from Traumatic Death

Patients may express guilt that they will be benefiting from another's tragic death and may be hesitant to accept a cadaveric graft. Empathetic discussion to explore such issues can reassure and ease anxiety.

Pretransplant Support

Pretransplant visits help to initiate a trusting and supportive relationship between the patient, the family and the transplant team. Support continues from the transplant nurse practitioner throughout the waiting time and the transplant itself.

DONOR AND RECIPIENT MATCHING

Immune System: Overview

The human body has a complex system of defences that can provide protection against infection and disease. This system has the ability to target, isolate and destroy potentially harmful invaders. This destruction is achieved in three stages – first by the recognition of structures on the invader (antigens) which are not present in the host. Antibodies and T cells that can recognise the antigens as 'foreign' are then produced. These antibodies and T cells then attach to the invader and destroy it both directly and by recruiting other mechanisms of destruction. Exactly the same happens to a transplant unless it is from an identical twin. The 'foreign' antigens on the transplant induce antibodies and T cells. These target the transplanted organ and do their very best to destroy it. The term 'transplant antigens' is used to describe those antigens which are most important in this regard. Only two are really important, the human leukocyte antigen (HLA) system and the ABO system (see below). In order to prevent rejection it is necessary to circumvent the immune system (matching and cross-matching) and to suppress the immunological response.

Components of the Immune System

Leukocytes (white blood cells)
These comprise the cells which produce the antibody (B lymphocytes), recognise the foreign antigens (T lymphocytes), directly destroy invaders (activated or killer T lymphocytes), or can be called in to help with the destruction process (monocytes, polymorphs and eosinophils). Thus, it can be seen that the lymphocytes play several roles and therefore have the major influence on graft acceptance.

Lymphocytes
These comprise 20% of the total white blood cell count (WBC) and are made up of several groups of cells with specialised functions. The term 'orchestra' is often used to describe the mode of operation. Each section of the orchestra is made up of individuals with similar but not identical characteristics. The overall result of the orchestra playing is a result of each section performing in concert with the others.

Lymphocyte types
- *T cells*. These have antigen recognition structures fixed to their surface.
- *B cells*. These have antigen recognition structures that can be secreted (antibodies).

T cells and B cells can be naive or activated. T cells can be activated to various functions, namely helper, killer or tolerant status. B cells can be activated to produce antibody or memory.

Each naive lymphocyte has an antigen recognition structure that is unique, for example different from other members of its section and thus capable of seeing a different antigen. In this way literally millions of 'foreign' antigens can be recognised. Each time a recognition event occurs a naive cell becomes activated and divides. Thus, even if a single cell recognises an antigen as foreign it keeps dividing until it forms a significant number of identical cells (a clone), all capable of recognising the antigen. Depending on influences from other sections, T cells can help B cells produce antibody (helper T cells), kill targets bearing the antigen directly (killer T cells), or become tolerant (i.e. capable of recognising the antigen but not producing a damaging response to it). B cells can produce antibody in around 8–10 days if they see it for the first time (naive B cells) or within 24 h if they have seen it before (memory B cells). B cells produce much more antibody if they get help from the T cells which can themselves see the same antigen.

One point about antibody production which is relevant to transplantation is that the process which produces it is long lived. This is very good news for vaccination programmes, where having antibody around for years and years is very beneficial. It is very bad news for transplantation.

ABO Blood Groups

The ABO system of human blood groups was described by Landsteiner in 1902. Blood group is determined by A and B antigens on the surface of the red blood cells. Each individual has one of the four basic blood group types O, A, B or AB.

Each individual has antibodies to the blood group antigens that they do not express (Table 11.2). Antibodies against the blood group antigens can cause hyperacute rejection and therefore matching of blood group between donor and recipient is vital. Blood group O organs can be transplanted into all groups; O is classified as the universal donor. Blood group AB recipients can receive organs from all groups; AB is classified as the universal recipient.

Table 11.2 The ABO blood group system

Blood Group	% of population	Antigens expressed	Antibodies expressed	Acceptable donor blood group
O	47%	None	Anti A, Anti B	O
A	42%	A	Anti B	O,A
B	8%	B	Anti A	O,B
AB	3%	AB	None	O,A,B,AB

Histocompatibility Antigens

A further set of proteins that can trigger the B and T cell response are the transplantation antigens or the histocompatibility antigens. The histocompatibility antigens can be divided into two groups, major and minor.

Major histocompatibility complex (MHC)

This system, first discovered in the mouse by Peter Gorer at Guy's Hospital in the late 1930s is, as the name suggests, the most important system in transplantation and indeed in immunity to infection. The human system is termed HLA (for human leukocyte antigen) and was identified by Dausset, van Rood and Payne in the 1960s (Klein, 1986). The sera from pregnant women were found to have antibodies that recognised lymphocytes from their partners and from some random blood donors. The reason for this is that pregnancy is in some ways like a transplant. Passage of blood from partner or child to mother results in killer T cells and antibody being produced to the foreign antigens on the blood cells. Since the most potent foreign antigens are those of the HLA system, most of the mother's response is directed against them and the long-lived antibody-producing cells remain in her blood. These antibodies can persist for over 40 years.

The HLA system is complex. There are four main series important for transplantation, A, B, C and DR. There are over 30 antigens in each series. Each person can have two from each series (one from each parent). The permutation on 2/30 from A, 2/30 from B, 2/30 from C and 2/30 from DR means that, outside of a family it is very rare for individuals to have identical HLA types. Luckily for matching in renal transplantation, DR is dominant. However, most of the antibody and T cell response is produced to A, B and C.

The rules for HLA and matching are not nearly so clear cut as the rules for ABO, but there are several strong guidelines:

- Transplantation of a kidney into someone who has antibodies directed to a foreign (mismatched) HLA antigen on that kidney will result in hyperacute rejection.
- Transplantation of a kidney into someone who has strong memory to a foreign (mismatched) HLA antigen on that kidney will result in very rapid rejection.
- Transplantation of a kidney with two mismatches at DR will have more rejection than one with one mismatch at DR, and both will have more rejection than a kidney with no DR mismatches. However, rejection episodes can be treated or mismatched patients given additional immunosuppression (Fig 11.2).

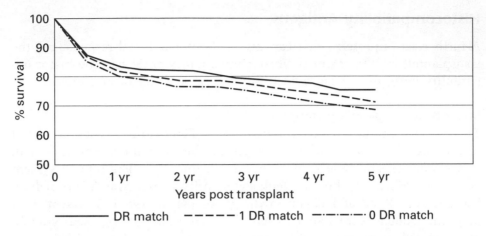

Fig. 11.2 *Influence of HLA-DR matching on renal allograft survival.*

Donor and Recipient Matching

The majority of organs for transplant come from cadaveric donors. It is essential to match for blood group and to achieve the best DR match possible. Since antibodies can be induced to pregnancies or transfusions or previous transplants and can be boosted by infection, regular screening of patients on the waiting list is necessary to maintain knowledge of their current antibody status. Donors are avoided if they contain any mismatch to which the recipient is responding to or has responded to.

Donor and recipient cross-matching
As a final check for current antibody and for the accuracy of past screening, a recent sample and selected past samples from the recipient are always checked against actual donor cells before transplantation.

UK matching system
Within the UK, each transplant centre has a local list of recipients awaiting transplant. There is also a national list held at the UK Transplant Support Services Authority (UKTSSA) in Bristol. Each cadaveric donor is tissue typed at the local transplant centre and one kidney is transplanted into a local recipient. The other kidney is offered to Bristol for a close tissue match elsewhere in the UK. Such a system helps to ensure close matching for a majority of transplant recipients.

Pretransplant cross-match
Prior to transplant, a cross-match test is performed in the tissue typing laboratory. A blood sample from the recipient is mixed with lymphocytes from the donor. If the donor cells react (die), the result is termed as a positive cross-match; the recipient is adversely reacting to the donor antigens.

In the presence of a positive cross-match, transplantation cannot proceed, as the transplant would be rejected.

Sensitisation

When there is a positive cross-match, the recipient is sensitised to that donor. The higher the level of sensitisation, the greater will be the difficulty in finding a transplant that will not reject.

Sensitisation can occur during pregnancy (partner's antigens), during blood transfusion and after transplantation. In order to reduce the risk of sensitisation it is important to minimise the giving of blood transfusions.

Some recipients may have a high level of sensitisation (highly sensitised). Many cross-matches are performed for each recipient. If the recipient does not react with the various donors tested then they are classified as unsensitised. If the blood reacts with 50% of donors they are 50% sensitised, and if blood reacts with 100% of donors they are highly sensitised.

Unfortunately, some highly sensitised candidates wait years for a compatible transplant.

CADAVERIC (HEART BEATING) DONATION

The majority of renal transplants result from cadaveric donation. Cadaveric donors are patients that have suffered irreversible brain stem damage (brain stem death) and are maintained on a ventilator within a critical care unit.

Causes of Brain Stem Death

The most common causes of brain stem death are listed in Table 11.3.

Cerebral swelling resultant from trauma or anoxia and intracerebral bleeding can cause raised intracranial pressure which forces the cerebral hemispheres through the tentorial hiatus thus compressing the brain stem and interrupting its blood supply. Such herniation of the cerebral tissue is usually described as 'coning' and results in irreversible damage to the brain stem.

Table 11.3 *Common causes of brain stem death*

- Intracerebral bleed or infarction
- Head trauma
- Cerebral hypoxia due to:
    respiratory arrest
    cardiac arrest
    smoke inhalation/carbon monoxide poisoning
- Cerebral tumour
- Drug overdose
- Intracranial infection

Brain Stem Functions

The brain stem is responsible for the capacity to breath spontaneously and the capacity for consciousness. If the brain stem is irreversibly damaged then there is loss of function and it is argued that the 'irreversible loss of the capacity for consciousness and the irreversible loss of the capacity to breath' constitutes brain stem death, which constitutes death of the person (Pallis, 1994).

Brain stem death diagnosed by signs of irreversible damage to the brain stem is an accepted concept in most countries of the world.

Brain Stem Death Diagnosis

Tests to diagnose brain stem death originated from the Harvard Medical School criteria (Harvard Medical School, 1968) which were published in the USA in 1968. A UK Code of Practice for the diagnosis of brain stem death was agreed by the Conference of Medical Royal Colleges in 1976, 1979 and 1991 (UK Code of Practice, 1991).

The clinical diagnosis of brain stem death involves three steps. The first step is to ascertain that the following *preconditions* have been met:

- the patient is deeply comatosed and on a ventilator;
- the patient has been maintained on the ventilator for sufficient time to ascertain that the brain damage is irreversible;
- there is a positive diagnosis of the cause of the coma.

The second step is to *exclude* other possible causes of coma:

- primary hypothermia (< 35 °C);
- drug intoxication or alcohol intoxication;
- metabolic and endocrine disturbances.

The third step is to perform testing to ascertain:

- absent brain stem reflexes;
- apnoea (loss of capacity for spontaneous breathing).

Tests for brain stem death: absent brain stem reflexes
- The pupils are fixed and dilated: no response to light.
- Absent corneal reflex; patient does not blink when cornea is stimulated.
- Absent: vestibulo-ocular reflexes: no eye movements during or after slow injection of 20 ml of ice cold water into each external auditory meatus.
- Absent cranial nerve response to pain: no response to stimulation of any somatic area.
- Absent gag reflex: no response to tracheal and bronchial stimulation by a suction catheter.

- No respiratory movements occur when the respiratory centre is stimulated (apnoea testing).

Apnoea testing No respiratory movements occur when the patient is disconnected from the ventilator for long enough to ensure that the arterial carbon dioxide level rises above the threshold for the stimulation of respiration. The method is as follows:

- ventilate the patient with 100% O_2 for 10 min;
- prior to disconnection the $PaCO_2$ should be above 6 KPa (45 mmHg) and should rise to 6.66 KPa (50 mmHG) during the test;
- disconnect the patient from the ventilator;
- administer 100% oxygen at 6 l min^{-1} via a narrow bore catheter down the endotracheal tube;
- observe the patient for signs of respiratory effort for 10 min and/or until the $PaCO_2$ is above 6.66 KPa;
- reconnect the patient to the ventilator.

Declaration of brain stem death
The UK Code of Practice recommends that brain stem death testing should be carried out by two medical practitioners 'who have expertise in this field'. One should be a consultant and the other a consultant or senior registrar. Neither of the doctors should be a member of the transplant team or associated with potential transplant recipients.

Repetition of testing
The Code of Practice also recommends that testing should be performed twice to ensure that there has been no observer error. The interval between the tests is normally at the discretion of the critical care staff who will also consider the needs and circumstances of the family.

Time of death
The time of completion of the second set of negative tests is legally the time of death, and this should be recorded as such on the death certificate.

Criteria for Organ Donation
- Age 0–75 years.
- The patient has suffered severe and irreversible brain damage resulting in brain stem death.
- The patient is maintained on a ventilator.
- The patient has no major untreated sepsis.
- The patient has no malignancy – except primary brain tumour.
- The patient is HIV and hepatitis B and C negative.

Patients from high-risk groups (as defined by the Department of Health) should also be excluded. Other diseases may preclude donation of specific organs; however, it is recommended that critical care staff consider organ donation in all brain stem dead patients and refer to the local transplant co-ordinator for a decision regarding medical suitability.

Requesting Donation

In the UK, the legal requirements for organ donation are contained in the Human Tissue Act 1961. The Act states that:-

> 'The person lawfully in possession of the body of a deceased person may authorise the removal of any part from the body for use for the said purposes, if having made such reasonable enquiry as may be practicable, he has no reason to believe:
>
> (a) that the deceased had expressed an objection to his body being so dealt with after death ... or
> (b) that the surviving spouse or any surviving relative of the deceased object to the body being so dealt with.

Therefore, in practice, it is the next of kin or the patient's executor who are usually approached to give permission for donation. If the patient has signed a donor card there is no statutory requirement to approach the family, but in practice the views of the family are always sought and if objections are raised donation does not occur.

If the next of kin cannot be notified, the body remains in the possession of the hospital. In such cases the hospital manager can give permission for donation as long as reasonable enquiries have been made and that 'there is no reason to believe that the deceased had expressed objections'.

Religious beliefs

As far as it is known, no major religious groups in the UK object to the principles of organ donation and transplantation. Some groups feel that it is only permissible if the donor themselves requested donation. These groups include, in particular, Orthodox Jews, Christian Scientists and some Hindu groups. The Jehovah's Witnesses have religious objections to blood transfusions, but feel that donating or receiving organs is a matter for each Jehovah's Witness to decide for themselves.

It is often thought that the Muslim faith does not support donation and anecdotal evidence suggests that British Muslims are, in general, reluctant to donate organs. However, recent legislation has approved donation and transplantation in Muslim countries such as Saudi Arabia. Also, a recent FATWA issued by the Muslim Law Council (a body that is to the Muslims what the Vatican is to the Catholics) has stated that Muslims may donate organs. They may carry donor cards and their next of kin may give permission for donating (Carlisle, 1995). Previous reluctance to donate may have been cultural rather than religious and therefore information and liaison with Muslims will be vital in order to encourage donation.

Fear of increasing the distress of the family

Critical care staff have expressed fears that offering donation may increase the distress of the bereaved (Wakeford and Stepney, 1989); however, experience suggests that offering the choice to donate, if performed with empathy, does not increase distress. Indeed, donor families report that the act of donation brings comfort and something positive in an otherwise negative situation (Buckley, 1989). American and UK studies have noted that a fundamental need for relatives during a 'crisis time' is 'to feel there is hope' (Molter, 1979; Coulter, 1989; Wilkinson, 1995). In the presence of a diagnosis of brain stem death there can be no hope for the patient but donation can be an option of hope with life for others.

Acceptance that death has occurred

It is crucial that the bereaved family have accepted the fact that death has occurred before donation is requested. In the case of brain stem death the acceptance of death is more difficult for the family as they are asked to accept a 'new concept of death'. The accepted concept and image of death involves a cold, lifeless body without a heartbeat; however, in the case of brain stem death the family are presented with an image of a warm patient with a heart beat who appears (due to the ventilator) to be breathing. Therefore, the visual message is one of life but the verbal message is one of death. In such cases denial is often enhanced and relatives must struggle to understand and accept the situation. Denial may be particularly acute in the case of an intracerebral bleed where there is no outward sign of injury or trauma.

Clear communications must ensue, the core message being that 'there is no hope of recovery'. Irreparable damage has occurred and the brain has died – death of the brain stem is death of the person.

When to offer donation

It is damaging to approach the family too early, as trust may be lost. A recent study to examine the reasons for relatives' refusal (Mori/UKTCA/ BACCN, 1995) notes that a refusal may have been because the family were 'approached too early by inexperienced staff'. This study also reports that 'Consent for donation rates are higher in cases where the request is made after the second set of brain stem tests'. Furthermore, a study from the USA noted that relatives were more likely to agree to donation if the explanation of brain stem death and the request for organ donation were clearly separated in time (Garrison et al., 1991). Thus it is important for the family to have accepted that death has occurred before donation is offered, also to inform the family of the death and to request donation at separate meetings.

Who should offer donation?

All studies report that the person who has established a trusting relationship with the family is the most appropriate person to offer donation. It is important that the requestee has a positive view of donation and can offer it in a positive way.

How to offer donation

There are no 'right' words; each situation is unique and families will have their own individual responses. The family should be asked if they have any objection to donation rather than for permission to proceed. Some families will require time to consider their decision. Many relatives will have additional questions concerning the process of donation and its implications at this time. It may be helpful for the family to meet with the transplant co-ordinator, who can answer specific questions. The family may require reassurance on the following issues:

● that the donor will feel no pain;
● that there will be dignity and respect throughout the donor surgery;
● that the body will not be grossly mutilated or disfigured;
● that the surgical wound will be sutured;
● that they can view the body after surgery and that the funeral will not be delayed.

The transplant co-ordinator will work closely with other health care professionals to answer further questions and to facilitate the wishes of the family. The co-ordinator can also reassure the family that she/he will be present throughout the surgery and at the end to oversee and continue care.

Continuing care after donation

Letters of thanks containing brief anonymous information concerning the transplant recipients are given or sent to the donor family after the donation. Further help and support is also offered. Many families state that the news of the successful transplants is a source of comfort.

Refusal to donate

A study by Gore *et al.*, (1989) reported that approximately 30% of relatives of potential donors within intensive care units refused consent. The Mori/UKTCA/BACCN (1995) study also reports a 38% refusal rate. The five most common reasons given for refusal were:

● the relatives did not want surgery to the body (24%);

- the patient had stated in the past that they did not wish donation to take place (21%);
- the relatives felt that the patient had suffered enough (21%);
- the relatives were divided over the decision (19%);
- the relatives were not sure whether the patient would have agreed to organ donation (18%).

Refusal rates of 30% represent a desperate lost potential. Therefore, it is vital that information programmes to allay fears and to present the successes of transplantation continue. It is also helpful to implement education for health care staff to examine the issue of requesting donation so that personnel will feel comfortable when offering this option of hope to the family.

If the family agree to donation, the ventilation continues and the preparations for the donor surgery are made, but if the family refuse donation then ventilation will cease.

Clinical Care of a Potential Organ Donor

Brain stem death results in changes to normal homeostatic mechanisms; such changes will ultimately result in cardiac arrest. Once permission has been given for donation it is important to stabilise the condition of the donor to ensure optimal condition of the organs for transplantation.

The major problem following brain stem death is hypotension. This is usually due to hypovolaemia, loss of antidiuretic hormone (ADH) leading to diabetes insipidus, loss of vasomotor control and other factors. Donor care may be encompassed into the rule of '100s' and '10s' (Table 11.4).

Table 11.4 *Donor care: rule of 100s and 10s*

- Systolic blood pressure > 100 mmHG
- Urine output > 100 ml h^{-1}
- Arterial PO_2 > 10 kPa
- Central venous pressure (CVP) > 10 mmHG

Strategies to achieve the rule of '100s' and '10s'
To maintain the blood pressure at 100 mmHG systolic:

- Fluid load to a central venous pressure (CVP) of + 10 mmHG – using two units of haemacel/gelofusin followed by alternating normal saline and dextrose 5%.
- If systolic blood pressure of 100 mmHG is still not achieved then commence dopamine at 10 µg kg^{-1} min^{-1} (if effective the dopamine can be weaned down to between 2 and 10 µg kg^{-1} min^{-1}).

- If the blood pressure remains unresponsive, dobutamine 5–10 $\mu g\,kg^{-1}$ min^{-1} should be commenced.
- If urine output exceeds 200 ml h^{-1} give DDVAP (desmopressin) 0.5–2.0 $\mu g\,kg^{-1}\,min^{-1}$ subcutaneously or intramuscularly.

Inotropic dosage use of adrenaline and noradrenaline
- Minimise the use of inotropic drugs, therefore *infuse i.v. fluids to maintain CVP of 10 mmHG*
- Both adrenaline and noradrenaline should only be used as a last resort to treat hypotension, as they will decrease the viability of the heart and lungs for transplant.

The Role of the Transplant Co-Ordinator

All renal transplant centres within the UK employ transplant co-ordinators. The transplant co-ordinators are senior practitioners (usually with a nursing background), who offer a 24-h service to intensive care units with regard to organ donation. The role of the transplant co-ordinator at the time of donation is to offer:

- advice regarding suitability of a potential organ donor;
- advice regarding donor clinical care;
- advice and/or help with the approach to relatives;
- organisation of the organ donation procedure and surgery;
- support of the family and staff.

Organisation of the organ donation procedure and surgery
The transplant co-ordinator will usually attend at the donor hospital to offer advice and support to the donor family and critical care staff. Organisation of the organ donation is complex and the transplant co-ordinator will attempt to make all arrangements with a minimum of distress to the donor family and the critical care staff. The majority of organ donations today are multiple donations and it is the transplant co-ordinator who organises the necessary blood and clinical tests, liaises with the heart, liver, renal and ophthalmic teams and arranges the donor surgery (Table 11.5).

Permission from the Coroner

If the case comes under the jurisdiction of the coroner (or procurator fiscal), then permission must be obtained to proceed to organ donation. Cases usually requiring the coroner's permission include:

- road traffic accident;
- suspicious deaths/suicide;
- deaths less than 12 h after surgery;

Table 11.5 *Organ donation: role of the transplant co-ordinator*

- Arrival at donor hospital
- Meet with critical care staff
- Assess potential donor suitability
- Advice regarding donor clinical care (if requested)
- Meet with donor family; offer advice and support (if requested)
- Permission from the coroner or coroner's officer
- Organise clinical tests and blood tests:

Clinical tests	Blood tests
12 lead ECG	ABO blood group
Chest X-ray	Biochemistry
Approx. size and weight of donor	Urea & electrolytes
Arterial blood gases	Liver function tests
	Full blood count
	Virology screen
	HIV
	Hepatitis B & C
	Cytomegalovirus (CMV)

- Contact UKTSSA re super urgent cases
- Liaise with heart, liver, renal and ophthalmic teams
- Liaise with theatre staff and obtain theatre time:
     accompany donor to theatre
     assist surgical teams
     support theatre personnel
- Final care of donor
- Contact with donor family offering information and/or support
- Information and thanks to donor hospital personnel

- traumatic deaths.

It is unusual for permission to be withheld except in the case of suspected murder.

Removal of Kidneys from a Multi-Organ Donor

It is most common now for kidneys to be taken out as part of an operation from a multi-organ donor. This requires careful co-ordination between the teams involved to make sure that there is no compromise to viability in any of the transplanted organs (Plates 2, 3 and 4).

The exact details of the operation vary from centre to centre, but the principles include a generous incision giving good exposure to the organs of interest with the heart still beating, and placement of cannulas for *in situ* perfusion and cooling.

- A bilateral subcostal incision with a mid-line sternotomy is a common approach. The heart and lungs are inspected and mobilised first to allow rapid removal at a later stage.

- A careful laparotomy is carried out before dissection of the major blood supply to the liver. The common bile duct is transected and the gall bladder incised and flushed to prevent biliary autolysis.
- Cannulae are placed into the aorta and portal vein for perfusion (Fig. 11.4). The distal inferior vena cava is for similarly treated drainage. Ventilation ceases when the aorta is cross-clamped. Perfusion starts simultaneously to minimise warm ischaemia.
- The organs are removed; first heart and lungs, followed by the liver and then the kidneys. Careful co-operation between teams is required to minimise damage to the various organs. Pancreas is used for transplantation with increasing success; concurrent retrieval with the above organs has not been associated with adverse outcome.

Before closure of the abdominal incisions specimens of donor lymph nodes and spleen are removed for histocompatibility and tissue typing.

Surgical Technique for Cadaveric Donor Nephrectomy

If the kidneys are to be removed alone, bilateral nephrectomy is accomplished through a long mid-line incision or a bilateral subcostal incision. The kidneys are either taken out *en bloc* or individually on patches of inferior vena cava and aorta. The technique preferred in this centre entails the removal of an individual kidney on a patch of aorta and inferior vena cava. The technique is as follows:

- Abdominal incision and laporotomy are performed as for multi-organ retrieval.
- The aorta is dissected up to the superior mesenteric artery and the inferior vena cava dissected above the renal veins.
- Slings are placed around the aorta and the inferior vena cava above the bifurcation ready for tying at a later stage.
- A catheter is passed into the aorta through an incision just above the bifurcation. The balloon of the catheter is distended with fluid and ties placed around the aorta distal to the balloon to hold it in place (Fig. 11.4). Care must be taken not to overdistend catheter balloons as this can obstruct the lumen of the catheter.
- A similar procedure is carried out with the inferior vena cava just above the confluence of the right and left common iliac veins, and the aorta and inferior vena cava below the catheters are tied off.
- The aorta is tied off in the upper abdomen and perfusion is started through the Foley catheter (Fig.11.3). As perfusion starts ventilation is discontinued.
- The kidneys begin to get cold at this stage and, while the perfusion fluid is running through into the kidneys and out through the renal veins, the kidneys should be surrounded by ice to assist cooling and prevent rewarming from the adjacent tissues.

- The inferior vena cava above the renal veins is ligated and the blood from the kidneys drains out through the catheter in the inferior vena cava.
- After 2 l of fluid has flushed through and the kidneys are cold they can be mobilised and the cannulas removed.
- The inferior vena cava is split up the middle and along the back, taking care not to divide the right renal artery. The aorta is also divided anteriorly and posteriorly, taking care to avoid damaging the left renal vein which crosses in front of the aorta and, having done this, each kidney is taken out with a section of aorta and inferior vena cava and placed in iced saline, where it is reflushed with preservation fluid.
- Normally, no further dissection is done at this stage, but the kidney is placed in sterile bags and sent at 4 °C to the receiving centre. Further dissection of the kidney is performed immediately before subsequent transplantation into the recipient.

Following removal, each kidney is examined for any surgical injury and unusual anatomy and is placed in a sterile bag with a small amount of perfusion fluid. This bag is then placed inside two further polythene bags to ensure sterility. The kidney is finally packed into a transport container with ice (Fig. 11.4).

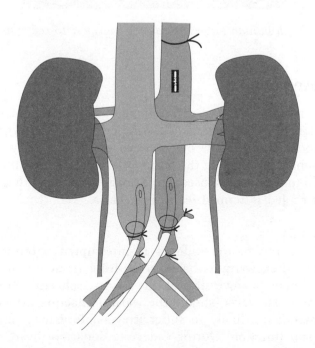

Fig. 11.3 *Perfusion catheters* in situ *for cadaveric donor nephrectomy.*

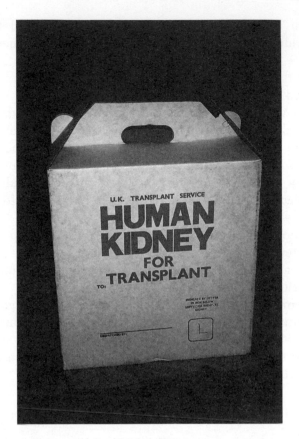

Fig. 11.4 Box with human kidney, ready for transport to the transplant centre.

Organ Preservation

The aim of preservation is to maintain the organ in an optimal condition until transplantation can occur. All living cells require oxygen to survive. Once the blood supply to the organ ceases, the lack of oxygen will result in cellular ischaemia. Cooling the organ will reduce the cellular metabolism and thus help to minimise subsequent damage. Ischaemia that occurs before the organ is cooled is termed warm ischaemia.

Warm ischaemia

If the blood supply to the kidneys is interrupted without cooling, the tubular cells suffer warm ischaemia resulting in acute tubular necrosis (ATN). ATN may be reversible if the warm ischaemia time is limited (approx. 45 min). However, should the warm ischaemia extend longer than 1 h the glomeruli are likely to suffer irreversible damage and the kidney may not regain function. During cadaveric donation (heart beating donation) the ventilation and blood supply continue until the perfusion system is in place. As perfusion with cooled fluid commences, the ventilation ceases. Thus, the kidney is immediately cooled and the warm ischaemia is limited to approximately 1–2 min only.

Cold ischaemia

The ice should maintain the kidney at approximately 4 °C, thus minimising ischaemic damage and enabling transport to the transplant centre. The time from the beginning of cooling to reperfusion and rewarming of the time of transplantation is termed the cold ischaemia time. Most kidneys can be stored for 24–48 h if necessary. However, recent studies suggest that prolonged cold ischaemia may reduce the function of the transplant, particularly if the kidney is from an elderly donor. Therefore, most transplant centres transplant kidneys within 24 h of removal when possible.

LIVING RELATED DONATION

An Oxford patient, Graham Frew, received a kidney transplant from his twin sister, Anne, 31 years ago (03.05.64) at the Hammersmith Hospital. At the time of the transplant Graham weighed less than 38 kg and was severely hypertensive and blind. Without the transplant, Graham would have died within days. Fortunately, his transplant was successful and continues to function well with a current creatinine level of 153 mmol l^{-1}. Graham's sister has had no long-term problems.

In the early days, such living related donor transplants were the only possible option but, with the advent of improved immunosuppressive regimens and cadaveric donation, there has been much debate surrounding the continuing need for living donation.

Ethical Issues

The core factors of the living donation debate involve the critical issue of a balance between 'doing good without doing harm' and also the concept of 'altruism'.

Physical well-being – doing good without doing harm

The donation will most certainly 'do good' in benefiting the recipient but may also 'do harm' to the donor, as the surgical procedure exposes the living donor to major clinical risks. Mortality from living donor surgery is difficult to assess because the statistics are not confirmed; however, donor deaths have been reported. On the basis of undocumented reports, a figure in the region of 1 in 4000 may be correct, with death from pulmonary embolism being the commonest cause (Allen and Chapman, 1993).

Early postoperative complications may also occur and may include chest infection, deep vein thrombosis, wound infection and postsurgical depression amongst others. Long-term complications have not been demonstrated, with follow-up studies of living related donors, for as long as 20 years, finding no functional abnormalities. Careful preoperative assessment, expert surgical teams and close postoperative monitoring have reduced the risks to a minimum in most centres. However, living donation is surgery which presents a potential for harm to the donor's physical well-being.

Psychological well-being – doing good without doing harm

Undoubtedly, many living donors gain psychologically from the act of giving. Studies suggest that donors describe the act 'as one of the most meaningful experiences in their lives' (Fellner and Marshall, 1968) and 'view themselves as more worthwhile because of donation' (Simmons *et al.*, 1971). The satisfaction of helping a 'loved one' return to a normal lifestyle is very rewarding for many. Indeed, it has been suggested that there may be psychological harm if a donor is prevented from giving (Simmons *et al.*, 1977). Thus, living donation presents physical risks but psychological gain for the donor.

Altruism

Altruism – the act of unselfishness – means giving freely without thought of reward. Much debate has surrounded this concept, with writers questioning the fundamental reasons for giving. Kemph (1966) reported that although donors were 'consciously altruistic' there was 'considerable unconscious resentment' towards the recipient and towards hospital personnel who requested or encouraged the donation. Other studies have suggested the presence of a degree of coercion or subtle familial pressure. Simmons *et al.* (1977) noted that the 'black sheep' of the family may donate in an attempt to be reinstated within the family and that others may donate because of a fear of family rejection if they refuse. There have also been reports of financial incentives or other 'material rewards' offered by recipients to donors to encourage donation.

The decision to donate is essentially personal and no-one can doubt that many offers are entirely altruistic, but some clinicians feel that the possibility of overt or covert coercion make living donation unacceptable.

Benefits for the Transplant Recipient

Although the ethical issues have been recognised and much debated, the decision to continue with living related donation has usually been based upon the very real benefits that ensue for the recipient. Living related donation has always demonstrated higher graft survival rates than cadaveric donation. Although recent advances in immunosuppression have narrowed the gap between the two groups (Fig.11.5), in most cases the living related

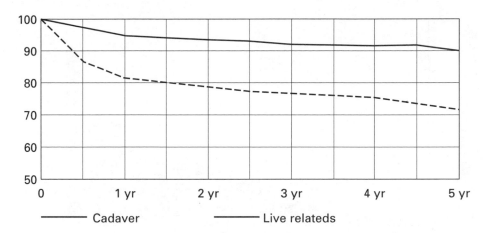

Fig. 11.5 *Cadaver allografts compared to live related allografts. Figures from Oxford transplants 1984–date.*

grafts still have a 10% better survival rate at 1 year and a significantly higher probability of function in the long term. The closer tissue match achieved with related donation usually results in fewer rejection episodes and a reduced amount of immunosuppression.

The living donation can be planned to take place at the most suitable time (medically and socially) for the recipient. As renal function deteriorates, transplantation can be planned for the predialysis phase, thus avoiding the physical and psychological stress of dialysis adjustments. Similarly, planning can minimise disruption to family and working patterns.

Such benefits have encouraged units to continue with living related donation. Indeed, with the increasing shortage of cadaveric organs, many centres are seeking to increase the numbers of living related grafts and are also considering living unrelated programmes.

Transplant Rates

Living related donation programmes vary throughout the world. Norway has the highest rate with 40% of the total transplant programme resulting from living donation. Sweden, the USA, Denmark and Greece also have relatively high rates. The UK has a low rate with only 5% of the total transplant programme resulting from living related donation (Fig.11.6).

Living unrelated donation (genetically unrelated – emotionally related)

In Norway, parents, siblings, adult children, uncles, aunts, grandparents and spouses are accepted as donors, but for ethical reasons volunteers outside the family are not accepted (Salter, 1988). Spouses are, of course, genetically unrelated but are recognised as 'emotionally related'. The Norwegian experience suggests that transplantation between spouses (partners) can

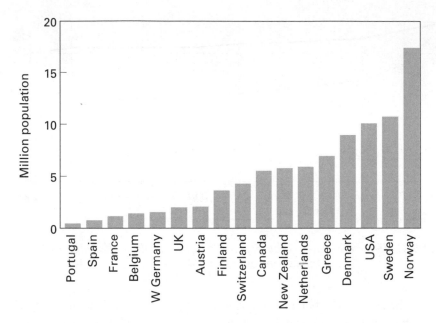

Fig. 11.6 *Live transplants per million population. Data from UKTSSA (Bristol) with permission.*

achieve graft survival rates identical to the best achieved with cadaveric organs. Similar results for transplantation between partners have been reported in the USA and these results are prompting some UK centres to investigate and utilise this previously untapped source of grafts. All centres stress that the donor must be well motivated and well informed and that the offer must be 'altruistic' and come from within a 'stable relationship'.

Buying and Selling of Organs

Living related and living unrelated transplantation in the UK is controlled by strict laws to prevent the possibility of illegal practices such as financial payments and coercion. However, the buying and selling of organs does occur in some of the third world countries and is an accepted practice. Indeed, some clinicians have suggested that a similar system, strictly controlled by legislation, could be introduced into the UK to increase transplant rates. The ethical and moral ramifications would be immense and at present such a concept is totally unacceptable to many.

Donor and Recipient Matching

Individual tissue type is inherited as half from each parent. Therefore, matching within a nuclear family unit will result in a potential donor who is (i) HLA identical; (ii) a one haplotype match; or (iii) a mismatch.

Immunological aspects (example as for donor-related (DR) matching)

Matching for the major histocompatibility complex will take place, however. Figure 11.7 demonstrates tissue type inheritance using the DR locus.

Therefore, potential donors may be

- HLA identical as with DR 1 : 3 (siblings);
- a one haplotype match as with: DR 1 : 3 and DR 1 : 8 (siblings)
                                    DR 1 : 4 and DR 1 : 3 (parent child);
- unmatched as with DR 1 : 3 and DR 4 : 8 (siblings).

The results of HLA identical and one haplotype matches demonstrate higher graft survival rates than cadaveric transplants. Therefore, parents and siblings are usually the most suitable living donors from a tissue-matching perspective. Donor and recipient must also be matched from an ABO blood group perspective.

Parents are usually very willing to donate but siblings may be ambivalent and experience a crisis of loyalties between the family of birth and the family of marriage.

Psychological Issues

The question of the possibility of living related donation may bring unity to a family group but it may also bring conflict. Parents will often offer early in the disease process and are extremely well motivated, but problems can arise if one parent is 'more suitable' due to tissue matching or physical constraints. The 'less suitable' parent may feel rejected and excluded from the donation and transplant process.

Siblings may be willing or ambivalent and it may be difficult to express ambivalent feelings because of societal concepts of family loyalty and love. A sibling of a patient at this centre expressed the wish that 'the request had never been made, as once verbalised it was impossible to refuse without feeling enormous guilt'. Married siblings may wish to donate but may encounter hostility from their partner who feels that the risks are too great and that responsibilities to the family of marriage are more important than loyalty to the family of birth.

Problems may also arise within the donor–recipient relationship following the transplant surgery. Cramond (1967) noted that an ambivalent relationship can occur between donor and recipient, with the donor seeking to 'overprotect' and the recipient resentful of the 'obligation' and the subsequent dependency relationship. Experience at this centre has noted such problems, particularly when the donor has been a parent and the recipient an adolescent child. Kemph (1966) reported unconscious resentment from donors which was enhanced if the recipient received more attention and degenerated, in some cases, into postsurgical depression. Also, recipients in this study expressed difficulty with the 'obligation' and an underlying

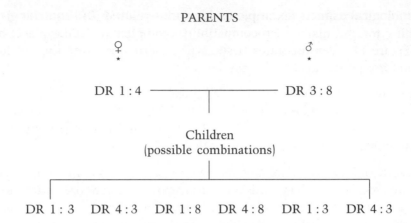

Fig. 11.7 *An example of tissue type inheritance.*

guilt that the debt could never be repaid. Obligation and guilt were expressed either by obsequious behaviour or hostility towards the donor. However, many studies report contrasting findings, with favourable outcomes and the donor and recipient relationships enhanced by the donation (Cramond, 1967; Bennett and Harrison, 1974; Hiras *et al.*, 1976; Smith *et al.*, 1986).

Ongoing psychological support is a necessary part of a living related programme. Donor and recipient must be well informed concerning the risks and benefits and also the psychological difficulties that may develop. Separate meetings, both for the donor and the recipient, with medical staff and nurse/counsellor should be planned so that feelings, fears and anxieties can be discussed with honesty. The motivation to donate should be explored and, if appropriate, the donor offered the opportunity to withdraw without guilt or family conflict.

Similarly, the decision to receive should be explored and the recipient offered the opportunity to refuse. Several patients at this centre have refused living donation, preferring to wait for cadaveric grafts so as not to 'inflict my disease on my family'. The dynamics of the donor and recipient relationship must be well understood so that help and advice may be offered if difficulties arise.

Assessment and Preparation of Donors

The living donor must be:

- well motivated;
- in excellent health with two normal kidneys and normal renal function;
- blood group and tissue match compatible with the recipient.

The assessment and preparation for living donation is extensive and is normally carried out in stages over several weeks or months. Different centres will conduct tests at different stages but most units complete the same catalogue of tests in order to ensure that the criteria are fulfilled. Usually the assessment involves three stages. At each stage the donor meets with medical staff and the nurse counsellor. Various tests are grouped together for each visit, thus minimising the disruption to the donor's working and personal life. Prior to stage I, the donor will have received written information regarding the risks and benefits and the pre- and post-operative experiences. Preliminary blood grouping and tissue typing may have occurred before the stage I visit (if not, they will be completed during this visit).

Stage I

The donor and recipient and other family members are invited to the transplant centre to meet with the transplant surgcon and the nurse counsellor. At this meeting the risks and benefits are explored, as are the forthcoming tests.

The donor and recipient have the opportunity to meet with the nurse counsellor alone, so that individual thoughts and anxieties might be explored in privacy. This is also an opportunity to explore the donor–recipient relationship. Such meetings help to initiate a trusting relationship with the nurse counsellor so that support can be available throughout the experience.

Assessment at stage I:

- *Age.* The donor must be above the age of consent and below the age of 60–65 years (age limits may vary in specific circumstances).
- *Informed consent.* The donor must be able to understand the risks that may ensue.
- *Preliminary medical history.* Exclude untreated hypertension; diabetes; other problems that would suggest anaesthetic risk to donor or recipient well-being.
- *Renal disease.* Familial renal disease may prohibit donation.
- *Allergies.* Exclude if anaesthetic risk.
- *Medications.* Contraceptive pill.
- *Social history.* Exclude heavy smoker; drug or alcohol abuse; female if planning an early pregnancy, as pregnancy may increase strain on renal system; hobbies or lifestyle that may suggest an increased risk of damage to the renal system.
- *Obesity.* Grossly obese may be asked to reduce weight prior to surgery.
- *Blood tests.*
- *Tissue typing.* T and B cell cross-match.
- *Urea, electrolytes and creatinine.*

- *Glucose.*
- *Liver function tests.*
- *Viral screen.* Cytomegalovirus (CMV), HIV, hepatitis B, hepatitis C, Epstein Barr virus.
- *Urine tests.*
- *Mid-stream urine (MSU).* Culture, microscopy.
- *Urinalysis.*

If the initial assessments are satisfactory and the donor still wishes to donate, stage II is completed by the unit nephrologist.

Stage II
Assessment at stage II:

- *Full medical history.*
- *Family history.*
- *Discussion regarding decision to donate and implications of the donation.*
- *Examination.* Full physical examination; blood pressure monitoring; chest X-ray; ECG; intravenous pyelogram; ultrasound scan.
- *Blood tests.* Full blood count; erthyrocyte sedimentation rate; clotting; lipids.
- *Repeat* urea; electrolytes and creatinine; glucose; liver function tests.
- *Urine tests.* 24 h urine analysis x 2.
- *Repeat* MSU culture and microscopy; urinalysis.

If the results of these tests are satisfactory the donor assessment will proceed to stage III.

Stage III
Assessment at stage III:

- *Glomerular filtration rate estimation.*
- *Renal angiography.*

Throughout the assessment programme the donor should be assured that it is possible to retract the offer to donate, should they so wish, and that if such a decision is made, support and advice will be given. It is important that the donor does not feel that they are on a rollercoaster that cannot be halted.

Renal angiography
Renal angiography is required to examine the vasculature of the kidneys. Most patients will have a single artery to each kidney; however, in some cases there may be multiple arteries. It is technically possible to transplant a kidney with more than one artery, but the surgical technique is simpler

and less hazardous if there is a single artery. If both kidneys are shown to have single arteries then the left will be chosen for the transplant as this kidney has a longer renal vein which facilitates the surgical anastomosis.

The donor is admitted for 24 h for the angiography to be performed. This admission offers a further opportunity for the donor to meet with the nurse counsellor and also the surgical team that will be performing the nephrectomy. The nurse counsellor can further explore any fears and anxieties and can also fully outline the pre- and postoperative procedures.

Two separate surgical teams are usually involved with a living related donation. A consultant urologist and team perform the nephrectomy and the transplant consultant and team perform the transplant. The urological team assume responsibility for donor care and the transplant team responsibility for recipient care. The donor and recipient are nursed in separate units which are closely linked for easy access for visiting. However, separation is not a fixed policy and donor and recipient may be together if that is their particular wish or if there are language problems or other difficulties.

During the renal angiography admission, the donor will meet with the consultant urologist, who will discuss the implications of the nephrectomy and will check the assessment tests. The donor will also visit the urological unit and meet the nursing team.

The recipient should also be offered the opportunity to meet with the nurse counsellor and the transplant surgeon to discuss pre- and postoperative care and any specific fears and anxieties. Many recipients are fearful both for the donor and themselves. Guilt is often expressed, as is the anxiety that should the transplant reject all will have been in vain. Discussion, exploration and the sharing of such thoughts can help to reduce tension and anxiety. Other family members, particularly parents if it is a sibling to sibling transplant, will require psychological support.

Providing all the assessment tests are satisfactory, the final tissue typing cross-match test will be performed the week prior to transplantation. The donor and recipient will be admitted on the day before transplant and will usually spend the day together in between the various preoperative procedures.

Preoperative Care for the Donor

The preoperative care for the living donor will be similar to that given to patients undergoing conventional nephrectomy and is listed below. However, particular attention should be given to psychological and social support.

Preoperative living donor assessment
Before surgery, certain tests performed during the assessment programme will be repeated. The preoperative assessment includes:

- *Medical history.*
- *Full examination.*
- *Blood pressure; pulse; temperature; weight.*
- *Allergy check.*
- *Blood tests:* Urea and electrolytes; full blood count; E–R clotting; cross-match; two units of blood.
- *Urine analysis and MSU.*
- *Repeat chest X-ray* (if necessary)
- *Repeat ECG* (if necessary)
- *Assessment*: by anaesthetist; urologist; physiotherapist.
- *Informed consent.*
- *Nil by mouth.*
- *Preoperative hygienic care.*
- *Premedication.*

Surgical Technique of Nephrectomy

Living related donor nephrectomy is always emotionally taxing surgery and can be technically difficult. This is the only time when a surgeon is operating on a person who is perfectly well and does not need surgery for their own benefit. From that point of view there are no advantages to the person who is undergoing surgery, except possible psychological benefits in giving a gift to a relative, and there are the inevitable potential complications of any major surgical procedure which involves a general anaesthetic. As discussed earlier, the estimated mortality from living related donor nephrectomy is 1 in 4000. Thus, while very rare, the risks are certainly not negligible and major morbidity or death is very traumatic not only for the relatives but for the members of the surgical team themselves.

The two approaches for removing a kidney from a live donor are either transabdominal, intraperitoneal, or via the loin over the 11th or 12th rib, either spreading or removing the 11th or 12th rib. The intra-abdominal approach is usually through a transverse incision in the right or left upper quadrant.

The kidney is carefully exposed and meticulous dissection is carried out with careful handling of the kidney and careful exposure of the renal vein and artery. The gonadal and adrenal tributaries of the renal vein are ligated and divided and often a posterior lumbar vein needs ligating and dividing as well.

The renal artery is cleaned and exposed at its junction with the aorta and the ureter is identified and dissected down to the pelvic brim or just below, where it is ligated and divided. It is very important to avoid too much dissection in the hilum of the kidney and it is also essential to avoid stripping the ureter of its adventitia. The blood supply to the ureter normally comes from the renal artery, branches from the gonadal vessels and the external iliac artery and branches of the superior vesicle artery. In a transplant kidney the blood supply to the ureter is entirely dependent on the renal artery and it is essential to keep a good amount of adventitia around the ureter to allow the blood to reach the distal ureter. One of the major complications after transplantation is ischaemia of the lower end of the ureter and this is normally due to stripping of the ureter at the time of the donor surgery.

When the kidney is free and attached just by the artery and the vein, the artery is ligated and divided first, followed by the vein. The kidney is removed and placed in iced saline where perfusion is started immediately and after careful inspection, any further dissection is carried out and a renal biopsy is taken.

Our practice is to then place the kidney in a sterile surgical glove, in which the fingers have been tied off, surrounded by iced saline as this allows it to be handled and kept cool at the same time. The vein is left protruding through a small incision in the glove ready for anastomosis into the recipient. After ensuring haemostasis in the donor, the abdominal wound is closed.

Postoperative Management: Living Donor

The postoperative care for the living donor is similar to the care given for a conventional nephrectomy. Nephrectomy is recognised as painful surgery requiring frequent analgesia in the early postoperative phase. Satisfactory pain control is essential to reduce patient anxiety to facilitate movement and adequate respiration, thus reducing the risks of early postoperative complications. In most centres, patient controlled analgesia using an opiate is utilised. Chest physiotherapy and mobilisation usually commence on the first postoperative day and stockings are in place to prevent formation of deep vein thrombosis.

Hydration: fluid and electrolyte balance
Paralytic ileus may occur as a result of the retroperitoneal dissection and the handling of the bowel. Therefore, the intake of oral fluids must commence slowly and only increase as ileus resolves and bowel sounds are evident. In practice, hydration is maintained by intravenous infusion for the first 24–48 h until oral intake is sufficient. Close monitoring of fluid and electrolyte balance is necessary until dietary intake is adequate.

The passing of urine may prove difficult due to the pain of movement and anxiety. However, the need for catheterisation is rare, and with adequate pain relief it should be possible for the female patients to be assisted on to a commode to facilitate voiding as naturally as possible. Regular MSU specimens should be obtained for microscopy, culture and sensitivity during hospitalisation.

Wound management

Wound management should include close monitoring to exclude complications of bleeding and infection.

Emotional support

During the early postoperative period emotional support should be offered, as should frequent information regarding the progress of the recipient. Donor and recipient should be re-united at the earliest opportunity and encouraged to spend time together. The donor may experience a feeling of anticlimax after the surgery due to a release of the preoperative tension and anticipation. Such anticlimax may combine with postanaesthetic 'blues' to form a mild depression with emotional lability. Staff should recognise the altruism of the act and offer understanding and reassurance.

Discharge

The majority of living donors will be discharged between the fifth and seventh postoperative day. It is recommended that they continue their postoperative recovery at home for approximately 6 weeks to 2 months. Return to work will be variable depending on type of employment and its physical and psychological demands. Physical monitoring may include two further assessments by the urologist. Long-term physical monitoring is not thought necessary in the absence of any complications. Emotional support should continue as appropriate, with help available if difficulties arise.

INCREASING DONOR ORGAN SUPPLY

Extending the living related and unrelated donation programmes will increase the supply of kidneys, livers and in some cases lungs for transplantation but it is also necessary to introduce alternative initiatives for increasing cadaveric organ supply.

Elective Ventilation

Research conducted at the Royal Devon and Exeter Hospital in 1989 reported that some patients who had suffered cerebrovascular catastrophes (CVA) and had died in the medical wards of the hospital would have been suitable organ donors. Multiple organ donation did not occur as these deaths were asystolic; however, it was postulated that donation would have been possible if death had taken place in an intensive care setting. Therefore, a protocol for increasing organ donation after cerebrovascular death was implemented (Feest et al., 1990).

This protocol stated that 'patients fulfilling the criteria as potential organ donors could be identified on the medical wards; once identified, the relatives could be approached with regard to donation and if permission was given, the patient moved to intensive care for ventilation to 'facilitate donation". (This practice became widely known as 'Elective ventilation'.) The programme proved successful and in 19 months the hospital reported eight such donations. It was suggested that these results, if replicated throughout the UK, would greatly increase the numbers of donor organs.

However, a legal ruling in 1993 described the act of 'elective ventilation' as 'unlawful' as 'the ventilation was deemed not to have been initiated for the benefit of the patient' (New et al., 1994). With the advent of this ruling the 'elective ventilation programmes' were discontinued, but discussions regarding the ethical and legal issues continue in the hope that solutions may be found. In the interim, some units have introduced asystolic donation programmes in order to facilitate renal donation.

Asystolic Donation (Non-Heart-Beating)

An initiative at the Leicester General Hospital suggests that asystolic (non-heart-beating) donation could become an increasingly important source of renal organs. Since 1992, Leicester have identified asystolic donors in the medical wards and the Accident and Emergency Department of the local hospital. At the time of asystole and following certification of death (providing that there are no medical contraindications to donation), an intra-aortic catheter is inserted and ice cold perfusion of the kidneys commenced. Such perfusion reduces the warm ischaemic damage and allows time for medical/ nursing colleagues to approach the family and the coroner for permission to proceed to donation. If permission is granted the kidneys must be removed within 40–45 min of asystole in order to avoid irreversible renal damage.

Ethical concerns about the insertion of the catheter before consent has been given were widely discussed with health personnel, the coroner and the general public, and all groups consented to the initiative, which has proved successful.

Initial results suggest a marginally higher rate of relative consent in asystolic donation than is usually achieved in brain stem death donation. This may be due to the skill of the staff requesting and also the fact that with asystole the patient appears 'dead' in the conventional sense (cold, pale and cyanosed), thus there may be less psychological denial for the family.

The insertion of the catheter requires surgical expertise, as kidneys may be lost if perfusion is inadequate. In practice, some ischaemiac damage does occur and there is a higher incidence of post-transplant non-function and ATN with these grafts. However, results of 26 transplants from asystolic donations show that the 'long term function and graft survival appear comparable with kidneys from heart beating donors' (Veitch, 1995).

Other centres including Guy's Hospital, London, have introduced asystolic donation programmes and it is hoped that they will provide a useful additional supply of kidneys. However, the limiting factors will be the need for a rapid response time from the retrieval teams and the need for catheter insertion expertise. Such factors may preclude donation from hospitals that are some distance away from the transplant centre.

Opting-in/Opting-out

Within the UK the general public are encouraged to 'opt-in' by making the voluntary decision to donate organs. This decision is supported by the carrying of a donor card and informing relatives of this wish. Thus, donation is a voluntary gift.

Research suggests that approximately 75% of the general public support donation but only 30% actually carry a donor card. The reluctance to actually sign and carry a donor card may be due to the fact that death remains a taboo subject within our society and also that many are somewhat superstitious and feel that signing a card may somehow be 'tempting fate'. Furthermore, few of us wish to consider our own mortality.

Additional problems with this system are that in practice the donor card may not be available at the time of death, or relatives may either be unaware of the donor's wishes or may choose to ignore them. Several groups, mainly patient groups, have pressed for the introduction of an 'opting-out' system, whereby everyone is deemed to wish to donate unless they have registered an objection. The opting out system has been introduced in Europe (namely Austria and Belgium), and appears to be successful. However, with a true opting-out system the wishes of the family are not considered. At present it is felt by the major health groups in the UK that the denial of the family's wishes is unacceptable practice. Therefore, the government has decided to continue to support opting-in with the introduction of a new national registry, whereby those wishing to donate can register their wishes on to the national computer. The computer can be accessed by critical care staff should death occur. However, relatives will still be asked for consent.

Such measures may increase donation rates but it is well recognised that with the growing waiting lists the demand for organs will always outstrip supply. The only solution to the problem in the long term may be the introduction of xenotransplantation.

Xenotransplantation (Transplant of Animal Organs into Humans)

There is too little space here to discuss in detail the ethical, moral and practical issues regarding the use of other species, and which species would be most suitable. From the point of view of the biology, closely related non-human primates such as chimpanzees would be logical, since there is no hyperacute rejection problem. However, it has been universally agreed that such species would be ethically unacceptable, impractical since they are endangered species, and dangerous to use because of the possibility of viral transfer or similar disasters. For practicality, the acceptable species would be those in current large-scale usage for food production, such as the pig.

The most obvious and immediate problem confronting the use of xenografts is the problem of hyperacute rejection. Connection of a suitably prepared pig kidney to the blood circulation of a dialysis patient initially results in normal perfusion of the kidney, which becomes pulsatile and pink and may even briefly produce urine. However, within minutes the pulsatility of the kidney lessens, and then ceases, the kidney becoming initially blue and finally almost black as the circulation ceases due to thrombosis. This typical pattern of rapid graft failure was initially described in human kidney allografts and was termed hyperacute rejection. The cause was subsequently shown to be the presence in the recipient of high titre antibody against the donor tissue, binding of the antibody causing complement activation and subsequent activation of the clotting cascade. Blood group ABO incompatibility was a potent source of antidonor antibody that was easily avoided, but some cases of hyperacute rejection still occurred even after blood group matching. In the case of human allografts it was possible to avoid this fairly rare occurrence by testing for the presence of antidonor antibody and avoiding transplantation when antibody was detected. However, in the case of xenotransplantation between distantly related species, antibody is always detectable despite matching for blood groups, and this antibody came to be known as heterophile or natural antibody.

Two fundamental recent discoveries are the basis for a number of new approaches to prevent xenograft hyperacute rejection, for example by blocking or removing the natural antibody or infusing human complement regulatory proteins. The recent advent of transgenic manipulation has also allowed the concept of developing herds of animals which express high levels of human complement regulatory proteins on their cells. Research is moving so rapidly that already herds of transgenic pigs have been produced and organs from these pigs are undergoing preclinical experimental studies with preliminary encouraging results.

It now seems likely that combinations of the above approaches will eventually allow transplantation of organs between species such as the pig and man, avoiding destruction of the graft by hyperacute rejection. However, this is likely to be only the first of several barriers to successful xenograft usage. From present evidence the processes of cellular rejection may well be entirely different to those seen in allograft rejection. Some argue that they may be easily overcome, but this remains to be proven in a preclinical model. There also remains the problem of species compatibility for crucial molecular and biochemical pathways, which is certain to be a problem for transplantation of the liver, since this organ is so intimately involved in many biosynthetic pathways. The animal rights movement may also promote heated debate on the moral acceptability of xenotransplantation.

More practical issues such as the danger of cross-species infection and production control may present stumbling blocks. Nevertheless, the rapidity with which knowledge is being accumulated and the ingenuity of the solutions proposed so far leads one to suspect that successful organ xenografts may be achievable within the next decade.

WAITING LIST

Once the pretransplant assessment has been completed and the tissue typing and blood grouping details are finalised, the name of the patient will be added to both the local and national waiting lists. Waiting time is impossible to predict.

It is important to explain to the patient that the transplant waiting list is very different from other hospital waiting lists in that they do not simply have to wait until their name reaches the top of the list to receive a graft. The transplant list is essentially a 'pool of recipients', and each transplant is allocated on the basis of the 'closest match', irrespective of time waiting. Therefore, their name will join the recipient 'pool' and they must wait for the 'best match' for them. This is a difficult concept to understand and some patients become distressed if another patient, who has waited less time, is transplanted before them.

It is also important that patients do not 'sit by the phone' all day waiting for 'the call', thus greatly restricting their lifestyles. Most centres have a supply of long distance pagers, given free by a telephone company, which potential recipients can carry to ensure contact. Patients are encouraged to keep as active and as healthy as possible whilst waiting and to continue as normal a lifestyle as possible. Some patients may still feel ambivalent about a transplant at this time. Specific fears and anxieties may need to be explored and support given within the context that the patient must be allowed the time to decide the best treatment for themselves. On-going contact with the transplant nurse practitioner is vital during the waiting time. In this centre the patients who are waiting are contacted every 3–4 months and offered support and reassurance. Support is especially important at times of additional stress such as when a fellow dialysis patient receives or rejects a kidney.

PREOPERATIVE MANAGEMENT FOR A RENAL TRANSPLANT RECIPIENT

'The Transplant Call'

Transplant recipients report mixed reactions of relief, excitement, anxiety and sadness when they receive the transplant phone call – relief that the waiting time may be over; excitement for the new life ahead; anxiety that the surgery may be difficult or that the transplant may fail; and sadness that a family elsewhere has experienced tragedy in order for the kidney to become available (Dubovsky and Penn, 1980).

During the telephone conversation the recipient is informed that a transplant may be possible and that they should travel to the transplant centre and have nothing further to eat or drink. Brief questions are also asked to clarify current health status and to exclude any infections or other problems that may prevent transplantation.

Some centres contact two recipients for each transplant so that should a positive cross-match occur for one, a second recipient is already prepared, thus minimising the cold ischaemia time. It has been found that contacting two recipients can lead to repeated disappointments, anger and depression, therefore often only one recipient is called to the transplant centre in the first instance.

Nursing Admission

Upon arrival, the recipient and family are welcomed by the nursing team and are helped to familiarise themselves with the unit. Brief information is given regarding the forthcoming blood and clinical tests, questions answered and anxieties explored during the nursing admission procedure.

Nursing admission procedure
- Blood pressure, pulse, temperature, respirations.
- Current weight : dry weight.
- Past medical history – renal disease.
- Dialysis history – current practice and date and time of last dialysis.
- Current health status – recent relevant health events (i.e. blood transfusions/infections).
- Normal urine output – (if any).
- Social information.
- Allergies.
- Name band applied.

Medical Assessment

Urgent medical assessment and blood tests are required to assess fluid and electrolyte status (as dialysis may be needed prior to surgery), also to complete the final tissue typing cross-match test, and therefore the medical assessment immediately follows the nursing admission procedure.

Medical assessment procedure
- Medical history.
- Renal disease history.
- Dialysis history.
- Current health status – recent relevant events.
- Allergies.
- Medical examination.
- Blood tests:
    urea and electrolytes;
    liver function tests;
    tissue typing cross-match;
    viral screen (as in pretransplant assessment);
    cross-match for two units of blood available for transplant surgery.
- Clinical tests:
    chest X-ray;
    electrocardiogram (ECG);
    mid-stream specimen of urine (MSU) urinalysis.

Preoperative Dialysis

The results of the medical assessment and blood tests will determine the need for dialysis. Fluid overload and electrolyte imbalance (particularly hyperkalaemia) must be corrected, as they represent an anaesthetic risk and may enhance post-transplantation difficulties.

Haemodialysis with minimal heparinisation (to avoid excessive bleeding) is often necessary to ensure optimal weight and reduce fluid overload and serum potassium levels.

CAPD patients may require rapid exchanges to achieve optimal fluid and electrolyte status. The peritoneal catheter exit site should be examined for any signs of infection and a swab taken for culture and sensitivity. Also, following the necessary exchanges the catheter should be drained and a fluid specimen sent for microscopy culture and sensitivity and then the catheter capped, leaving the patient empty of fluid.

Information and Emotional Support

During the dialysis time it is often possible to explore individual fears and anxieties and offer emotional support and information regarding postoperative medications and procedures. A booklet may be available and questions can be answered and further information offered as required. Recipients are often emotionally labile at this time ('tears and laughter') and require much emotional understanding and support.

Immediate Preoperative Care

It is usual for the physiotherapist to visit to commence chest physiotherapy and advise regarding postoperative mobility and for the anaesthetist to perform an assessment. Once the tissue typing cross-match has proved negative the final preoperative preparation begins:

- skin swabs/nose and throat swabs – for viral, bacterial and MRSA screening;
- swabs and dressings to other dialysis lines (i.e. permacaths);
- suppositories (if required);
- bath/shower/hair wash;
- operation gown;
- marking and dressing (to protect) arterovenous fistula from inadvertent use of invasive monitoring (e.g. i.v. lines, blood pressure cuffs) plus to maintain warmth, thus avoiding clotting.

Preoperative medications

Medications 4 h preoperation
- Cyclosporin
- Azathioprin
- Prednisolone
- Aspirin (unless contraindicated).

Medications immediately preoperation
- Premedication
- Diabetics: sliding scale insulin as appropriate.

SURGICAL TECHNIQUE FOR RENAL TRANSPLANTATION

Before transplantation begins a catheter is placed into the bladder. This allows drainage of the bladder during the transplant operation and also allows the bladder to be filled with solution containing antibiotics to facilitate later identification of the bladder for reimplantation of the ureter. The right or left iliac fossa is the normal site for the transplant (Fig.11.8).

- An incision is made curving from just above the pubic symphysis to just above the iliac crest.
- The inferior epigastric vessels are ligated and divided and an extraperitoneal approach is made down on to the iliac vessels.
- The external iliac artery and vein are freed and small branches or overlying lymphatics are ligated and divided.
- Clamps are applied to the external iliac vein and the renal vein is anastomosed to the external iliac vein with continuous 5.0 prolene sutures.
- Clamps are then applied to the external iliac artery and the renal artery on its patch (known as the Carrell patch) is anastomosed with continuous 5.0 proline to the external iliac artery (Fig. 11.9).
- Once the anastomoses are complete, the clamps are released, taking the venous clamps off first, and the kidney normally perfuses quickly and one is often able to see immediate urine production.
- The bladder is then filled through the catheter and the ureter put into the bladder and then tunnelled submucosally to prevent urinary ureteric reflux (the Leadbetter–Politano technique). Some centres may use an extra vesicle technique which involves splitting the muscle, laying the ureter just above the bladder mucosa and so into the bladder, and closing the muscle over the top. If the bladder has been opened it is closed with two layers of vicryl.
- The wound is closed in the usual fashion and the bladder washed out at the end of the procedure.

RENAL TRANSPLANT REJECTION

There are three types of renal transplant rejection:

- hyperacute rejection
- acute rejection
- chronic rejection.

Hyperacute Rejection

Hyperacute rejection (Fig. 11.10) occurs rapidly within minutes or hours of revascularisation of the transplant. It is caused by:

- The presence of preformed cytotoxic antibodies in the recipient's blood (resultant from previous failed transplants, blood transfusions or pregnancies) reacting against the donor's histocompatibility antigens.
- ABO incompatibility between the donor and the recipient.

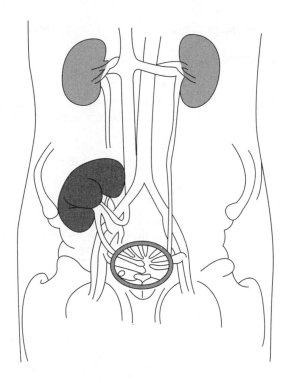

Fig. 11.8 *Position for the transplant kidney.*

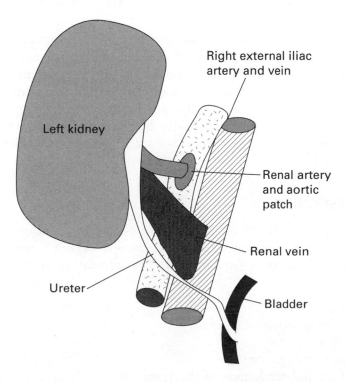

Fig. 11.9 *The surgical technique for renal transplantation.*

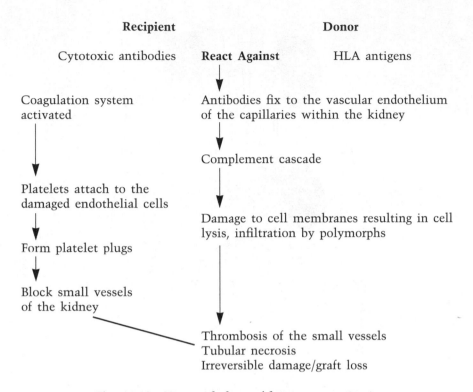

Fig. 11.10 *Histopathology of hyperacute rejection.*

The final lymphocytotoxic cross-match prior to transplant should demonstrate that cytotoxic antibodies are present and transplantation should not take place, thus a hyperacute rejection is a rare phenomenon today.

Hyperacute rejection may be observed during the transplant surgery. Instead of the kidney becoming distended and pink as the arterial and venous clamps are released, as is usual with hyperacute rejection the kidney will remain flaccid and become blue. Damage is almost always irreversible and the graft is lost.

Acute Rejection

Acute rejection (Fig. 11.11) is usually a combination of cellular and antibody medicated rejection which most usually occurs between 4 days and 2 months following transplantation. The clinical signs of acute rejection may include:

- pyrexia
- renal dysfunction
- weight gain
- fall in urine output
- swelling and tenderness of the transplant

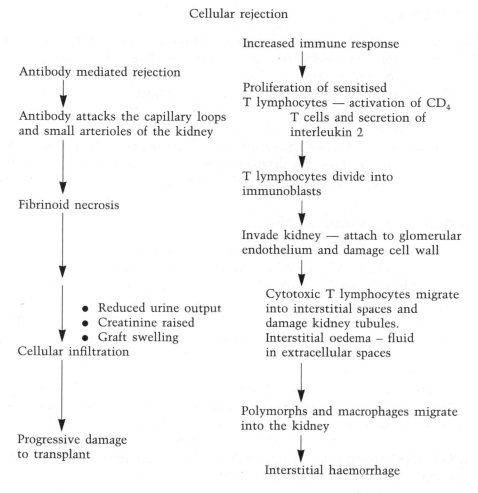

Fig. 11.11 *Histopathology of acute rejection.*

- ankle oedema
- flu-like symptoms.

Acute rejection can usually be controlled by increased immunosuppression; however, a severe rejection may result in some loss of overall graft function.

Chronic Rejection

Chronic rejection usually occurs over months or years but may occur at 10 days post-transplantation. There is a gradual occlusion of the lumen of the arteries of the kidney with interstitial fibrosis which destroys the graft. The exact mechanisms involved in chronic rejection are still unclear and may be immunological or non-immunological. The first signs of chronic rejection are usually a gradual worsening of renal function with proteinuria.

Graft Loss

The majority of recipients experience feelings of profound loss if their kidney transplant fails. Denial may be the initial response, followed by sadness, anger and depression (Galpin, 1992). At this time, empathetic understanding should be offered and the opportunity given for recipients to express their emotions freely. Recipients can be helped to understand that the loss of the graft is not the end and that there is hope for further transplants. In most cases the return to dialysis is gradually and success-fully negotiated and as the disappointment subsides, the majority very quickly ask to go back on the transplant waiting list.

Immunosuppression Regimens

Within the UK the most commonly used immunosuppression is a 'triple therapy' regimen involving cyclosporin (sandimmun), azathioprine (imuran) and prednisolone medications. Monoclonal (OKT$_3$) and polyclonal (anti-lymphocyte globulin) may be added in cases of high sensitisation or recal-citrant acute rejection which has not responded to additional steroid therapy.

All these drugs are discussed in detail in Appendix One, and therefore only brief clinical references are outlined in this section.

Cyclosporin (Sandimmun cyclosporin)

Cyclosporin is a natural peptide found in two strains of fungi. It was first introduced into clinical immunosuppression in 1983.

Action Cyclosporin inhibits interleukin 2 and interferes with the growth and activation of T lymphocytes (see Fig. 11.11).

Side-effects Usually side-effects are dose dependent and responsive to dose reduction. The commonest side-effects include:

- nephrotoxicity – decreased glomerular filtration rate (GFR)
- hypertension
- hyperlipidaemia
- gum hypertrophy
- hepatic dysfunction.
- hyperkalaemia
- hypomagnesaemia
- hirsutism
- hyperuricaemia
- hypertrichosis
- tremors

Other less common side-effects include:

- muscle weakness
- thrombocytopenia.

Cyclosporin may be started immediately prior to transplant but because of the known nephrotoxicity it may be withdrawn for the preliminary phase in the presence of primary non-function due to ATN.

Absorption Cyclosporin is absorbed with variable efficiency by different individuals; therefore, regular monitoring of whole blood levels must occur. The usual therapeutic range is 200–400 µg mol l⁻¹ during the first 6 months of transplantation, with maintenance doses aimed at levels of 100–200 µg mol l⁻¹. Generally, patients who reject due to inadequate cyclosporin levels usually have levels less than 100, patients with cyclosporin nephrotoxicity usually have levels greater than 500 – but it is an individual response.

Azathioprine

Azathioprine is a derivative of the anticancer drug 6-mercaptopurine and was introduced into clinical practice in 1962.

Action Azathioprine inhibits both DNA and RNA synthesis and prevents growth of the lymphocytes (see Fig. 11.11).

Side-effects The main side-effect is neutropenia. If the white blood cell count (WBC) drops to below 3.5×10^9 l⁻¹ the dose should be reduced. If the WBC drops below 3.0×10^9 l⁻¹ the drug should be stopped temporarily.

Other side effects include:

- alopecia
- malignancy
- cholestatic jaundice (rare).
- general malaise
- pancreatitis (rare)
- muscular pains
- altered liver function

Because of the risk of neutropenia, blood counts must be checked at intervals of not longer than 3 months.

Prednisolone (corticosteroids)

Action The action of corticosteroid preparations is complex and involves anti-inflammatory responses with blocking of T cells and blocking of interleukin 1 (see Fig. 11.11).

Side-effects
- cushingoid appearance (facial swelling, swollen abdomen)
- fluid retention
- glaucoma
- increased appetite.
- hypertension
- psychosis
- peptic ulceration
- increase in blood sugar levels

Side-effects with long-term treatment
- subcapsular cataract
- pancreatitis.
- skin thinning
- osteoporosis

Many centres start steroid reduction at 2 months post-transplant and aim to remove steroid therapy at 1 year post-transplant because of the long-term side-effects.

Acute Rejection

Rejection treatment consists of an increase in the dose of corticosteroids. Usual practice is to administer three bolus doses of 1 g intravenous methyl prednisolone over a 3-day period (one bolus each day).

Orthoclone (OKT3) monoclonal antibody

Action   Antibody that reacts with CD-3 molecules on the lymphocytes and depletes them.

Side-effects

- chest pain
- pulmonary oedema
- gastrointestinal disturbances.
- fever
- chills
- dyspnoea
- infections

This drug can cause rapid pulmonary oedema and therefore it is essential that the patient is evaluated for volume overload and diuresed if necessary prior to administration of the drug.

Antilymphocyte globulin – polyclonal antibody

Action   Inhibits and destroys circulatory lymphocytes through antibody action.

Side-effects

- rash
- thrombocytopenia/leukopenia
- fever/chills
- anaphylaxis
- myalgia.

POSTOPERATIVE CARE AND COMPLICATIONS FOR THE RENAL TRANSPLANT RECIPIENT

In most cases the anaesthetist will insert a triple lumen central venous line via the internal jugular vein immediately prior to surgery. This line facilitates monitoring of fluid status and central venous pressure (CVP) and allows infusion of fluids and medications during surgery and the early post-operative phase.

Aims of Care

The aim of postoperative management is to provide the appropriate care to support primary transplant function and to aid optimal recovery. Initial care involves close monitoring of physical and psychological health, with frequent assessments and adjustments in response to changes in health status. During the first 24 h following the transplant the nursing care will be 'wholly compensatory' (Orem, 1991).

Immediate Postoperative Care

Cardiorespiratory status

Immediate base-line observations should be recorded, including blood pressure, pulse, respirations and temperature. Such observations should continue every 30 min until stable and thereafter hourly or as appropriate. Twenty-four hour ECG monitoring may be routine; however, in some centres such monitoring may only be used for patients in high-risk categories. Close monitoring of respiratory status is essential, as anaesthetic drugs and analgesia may be poorly excreted due to the reduced transplant function, thus depressing respiratory effort and increasing the risk of pulmonary complication. Early chest physiotherapy should be encouraged.

Pain management

The experience of pain is unique to each individual and therefore the use of patient-controlled analgesia is a suitable therapy as it will provide satisfactory pain management, reduce recipient anxiety and facilitate deep breathing and movement. An opiate derivative, such as morphine, is commonly used. Pethidine is avoided because of the possible accumulation of metabolites in the presence of reduced renal function. Recipients often report that the presence of the urinary catheter causes the greatest discomfort.

Hydration: fluid and electrolyte balance

Inadequate hydration may adversely affect transplant function; therefore, the maintenance of an acceptable venous pressure without the complication of fluid overload is an integral element of care. Fluid intake is usually administered through the central venous line. CVP measurements, recorded hourly, and urinary output measurements, recorded hourly, are used as a guide to appropriate fluid intake.

> Fluid intake protocol usually involves fluids being administered through an infusion pump with hourly intake equal to the previous hour's output plus 50 ml, with the aim of achieving a CVP level of approximately + 5 cm to + 10 cm of H_2O.

Peripheral line perfusion must also be included in the intake total. Infusion of dopamine may be introduced to help maintain pressure and improve transplant perfusion by reducing vasoconstriction of the smaller renal vessels. Monitoring of serum biochemistry and haemoglobin levels is on-going and the results will determine the type of intravenous fluid given. Often 5% dextrose is alternated with normal saline. Blood transfusion is rarely required.

Oral fluids are usually introduced within the early postoperative phase (as paralytic ileus is rare) and are gradually increased as appropriate. In uncomplicated cases the CVP line is removed after 48 h and nutrition introduced.

Urine output: catheter care

A urinary catheter will be *in situ* following the transplant surgery, and the urine may be blood stained due to the surgical procedures to the bladder and ureter. Clot formation may occur, resulting in pain and anuria. Gentle sterile bladder washouts should be performed to alleviate the problem and re-establish urine flow.

Twenty-four hour urine output should be recorded and it is, of course, important to note the volume of urine passed from the native kidneys pretransplantation when assessing urinary totals. Daily urine analysis and biochemistry should be noted and daily catheter specimens obtained for microscopy, culture and sensitivity. The catheter is usually removed on the fifth postoperative day. Some recipients may experience difficulty with voiding and also may have very limited bladder capacity due to pretransplant bladder atrophy. Reassurance and bladder 'retraining' strategies usually help to solve these problems.

Wound management

A wound drain may be present and drainage should be monitored. Observation and aseptic dressing of the wound will be given as appropriate and the sutures removed when healing has occurred. The immunosuppression regimen and other contributory factors such as diabetes or malnutrition may impede the healing process.

Infection control

In the past, transplant recipients were subjected to reverse barrier nursing techniques, to prevent cross-infection. With the introduction of less suppressive and more specific immunosuppression, such precautions are no longer considered necessary. However, recipients are immunocompromised and therefore infection control procedures should be strictly followed. Hand washing should take place before and after each nursing and medical procedure and visitors should be monitored for infections. Medications should include prophylaxis against infection and additional treatments commenced if infection is suspected.

The recipient should be helped to achieve personal and oral hygiene of a high standard and aseptic techniques utilised with regard to wound, peritoneal catheter site, urinary catheter and CVP line care. Catheter tips should be cultured for microscopy and sensitivity when removed.

Postoperative medications

- *Cyclosporin.* Immunosuppression to prevent rejection.
- *Azathioprine.* Immunosuppression to prevent rejection.
- *Prednisolone.* Immunosuppression to prevent rejection.
- *Co-trimoxazole (septrin).* Antibiotic to prevent infection/chest infection, particularly pneumocystis.

- *Ranitidine.* Reduces gastric irritation caused by steroids. Prevents gastric bleeding.
- *Nystatin pastilles.* Prevents oral infection (*Candida*).
- *Aspirin.* May be used in some centres to reduce the risk of thrombosis.

Continuing care

Nursing care requirements quickly change from 'wholly compensatory' during the early postoperative period to 'partly compensatory' over the following days. Recipients usually recover quickly from the anaesthetic and begin early mobilisation to prevent complications.

Diet is introduced as 'bowel sounds increase'. Constipation may be a problem due to anaesthetic, immobility and analgesia, and gentle laxatives or suppositories may be needed. Self-care is usually achieved by the fifth postoperative day.

Emotional support

Many recipients report a feeling of 'rebirth' in the early postoperative period with a rapid return of their '*joie de vivre*' (Frey, 1990). Emotions may be labile, with peaks of happiness intermingled with some sadness and anxiety; these feelings are often intensified by the steroid therapy.

Sadness may be linked to thoughts of the donor family and grief and guilt may be expressed that the transplant has resulted from 'another's tragedy'. It is often helpful to give the recipient anonymous details such as age, sex and cause of death of the donor, and to offer them the opportunity to write a letter of thanks to the donor family. The expression of thanks usually enables the recipient to accept the gift of the organ and to move forward to their new lifestyle.

Anxiety is usually linked to the fear of complications such as rejection, infection and graft loss. Recipients and their families require considerable support, understanding and in-depth information during the early postoperative phase, particularly if difficulties occur.

Complications of Renal Transplantation

Renal dysfunction – ATN

The most common cause of initial non function after renal transplantation is ATN, which may be due to prolonged hypotension in the donor or difficulties with ischaemia during the donor or recipient surgery. Dialysis support may be required until adequate transplant function is achieved. Haemodialysis, with reduced heparinisation, can be undertaken as necessary (a frequent clotting screen will be required), and CAPD recommended as long as the peritoneum has suffered no surgical damage.

Cyclosporin is known to be nephrotoxic and may therefore prolong ATN. Some units may reduce the cyclosporin dosage or withdraw cyclosporin therapy until the ATN is starting to recover. OKT3 or antithymocyte glob-ulin (ATG) may be utilised instead of cyclosporin if ATN is thought to be a potential problem.

Acute rejection (Histopathology of acute rejection, see p. 434)
Most transplant recipients will experience at least one episode of acute rejection. Acute rejection is usually a combination of cellular and antibody-mediated rejection which most usually occurs between 4 days and 2 months following transplantation.

The clinical signs of acute rejection may include:

- pyrexia
- fall in urine output
- rise in serum creatinine
- swelling and tenderness of the transplant
- weight gain
- flu-like symptoms
- ankle oedema.

The diagnosis of acute rejection is usually confirmed by a needle biopsy (see Chapter 6), and treatment is commenced immediately with a daily intravenous bolus of methyl prednisolone for 3 days. In severe cases anti-lymphocyte globulin (horse)/antithymocyte globulin (rabbit) (ATG/ALG) or OKT3 may be commenced. The rejection is usually controlled by the increased immunosuppression; however, a severe rejection episode may result in some loss of overall graft function.

Vascular complications

Transplant renal artery and renal vein thrombosis   Thrombosis of the renal artery or renal vein is a rare complication. Clinical signs of graft throm-bosis usually include renal dysfunction, anuria and hypotension. Diagnosis may be confirmed by ultrasound scanning (see Chapter 6). Immediate surgical exploration should be undertaken. In the majority of cases the transplant will be lost.

Transplant renal artery stenosis   Renal artery stenosis usually occurs between 6 and 12 months after transplantation. Signs include graft dysfunc-tion and severe hypertension with a bruit on auscultation over the transplant. Diagnosis is confirmed by angiography (see Chapter 6). In severe cases intervention may be required either by percutaneous transluminal angioplasty or surgery.

Urological complications

A major urological complication which may occur is avascular necrosis of the distal end of the transplant ureter, resulting in leakage of urine. Surgical reimplantation of the ureter will be required in most cases, using an internal ureteric stent.

Infections

Bacterial infections

Immunosuppression reduces the ability of the transplant recipient to mount a normal response to infection and predisposes the recipient to 'opportunistic infections' with organisms that are not usually pathogenic in non-immunosuppressed individuals. Hence, any sign of infection must be investigated and treated immediately.

The clinical signs of rejection are similar to those of infection (pyrexia, tachycardia, flu-like illness), therefore it is important that both possibilities are considered and investigations undertaken to exclude either cause.

Chest infections may result from *Pneumococcus*, *Haemophilus influenzae*, *Klebsiella* and *Pneumocystis* (septrin is often given as prophylaxis for *Pneumocystis* during the first 6 months post-transplant). Infection may develop rapidly, resulting in the need for ventilation. Early treatment with appropriate antibiotic therapies is essential.

Fungal infections

Oral candida is common and many centres use nystatin as prophylaxis for the first 2 months following transplant. Oral hygiene of a high standard should be encouraged.

Vaginal candida may also occur and recipients may be reluctant to report this problem, particularly to a male clinician in an outpatient setting. Recipients should be informed that candida is a potential problem and that treatment will be required. The opportunity to discuss such an issue with a female clinician or nurse should be provided so that reassurance and treatment can be offered.

Viral infections

Cytomegalovirus Cytomegalovirus (CMV) infection is usually acquired during childhood and early adulthood and is a minor flu-like illness. However, this minor illness can cause major complications in the immunosuppressed transplant recipient. CMV disease, after transplantation, may occur because of:

- Reactivation of latent disease in a CMV-positive recipient. Such reactivation is generally classed as 'secondary CMV'.

- Transmission of CMV from a CMV-positive donor to a CMV-negative recipient through the transplanted organ. Classed as 'primary CMV'.

CMV may also be transmitted through whole blood transfusions, hence many centres require that all renal patients receive CMV-negative blood.

CMV vaccinations for all transplant recipients in the pretransplant phase would be an ideal solution to this problem but, as yet, no clinically acceptable vaccines have been formulated. Also, matching so that CMV-negative recipients receive CMV-negative grafts would help to minimise the difficulties experienced, but such matching is not always possible in practice. Therefore, primary CMV disease does occur and can cause morbidity and mortality.

The usual time for manifestation of CMV disease is 4–8 weeks posttransplantation. Clinical signs include swinging pyrexia, rigors, malaise and, in extreme cases, pneumonitis, retinitis, gastroenteritis and encephalitis may develop.

Some centres use acyclovir as prophylaxis in all high-risk recipients (such as CMV-negative recipients receiving CMV-positive grafts). Other centres monitor serological progress and treat as appropriate. With primary disease, admission to hospital and treatment with gancyclovir is often necessary.

Herpes simplex and varicella zoster virus   Herpes simplex (type I and type II) commonly cause problems in the first months following transplantation. Oral and anogenital lesions may occur. Recipients may be reluctant to report such problems due to anxiety and embarrassment. Therefore, recipients should be aware that these lesions may arise and that they occur because of reduced immunity, not because of other social issues. Sympathetic and understanding care should be offered and treatment with acyclovir may be required.

Reactivation of the latent varicella zoster virus may also occur and present as classical 'shingles' lesions. Treatment with acyclovir is often necessary to prevent systemic complications. Disseminated varicella zoster (chickenpox) can be dangerous in immunosuppressed patients, resulting in some cases of severe illness with encephalitis, pneumonitis and meningitis. The recipients must be aware of the problems associated with such viral infections and should be encouraged to report signs and symptoms or contact with infected 'others'.

Common Diagnostic Tests Used to Investigate Renal Dysfunction

Ultrasonography (ultrasound scan) – see Chapter 6
A non-invasive investigation which can demonstrate non-immunological causes of renal dysfunction, such as vascular and urinary complications.

Transplant biopsy (needle core biopsy) – see Chapter 6

An automated 'biopsy gun' is used to obtain a core of cortical tissue from the upper pole of the transplant. This specimen of tissue is stained and examined for histological changes such as rejection. Needle-core biopsies may be performed routinely in order to provide a base-line histology picture and also to monitor the progress of the transplant. Such biopsies are also performed at times of renal dysfunction, particularly if rejection is suspected (Fig. 11.12).

RECIPIENT DISCHARGE FROM HOSPITAL AND CONTINUING CARE

If recovery has been uncomplicated the transplant recipient may be discharged home on the tenth postoperative day. During hospitalisation nursing interventions will have developed from (i) wholly compensatory; through (ii) partly compensatory; to (iii) educative and developmental (Galpin, 1992).

The educative and developmental intervention is very important for transplant recipients. They must have sufficient knowledge to monitor their health status, be compliant with medication regimens and report problems if they arise. Assessment of learning difficulties should be completed soon after transplant so that relevant interventions may be implemented to aid learning, knowledge and eventual independence. Physical barriers such as impaired sight and hearing can be aided by electronic blood pressure monitoring equipment. Language and literacy difficulties can be resolved with diagrammatic information, translations and medication presented in daily 'dosette' boxes, all promoting personal independence, although family members may be included in teaching sessions as appropriate.

The 'named nurse' may assess learning abilities (with an informal, non-threatening discussion) post-transplant and plan a teaching information programme, implement this programme and evaluate progress. Written information is given as appropriate both verbally and in the form of a written information booklet and at the time of discharge the recipient is able to:

- record and report changes in:
    pulse
    temperature
    respirations
    weight
    blood pressure
    and understand the relevance of such changes;
- measure and record 24 h urine output;

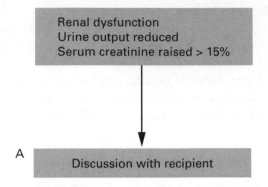

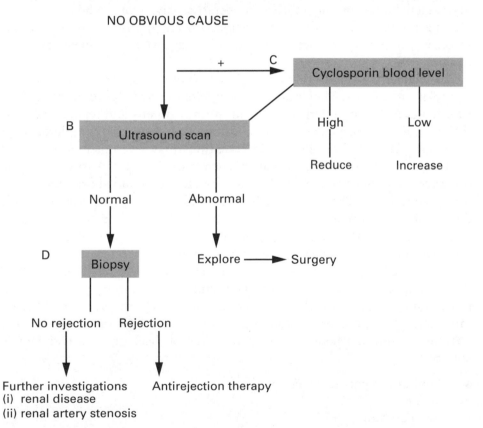

Fig. 11.12 *Assessment and tests completed in the presence of renal dysfunction during continuing care.*

- understand the action, dosage, side-effects of medication and the need for compliance;
- recognise the signs of rejection;
- recognise the signs of infection;
- telephone numbers of the transplant centre and how to contact staff;
- recognise the need to alert transplant personnel in light of any of these changes.

(Drug charts and monitoring booklets should be utilised as part of a self medication programme introduced on the second postoperative day.)

Immediately after discharge, recipients will be seen very frequently in the outpatient clinic and it is important that nursing intervention identifies developmental needs so that the recipient's knowledge base continues to expand and psychosocial care is offered. Reports suggest that some recipients feel that only the renal function and transplant progress is monitored, not the rehabilitation of the 'whole person'. Therefore, holistic care is essential, addressing psychosocial needs with physical needs; such care may be most appropriately offered by a transplant nurse practitioner, who can offer continuity of care as well as understanding and support.

The aim of on-going care is to 'empower' the recipient to achieve optimal individual rehabilitation. It is essential to help the recipient achieve a balance between monitoring health and gaining 'normality'. One of the most important post-transplant psychosocial tasks that the recipient needs to accomplish is the gradual relinquishing of the sick role and the eventual return to non-patient status (Christopherson, 1987). Medical and nursing staff can give a confusing message by referring to recipients as patients and demanding strict adherence to rigid health protocols, whilst at the same time insisting that transplantation offers a return to 'normality'.

Flexibility of care, understanding and encouragement are required to enable the recipient to take control of their lives and achieve the highest quality of life possible. On-going health monitoring will continue and problems may occur, but advice and support should be available throughout the complete transplant experience.

On-Going Care: Information and Support for Transplant Recipients

- *CAPD catheter.* If transplant function is satisfactory, the CAPD catheter is removed at 3 months post-transplant.
- *Diet.* Normal diet, but care with weight gain due to increased appetite and freedom from the renal diet. If cholesterol or lipid levels are raised dietary restrictions may be necessary.
- *Vaccinations: travel.* Transplant recipients should not receive 'live vaccines'. Therefore, it is important to consult the transplant centre

before travel immunisations are given. Foreign travel is encouraged but recognition of possible infection sources is necessary so that suitable precautions may be taken.

- *Skin care*. Immunosuppression predisposes recipients to skin damage from trauma and sun and increases the risk of skin malignancies. Therefore, dermatological monitoring and advice should be given and recipients should use 'factor 15 sun block' during sun exposure and report any skin lesions.
- *Fertility*. Female patients should be aware of fertility issues and be given advice with regard to birth control measures. Intrauterine devices are not recommended because of the risk of infection. Condoms or the 'mini pill' are the most appropriate therapies. Recipients should, ideally, wait at least 1 year before considering pregnancy. Advice should be available with regard to pregnancy risks in individual cases. Recipients cannot breast feed after delivery as the immunosuppression may transfer to the baby.
- *Employment*. Recipients may return to work as soon as they feel able as long as graft function and health are satisfactory and employment does not put either at risk. Help should be available for those recipients seeking employment.
- *Health education*. Smoking is discouraged due to the risk of enhanced cardiorespiratory and vascular complications. Exercise and activity is encouraged, although contact sports such as rugby or karate may put the graft at risk. Female patients should have regular cervical smears and breast examinations because of the increased risk of malignancy. Male patients should be monitored for potential malignancies and encouraged to perform testicular self examination.
- *Psychological health*. Psychological support should be available to help with sexual problems, body image problems and marital problems.
- *Social needs*. Help and advice should be available for social needs such as benefits, housing and return to work.

SUMMARY

A successful renal transplant can provide the best quality of life for ESRF patients. Janet Mosely (Fig. 11.13) was diagnosed ESRF aged 5 years (1972) and was on dialysis from 1972 to 1976. She received a cadaveric renal transplant in 1976 (aged 9 years). The kidney continues to function well to date, 19 years after transplant. Janet has pursued a successful music career, married and has two sons, Gregory and Daniel. Janet says 'It is amazing that the special gift from the donor has enabled me to achieve my career and personal goals and has resulted in the creation of a new family, a gift for generations to come'.

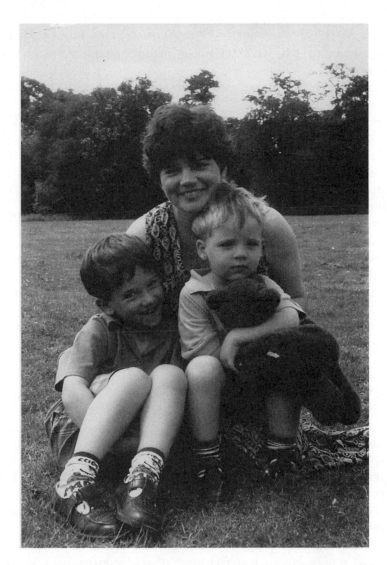

Fig. 11.13 *Janet Mosely with Gregory and Daniel.*

REFERENCES

ALLEN, R.D.M. AND CHAPMAN, J.R. (1993) *A Manual of Renal Transplantation.* Edward Arnold, London.

BENNETT, A.H. AND HARRISON, J.H. (1974) Experience with living familial renal donors. *Surg. Gynecol. Obstet.*, **139**: 894.

BLOGG, C.R., ANDERSON, M., SHODDLE, C. *et al.* (1973) Rehabilitation of patients treated by dialysis or transplantation. *Proc. Dial. Transplant. Forum*, **3**: 181.

BUCKLEY, P.E. (1989) The delicate question of the donor family. *Transplant Proc.*, **21**: 1411–2.

CARLISLE, D. (1995) Life-giving FATWA. *Nursing Times*, July 19, **91**: 2.

CHRISTOPHERSON, L.K. (1987) Cardiac transplantation: A psychological perspective. *Circulation*, **75**: 57.

CHURCHILL, D.N., MORGAN, J. AND TORRANCE. G.W. (1984) Quality of life in end stage renal disease. *Periton. Dial. Bull.*, **4**: 20.

Conference of Medical Royal Colleges and their faculties in the United Kingdom (1976). *Br. Med. J.*, **ii**: 1187–8.

Conference of Medical Royal Colleges and their faculties in the United Kingdom (1976). *Lancet* **ii**: 1069–70.

Conference of Medical Royal Colleges and their faculties in the United Kingdom (1979). *Br. Med. J.*, **i**: 32.

Conference of Medical Royal Colleges and their faculties in the United Kingdom (1979). *Lancet* **i**: 261–2.

COULTER, M. (1989) The needs of family members in ICU's. *Intensive Care Nursing*, **3**(1): 4–10.

CRAMOND, W.A. (1967) Renal homo transplantation – some observations on recipients and donors. *Br. J. Psychiatr.*, **133**: 1223.

DUBOVSKY, S.L. AND PENN, I. (1980) Psychiatric considerations in renal transplant surgery. *Psychosomatics*, **21**: 481.

EVANS, R.W. (1990) Quality of life assessment: a review. *Transplantation Reviews*, **4**(1): 28–51.

EVANS, R.W., MANNINEN, D.L., GARRISON, L.P. JR. *et al.* (1985) The quality of life for patients with end stage renal disease. *N. Engl. J. Med.*, **312**: 553.

FEEST, T.G., RIAD, H.N., COLLINS, C.H. *et al.* (1990) Protocol for increasing organ donation after cerebrovascular deaths in a district general hospital. *Lancet*, **335**: 1133.

FELLNER, C.H. AND MARSHALL, J.R. (1968) Twelve kidney donors. *JAMA*, **206**: 2703.

FREY, G.M. (1990) Stressors in renal transplant recipients at six weeks after transplant. *ANNA J.*, **17**: 443.

GALPIN, C. (1992) Body image in end stage renal failure. *Br. J. Nurs.*, **1**: 21.

GARRISON, R.N., BENTLEY, F.R., RAGUE, G.H. *et al.* (1991) There is an answer to the shortage of organ donors. *Surg. Gynaecol. Obstet.*, **173**: 391–6.

GORE, S.M., HINDS, C.J. AND RUTHERFORD, A.J. (1989) Organ donation from intensive care units in England. *BMJ*, **299**: 1193–7.

Harvard Medical School (1968) Report of the ad hoc committee of Harvard Medical School to examine the definition of brain death. Definition of irreversible coma. *J. Am. Med. Assc.*, **205**: 337.

HIRAS, J., ENCKELL, M., KUHLBECK, B. AND PASTERNACK, A. (1976) Psychological and social problems encountered in active treatment of chronic uremia. The living donor. *Acta. Med. Scand.*, **200**: 17.

HUDSON, K. AND HION, K. (1966) Coping with paediatric renal transplant ejection. *ANNA J.*, **13**: 261.

KEMPH, J.P. (1966) Renal failure, artifical kidney and kidney transplant. *Am. J. Psychiatr.*, **122**: 1270.

KLEIN, J. (1986) *Natural History of the Major Histocompatibility Complex.* John Wiley, New York.

MILLER, J.F. (1983) *Coping with Chronic Illness: Overcoming Powerlessness.* F.A. Davis, Philadelphia.

MOLTER, N.C. (1979) Needs of relatives of critically ill patients. A descriptive study. *Heart Lung.*, **8**: 332.

MORI/UKTCA/BACCN (1995) Report of a 2 year study into the reasons for relatives' refusal of organ donation. Obtained from UKTCA Secretariat. Royal Victoria Infirmary, Newcastle Upon Tyne NE1 4LP.

MORRIS, P.L.P. AND JONES, B. (1988) Transplantation versus dialysis – a study of quality of life. *Transplant Proc.*, **20**: 23.

NEW, W., SOLOMON, M., DINGWALL, R. AND MCHALE, J. (1994) *A question of give and take.* Research Report No. 18. The Kings Fund Institute.

OREM, D.E. (1991) *Nursing: Concepts of Practice*, 4th edn. Mosby Year Book.

PALLIS, C. (1994) Brain stem death: The evolution of a concept. In *Kidney Transplantation, Principles and Practice*, 4th edn. (ed. P.J. Morris). W.N. Saunders, London, pp. 71–85.

PERETZ, D. (1970) Development, object relations and loss. In *Loss and Grief: Psychological Management in Medical Practice* (eds B. Schuenberg, A.C. Carr and D. Peretz). Columbia University Press, New York, p. 5.

PETRIE, K. (1989) Psychological well-being and psychiatric disturbance in dialysis and renal transplant patients. *Br. J. Med. Psychol.*, **62**: 91.

PRICE, B. (1990) *Body Image: Nursing Concepts and Care.* Prentice Hall, London.

SALTER, M. (1988) *Altered Body Image: The Nurses' Role.* John Wiley, Chichester.

SIMMONS, R.G., HICKLEY, K., KJELLSTRAND, C.M. AND SIMMONS, R.H. (1971) Donors and non donors: the role of the family and the physician in kidney transplantation. *Semin. Psychiar.*, **3**: 102.

SIMMONS, R.C., KLEIN, S.D. AND SIMMONS, R.L. (1977) *The Gift of Life: The Social and Psychological Impact of Organ Transplantation.* John Wiley, New York.

SIMMONS, R.G., ANDERSON, C. AND KAMSTRA, L. (1984) Comparison of quality of life on continuous peritoneal dialysis, haemodialysis and after transplantation. *Am. J. Kidney Dis.*, **4**: 253.

SMITH, M.D., KAPPELL, D.F., PROVINCE, M.A. *et al.* (1986) Living related kidney donors: A multicentre study of donor education, socioeconomic adjustment and rehabilitation. *Am. J. Kidney Dis.*, **8**: 223.

SURMAN, O.S. (1989) Psychiatric aspects of organ transplantation. *Am. J. Psychiatry*, **146**: 972.

UK Transplant Co-ordinators Association (1993) Guidelines for Organ Donation. Obtainable from Secretariat: UKTCA, Royal Victoria Infirmary, Newcastle Upon Tyne, NE1 4LP.

UK Code of Practice (1991) Cadaveric Organs for transplantation: a code of practice. Her Majesty's Stationery Office (833/88), UK.

VEITCH, P. (1995) Asystolic donation. In *Transplantation '95. The Outlook of Transplantation Towards 2000.* Royal Society of Medicine, London.

VOEPAL-LEWIS, T., KETAFIAN, S., STARR, A. AND WHITE, M.J. (1990) Stress, coping and quality of life in adult kidney transplant recipients. *ANNA J.*, **7**: 427.

WAKEFORD, R.E. AND STEPNEY, R. (1989) Obstacles to organ donation. *Br. J. Surg.*, **76**(4): 35–9.

WEEMS, J. AND PATTERSON, E.T. (1989) Coping with uncertainty and ambivalence while awaiting a cadaveric renal transplant. *ANNA J.*, **16**: 27.

WHITE, M.J., KETAFIAN, S., STARR A.J. AND VOEPAL-LEWIS, T. (1990) Stress, coping and quality of life in adult kidney transplant recipients. *ANNA J.*, **7**: 421.

WILKINSON, P. (1995) A qualitative study to establish the self perceived needs of family members of patients in a general intensive care unit. *Intensive & Critical Care Nursing*, **11**: 77–86.

CHAPTER 12

COMMUNITY NURSING IN RENAL CARE

INTRODUCTION

In this chapter the reader gains an understanding of the complex nature of community nursing and the breadth of role the community renal nurse has in the care and management of the dialysis patient and family at home. The inseparable nature of health and social care is also highlighted.

The many factors involved in the success of home-based dialysis treatment in reducing patient morbidity are discussed, and central to this is the role of the nurse. The family and other carers are acknowledged as playing a vital role in caring for patients on home dialysis. The need to include other members of the primary health care team is recognised as an essential component to safe, effective dialysis in the community.

THE NATURE OF COMMUNITY AND COMMUNITY CARE

Many authors have sought to define the terms 'community' and 'community care' (Barnes, 1987; Booker and Simmonds, 1989; Heginbotham, 1990). 'Community' implies a group of people all of whom share something in common, which could be race, work, religion, a social activity or simply the area in which they live. A community gives care and support to those within it (Barnes, 1987; Skidmore, 1994). This liaison with family and friends means that they are relied upon to give support, comfort and help during stressful times. This traditional support is continued through the length of the illness.

It has been argued that planners and providers of health care require to understand the nature and function of a community in order to ensure the particular needs of those people living within it are met appropriately and sensitively. Nurses working in community settings must understand the community in order to plan and implement nursing care (Walton Spradley, 1991).

The Move to the Community

The provision of care in the community underpins one of the main philosophies of the National Health Service (NHS), namely enabling patients to live longer, as independently as possible, and to enjoy a better quality of life (DOH, 1990).

In the latter half of the twentieth century there has been a rapid technological expansion. Alongside this, there has been a return to care in the community. The increased sophistication of primary care, community nursing and outreach services means that patients with a chronic illness can be cared for at home (Beardshaw and Robinson, 1990).

The development of home haemodialysis (HD) programmes during the 1960s and 1970s and increase in use of continuous ambulatory peritoneal dialysis (CAPD) in the late 1970s further changed the emphasis of home dialysis, and with this came an introduction of community dialysis nurses working within renal units. Marks (1991) argues that providing care at home for dialysis patients is an excellent example of a clinically safe, organisationally feasible and financially viable alternative to hospital-based care. It is also recognised as an effective means to minimise hospital admission (Miller, 1990; Marks, 1991; Naylor, 1992). Above all, what must remain paramount is the preference the patient has for the location of the treatment and nursing care.

It is not until the patient is discharged home from the training programme that the unsupervised self-administration therapy commences. Until this point, the patient will have been closely supervised during the learning process and will always have had a renal nurse available to ask and assist in problem-solving situations and to answer any questions. After this level of input from the renal team, going home to be in charge of the dialysis treatment can be a worrying and frightening time for the patient and the family or carers. This is where the community renal nurse has such a vital role.

THE ROLE OF THE COMMUNITY RENAL NURSE

Community nurses have a different relationship with patients and the family compared to hospital nurses. In hospital, patients learn to abide by the rules, as it is the undisputed territory of the staff (Brindle and Brown, 1991). In the community this role is reversed; the patient's home is their territory and the nurse is a guest. The nurse is expected to abide by the 'rules of the house', showing due respect and consideration for the patient's customs, creed and culture.

The patient's home may often be ill suited to the provision of care and carrying out dialysis. With predialysis assessment visits, many of the initial environmental problems encountered can be overcome. This is discussed further below. The community renal nurse must accept the patient's norms and values and continue to nurse the patient in a non-judgemental manner, regardless of the home conditions. Working within these values, the community renal nurse can be a more effective provider of care (Humphrey and Milone-Nuzzo, 1991).

By the nature of the illness and treatment needed, it is acknowledged that patients receiving HD and peritoneal dialysis (PD) need long-term follow-up care (Wilson-Barnett, 1988). The spectrum of potential complications associated with dialysis therapy and the need for on-going education and training requires expert nursing care and is best provided where the patient carries out the treatment. As such, the role of the community renal nurse is an exciting and challenging one. It can be the cornerstone of the team by occupying the privileged position of knowing the patient, family, home life and other factors involved in the patient's day-to-day lifestyle.

Renal nurses can facilitate this supportive and educative network by bringing together the patient, family, community and other members of the multidisciplinary team to maintain optimum health and independence of the patient (Stewart, 1991). Enthusiasm and commitment to this approach is essential for the success of any renal replacement programme (Uttley and Prowant, 1994).

The primary aim of community nursing care for dialysis patients is to provide activities of daily living where appropriate, teaching patients about their dietary and fluid allowances and compliance with their dialysis therapy (Jaffe and Skidmore-Roth, 1993). Although these are essential components to home dialysis success, this statement fails to acknowledge the wider aspect of the role in the social, environmental, cultural and family influences on the patient's health and well-being.

DHSS (1986) recommends that specialist nurses working in the community should use expert knowledge and skill to care for patients and pass on that skill to other nurses by teaching and demonstration. Brindle and Brown (1991) outline the five aims of a nurse specialist which can be applied to the role of the community renal nurse and the holistic role in the care and management of home dialysis patients:

- control symptoms
- support and advice
- co-ordinate care
- meeting practical needs
- education and training.

Control Symptoms

Patients dialysing at home are in charge of the therapy and it is therefore essential to both the patient and carer that the patient remains asymptomatic of uraemia, fluid overload, dehydration and anaemia.

After the initiation of treatment, patients usually feel significantly better and are convinced that the renal replacement therapy is necessary and of great benefit. However, those involved in the care of renal patients would not deny that the treatment is monotonous and time consuming and, as such, technique and skills can become slack. The community dialysis nurse, with other members of the renal team, must try to maintain the patient's enthusiasm and motivation to continue the treatment as prescribed in order to ensure the patient stays well and symptom free for as long as dialysis continues.

On the first home visit following initiation of dialysis it is important that the nurse establishes some base-line observations with the patient, including the patient's target weight, state of hydration, peripheral oedema, blood pressure (BP), urine output as well as exercise tolerance level. The patient should always be aware of their target weight and the ensuing symptoms and any potential complications should this vary. Some patients may not feel confident enough to to change their CAPD regimen by using different strength bags or increasing or decreasing their fluid intake without first consulting the named nurse. As such, patients should be encouraged to understand the importance of BP recordings and the pattern of their weight so that over time they may feel confident and thus more 'in charge' of the treatment. The community renal nurse must take on the responsibility of empowering patients to do this.

On subsequent home visits, base-line targets previously set with the patient should be checked and revised as required. As a patient begins to feel better, appetite may improve and the taste sensation return. A weight increase is expected and in this situation an accurate fluid and weight assessment will be carried out on each home visit and a new target weight agreed. Feedback to the hospital renal team is vital as any difficulties a patient may be experiencing with the dialysis may indicate the need to arrange a peritoneal equilibration test (PET), adequacy studies or urea kinetic modelling (UKM) (see Chapters 7 and 8).

The control of uraemic symptoms can be enhanced by adhering to the diet advised by the renal dietitian. Advice previously given is reinforced and can be further explained. A practical example of this could be if a patient experiences itching. In this situation the nurse may think it appropriate to take a blood sample to check the patient's serum phosphate and calcium levels. Advice regarding the importance of taking phosphate binders with meals should be offered. Feedback can then be given to the dietitian, highlighting problems encountered and re-referring patients back to the dietetic service as necessary.

Jaffe and Skidmore-Roth (1993) argue that it is the community nurse's responsibility to reinforce the awareness of when and how to take the prescribed medication. By providing information about the indication for medication the patient is more likely to be aware that drug therapy is an integral part of dialysis success.

Another vital aspect of symptom control is the management of the patient's anaemia. The anaemia of chronic renal failure is a well-documented occurrence and imposes many restrictions on a person's activity level and way of life.

Active involvement in co-ordinating the prescribed erythropoietin (EPO) administration will ensure the correct dose, route and potential side-effects will be minimised, therefore keeping the patient's safety paramount (UKCC, 1992). The community renal nurse may need to involve district and practice nurses in the administration of the EPO in situations where the patient or carer does not wish to or when it has been assessed as inappropriate. Teaching community nurses about EPO ensures safe and effective patient care as well as promoting optimum health and well-being for the patient. The provision of up-to-date literature for nurses and patients is an important aspect of care.

Collection of blood samples will be required to monitor the patient's haemoglobin levels. Any adjustments in the EPO dose need to be discussed with the renal team and fed back to the patient and the community nurse involved. Periodically, blood sampling for control of uraemia may be necessary. Discussion of test results must first take place with the medical staff before any action deemed necessary is followed through. The patient should be informed of results to encourage involvement in care and also to avoid unnecessary worry.

Support and Advice

This is undoubtedly the foremost role of the community renal nurse. Patients and the family will require frequent help, guidance and support before commencing, and for as long as peritoneal or haemodialysis is used. Good-quality home support, prevention and early detection of problems that a patient may encounter can reduce the number of hospital inpatient episodes or attendances in the outpatient clinic (Naylor, 1992; Uttley and Prowant, 1994). Wilson-Barnett (1988) and Stewart (1991) argue that patients with chronic illnesses may well have increased mortality and morbidity if care and supervision in the community is denied to them. Preventing patients from being admitted to hospital for a dialysis-related problem should be one of the key objectives of providing a home visit service. The community team should audit this aspect of the role in order to prove its effectiveness.

Part of the role of providing support is acting as an advocate to the patient. This has been described by Kohnke (1980) as 'the act of informing and supporting a person so that he can make the best decisions possible for himself'. Patients may need to be supported through their decision and choice of renal replacement therapy and beyond.

Ideally, any prospective patient and family should have met the hospital and community renal nursing teams prior to commencing therapy. Seeing the patient and family at home before dialysis commences can gain the patient's trust and provide information and support. In this way, the patient and family can begin to establish a relationship before dialysis is required. Support and advice to the patient and family should begin at the first point of referral. There is often only a short amount of time available for nurses and other team members to prepare the patient and family for what could be life-long treatment (Uttley and Prowant, 1994).

It is acknowledged that choosing between two dialysis options is a highly complex process. When a patient is uraemic this choice may seem even more difficult to make, as they may find it hard to concentrate and under-stand the implications of the decisions. This process involves helping others to:

- weigh up the pros and cons of peritoneal and haemodialysis;
- consider the likely effect of pursuing each treatment method;
- decide which type of dialysis will be best (Ewles and Simnett, 1985).

Factors such as the patient's lifestyle, employment and existing support at home and in the community are involved in the choice. The choice of dia-lysis treatment by the patient and family makes acceptance easier and success more likely (Rivetti et al., 1993). Having made a decision on the preferred method of renal replacement therapy based on their own values, the patient will need further support to carry the choice through.

Jaffe and Skidmore-Roth (1993) highlighted 'ineffective family coping' as one of the major problems for carers. A patient's chronic illness can often exhaust the supportive capacity of the carer. Family members have been expected to be involved with home dialysis since the mid-1960s and although patients are taught to dialyse themselves, the spouse or other carer will become involved in the treatment and can experience considerable stress (Brunier and McKeever, 1993). Various studies have shown that women carers have recalled feelings of depression before the onset of home dialysis and the pattern of communication and dynamics of the relationship had changed. Psychosocial aspects of renal failure and dialysis are discussed more fully in Chapter 3. Anger and hostility are both factors which hinder adaptation to home dialysis. Good assessment skills are required to so that the effects of these problems are minimised. This ensures nursing care is focused on the individual patient and family needs. The well-being of any carer is paramount to the patient as well as to the health service as a whole (Hull *et al.*, 1989).

A variety of strategies to avoid crisis scenarios within a family can be initiated:

- assessing the family's need for help in the home and referring any identified needs on to the appropriate service;
- encouraging and referring families to use home care and other community resources instead of relying solely on relatives and friends;
- advocating the use of respite services to lessen the workload on caregivers;
- any communication with patients and carers needs to be in understandable language, avoiding jargon and unfamiliar words.

An example of this would be when the patient is told in clinic that there is a need to lose 'a couple of kilos'. The patient might mistake the instruction as meaning they are overweight rather than overloaded with fluid and not realise the intention is for an alteration in strength of PD fluid or to restrict fluid and salt intake.

Caring at home puts a strain on family relationships. The burden of the care may fall on one family member, imposing physical, mental and emotional strain (Hull *et al.*, 1989). Many restrictions are imposed on partners of patients using HD at home, as they have to be present throughout the dialysis session. The nurse can then introduce a range of interventions, primarily by providing accurate information about the treatment regimen, the likely progress and outcome, thus alleviating any fears and anxieties. It is essential to allow time for questions, answers and clarifications on each visit. In the non-threatening environment of the home, the family, carers and the patient should be encouraged to discuss the available options for change should they be unhappy with the treatment. More sensitive subjects can be more easily discussed (Uttley and Prowant, 1994). There is no pressure on the patient to hurry and the nurse will not be called away to another task.

Some of the perceived benefits to the patient and family from provision of support in the community are identified (Stewart, 1991):

- Deficits in knowledge and skill in dialysis technique can be identified and corrected by the nurse, which may help with the prevention of infections and the 'knock-on' complication of ill health and hospital admission.
- The patient and family's ability to adjust to the demands of dialysis can be monitored and referrals made to appropriate services as necessary.
- Family members and the patient have an opportunity to air problems and seek answers to physical, psychological, sexual and emotional needs away from the hospital environment.
- Patients and families will feel supported and less isolated.

Patients may benefit from support from each other. The community renal nurse can facilitate this by introducing people in similar circumstances by encouraging membership of the local the kidney patient's association attached to the renal unit. As supportive as renal staff are, they are no substitute for direct experience of life on dialysis that other patients and carers can offer.

An area where the community renal nurse can offer expertise and skill is in the terminal care of patients who withdraw from treatment. The decision to withdraw from or to terminate dialysis involves the patient, family and all members of the team. Psychological aspects of treatment withdrawal are discussed in Chapter 3.

Once a decision has been made to cease dialysis, the patient needs to be reassured that staff will continue to provide appropriate comfort and care until death, and to the family and carers afterwards (Oreopoulos, 1994). At this stage it is the duty of the nursing staff to provide terminal care to the dying patient with pain relief, advice on fluid control, support and reassurance. When a patient chooses to die at home, support from district nurses and other services for care and terminal support at home can be arranged. A link to the hospital can be maintained by the continuation of home visits.

Co-Ordinate Care

The role of co-ordinator is frequently used by nurses working in community settings. The community renal nurse is likely to be the patient's named nurse for home treatment. As many agencies, both health and social, are often involved in supporting patients at home, a care co-ordinator requires a familiar knowledge of the community in which the patient lives. The primary benefit of well co-ordinated community services is good quality health care delivered to patients (Burgess and Chatterton Ragland, 1983). Co-ordinated services avoid unnecessary duplication and foster patient-focused sensitive care.

The co-ordination of home care services has become increasingly important and complex as new technology and treatment methods are developed. Elderly people who may not have been offered dialysis 10 years ago are now being taken on for renal replacement therapy, most commonly PD. The elderly will often require more nursing and social care input as the dependencies increase. With the complex and inseparable nature of health and social care, it is important that a referral network has been established. This ensures that patients receive appropriate services with the minimum of delay.

In the predialysis period the patient will have been given information about the change dialysis will make. This period should be used as one of adjustment. Other members of the renal team will be involved, such as the social worker and predialysis counselling nurses. Patients have the benefit of practical advice from the nurse, who can demonstrate the amount of space required for storage of PD supplies and suggest the most appropriate place for doing exchanges. For patients using PD, any adjustments required in the home can be discussed and planned before the first fluid delivery arrives.

Although covered in the training programme, patients may need information reinforced and help to adjust to the home conditions. A flat, cleanable, surface for CAPD exchanges and a sink for hand washing should be available and somewhere located to hang the bag up for draining the fluid in. The patient needs to be made aware of a suitable place to warm CAPD fluid by way of an electric bag warmer and that scales for daily weight will be required. These are often supplied by the hospital.

Complex home care regimen

For patients who have many professionals involved in their care, confusion can arise if roles and responsibilities are not clearly defined. Well co-ordinated community services will avoid this.

A home visit shortly following discharge will support the patient whilst adjusting to dialysis at home. Ideally, the nurse should be present for the first CAPD exchange or HD session. Sensible planning is needed to ensure that a patient is not discharged from the training programme until all parties involved, including the patient, are ready and any community care requirements are in place. Examples of problems and their solutions that a patient may experience are:

- lack of knowledge of any part of the treatment regimen;
- unavailability of the community nurse for initial support;
- significant alteration in customary lifestyle.

Starting home PD and HD has a major impact on family life. Others involved should be made aware of the patient's new treatment and aspects of care involved. Any additions to the existing package of care need to be made explicit to the person responsible and added to the care plan. This may include the home carer breaking up the empty boxes from the CAPD fluid or putting out the patient's clinical waste for collection. Although these tasks may seem trivial, they are vital to a patient who is not able to do them.

Meeting any carers involved together with the patient is an excellent opportunity for the professionals to meet and discuss the individual roles and agree on a common aim – well co-ordinated seamless care to meet the patient's individual needs.

As a co-ordinator, the community renal nurse is in a perfect position to keep all members of the renal team informed of the patient's progress and ability to continue with the demands that dialysis imposes. Feedback is vital to the hospital team as well as to the patient's general practitioner (GP). The community renal nurses liaise with GPs regarding the patient's on-going condition and ability to continue the dialysis and any alterations in treatment (Wilkie and Brown, 1994). Informing all professionals involved with the patient fosters a cohesive team approach which is so vital in the care and management of patients on dialysis.

Care Planning

Under the present Patient's Charter, patients are entitled to a needs assessment carried out to a high standard. The community care plan should include the following:

- patient's own description of their needs and how they can best be met;
- The opportunity to have an advocate present – this could be a friend or relative;
- assistance for people whose first language is not English;
- listening to carers' views and ideas;
- taking account of carers' ability and willingness to participate in care;
- co-ordinating the involvement of different agencies to provide the most comprehensive assessment;
- giving accurate information (DOH, 1994).

The document *A Framework for Local Community Care Charters in England* sets out the entitlements a patient can expect from a care plan:

- it is in writing;
- it is shared with users and their carers;
- it covers all services when more than one agency is involved;
- it gives contact points;
- a statement of when the assessment and care plan will be reviewed to ensure they are still appropriate (DOH, 1994).

When formulating a care plan the community renal nurse must take the above points into account. It is important that prescribed nursing care is evaluated at agreed intervals to ensure that the care plan remains pertinent to the patient's current needs.

Nursing care plans and notes need to be accessible to all members of the renal nursing staff, especially for the out of hours service when a patient may require treatment. This ensures that patients receive individualised nursing care according to the prescribed plan.

Example 1

Mrs X aged 72 years	Diagnosis: chronic renal failure – cause unknown
Dwelling	Terraced house. Lives with husband
Helper	Husband
Treatment	CAPD for 3 months
Status	Married. Retired

Example 2

Mr Z aged 32 years	Diagnosis: chronic renal failure – polycystic kidney disease
Dwelling	3 bed semi-detatched. Has a bedroom converted for haemodialysis which is not used for any other purpose. Lives with mother
Helper	Mother
Treatment	Home haemodialysis for 6 months. Dialyses in the evenings
Status	Single. Works full time

Meeting Practical Needs

Although patients at home using dialysis are self-caring, the nurse has a practical role in maintaining the patient's health with effective dialysis therapy. During routine visiting the community renal nurse may encounter problems which require prompt nursing action. The patient, however, may not be forthcoming with information. With experience and sensitive questioning, the nurse can discover any difficulties patients could be having with the dialysis.

With PD the importance of exit site care must be reinforced to the patient and carer and this should be discussed on each home visit. It may be necessary to take a swab from the exit site for culture if it has become inflamed and is discharging. According to the individual unit policy, oral antibiotic

Community Nursing Assessment

Name _____ *MRS X* _____ Health Centre/Clinic *General Hospital*

Address *16 Cavendish Street* _____ Date _____ *1-6-97* _____

_____ *Oakham* _____

---

1. Patients perception and expectation of illness/condition.
   Mrs X has an established understanding of the need for peritoneal dialysis and it will be a lifelong treatment. Although she is aware that transplantation is an option but does not want to consider one at present.

---

2. Carers perception and expectation of illness/condition
   Mr X attended the training programme with his wife. He is supportive and takes an active role in the CAPD and is aware that his wife's kidney failure is irreversible.

---

3. Mobility
   Mrs X is fully mobile around her home but finds walking upstairs tiring as her legs are weak. She cannot walk further than 150 metres and holds onto her husband's arm for support

---

4. Personal Hygiene
   Mrs X is independent with washing. She showers daily and redresses her exit site immediately afterwards.

---

5. Hair   *Good condition with a healthy scalp*

   Skin   *Intact, occasionally gets itchy skin especially on her abdomen.*

---

6. Ability to dress/undress
   Mrs X is able to dress and undress independently

---

7. Language   *Speaks English clearly*
   Difficulty with words/sentences   *Articulates well*
   Body language   *At ease*
   Hearing:-   *Hears well*   Vision:- *Wears glasses for reading*

---

8. Breathing   *Mrs X gets short of breath when walking and climbing the stairs*

   Smoking   *Non smoker*

---

9. Weight   *Target weight 55Kg.*   Urinalysis
   Temperature
   Pulse   Blood Pressure

Community Assessment 1a

10. Home Safety
   Mrs X has a proven understanding of the need to have a separate clean area in which to carry out her CAPD.

11. Health Promotion
   Mrs X appreciates the need to take her medication and adhere to a renal diet and fluid allowance in order for her to remain well.

12. Sleep
   Mrs X sleeps well at night and finds that she sleeps during the day for short periods

13. Pain
   No pain

14. Orientation and memory
   Fully orientated

15. Emotional Status
   Mrs X is aware that her kidney failure is a lifelong medical condition. She says she is less worried now CAPD has now started and is happy the treatment has made her feel much better.

16. Body Image
   Says she is not bothered by the tube.
   Mrs X says she does not feel self conscious about the tube.

17. Medication *Erythropoietin 200 iu s/c x 2 week*
   Amlodipine 10mg OD
   Calcichew ī TDS
   Ferrous sulphate 200mg TDS

18. Eating and Drinking
   Eats well and has an improved appetite since CAPD started
   Says she finds it hard to adhere to 1000ml fluid allowance

19. Urinary function   *Passes approximately 400ml urine a day*

   Bowel Function   *Mrs X says her bowel habit is regular although is prone to constipation.*

20. Comments
   Mrs X is coping well with her dialysis and her husband is acting as a good support

Signature *Betty Elliott*

Community Asessment 1b

Community Nursing Assessment

Name _____ *MR Z* _____ Health Centre/Clinic *General Hospital*

Address ___ *22 The Street* _____ Date *1-5-97* _____

_____ *Kingswater* _____

---

1. Patients perception and expectation of illness/condition.
   Mr Z is on the active transplant list and hopes soon to receive a kidney. He is positive about home haemodialysis but likes to think he will not be doing it for years

---

2. Carers perception and expectation of illness/condition
   Mr Z's mother finds the haemodialysis a responsibility but says she is confident in her son's ability to do his dialysis properly. She hopes he will have a transplant soon.

---

3. Mobility
   Mr Z is fully mobile but does tire easily when he walks long distances.
   He is no longer able to play football.

---

4. Personal Hygiene
   Independent with washing

---

5. Hair   *Hair healthy*

   Skin   *Intact. No problems with pruritis*

---

6. Ability to dress/undress
   Fully independent with dressing and undressing

---

7. Language   *Speaks English*
   Difficulty with words/sentences   *none*
   Body Language   *Confident manner*
   Hearing:-   *Hears well*   Vision:- *Does not require glasses*

---

8. Breathing   *Occasionally gets short of breath*

   Smoking   *Mr Z classes himself as a 'social smoker'*
                  He will have a few cigarettes in the pub when with his friends

---

9. Weight   *Target weight 70KG*
   Temperature *Takes his temperature*
   Pulse   *pre + post haemodialysis*   Blood Pressure   *Mr Z takes his own BP*
                                                                pre and post dialysis

---

Community Nursing Assessment 2a

10. Home Safety
Mr Z has an emergency call bell so he can alert his mother of any problems during his dialysis.

11. Health Promotion
Mr Z has been advised about smoking and his health as he does not class himself as a 'real smoker' he does not see it as a danger to his health.

12. Sleep
Sleeps soundly.

13. Pain
Mr Z has pain only when inserting his fistula needles.
He uses topical emla cream for this
Occasional cramp at the end of haemodialysis

14. Orientation and memory
Fully orientated.
Retains information well.

15. Emotional Status
Mr Z says he is happier now he is on home haemodialysis and does not have to travel to hospital & can dialyse at his own convenience. He is now working full time

16. Body Image   *Says his fistula does not bother him at all*

17. Medication   *Calcichew ī TDS*
Nifedipine LA 90mg OD

18. Eating and Drinking
Mr Z says he only finds his fluid allowance a problem when going out for drinks with his friends
He enjoys a treat when on haemodialysis but says he is otherwise used to his dietary restrictions.

19. Urinary function
Passes approximately 1 litre a day

Bowel Function
Bowels regular - at least daily

20. Comments
To be advised re smoking before transplantation

Signature ___ *Jane Smith* _____

Community Nursing Asessment 2b

therapy can be initiated. Should the patient have an exit site infection it may be possible to discover the likely cause so this can be avoided in future. A demonstration of the correct exit site care and catheter immobilisation technique can be given to the patient. Observation of carrying out the procedure and an explanation of modifications to technique are necessary.

Peritonitis remains the most common and serious problem to patients using PD. Apart from the preventive role, practical skills are required in its diagnosis and nursing management. In many units the standard policy for the diagnosis and treatment of PD peritonitis is nurse led. Having established that a patient has peritonitis, an experienced renal nurse can decide whether the patient is unwell and requires medical attention and possible hospital admission. If the patient remains clinically well, the community nurse will take specimens of dialysis effluent and administer antibiotic therapy according to the renal unit's protocol. It may be necessary to teach the patient or carer to inject the PD bags or involve the district nurses, depending on the treatment protocol.

Follow-up visits during episodes of peritonitis may be necessary to ensure the fluid is clearing and the patient remains well.

In conjunction with the renal dietitian it may be appropriate to give the patient protein supplementation in the form of sip feeds to combat protein loss during the peritonitis episode (see Chapter 8).

Patients using HD at home have different needs requiring practical help. Difficulties with needling may be encountered, and the patient will require assistance and education regarding inserting needles correctly and identifying new sites to use. Visiting during a dialysis session is an excellent opportunity to observe the patient and carer's technique of setting up and commencing treatment or completing dialysis. Reinforcing fistula care is a necessary part of continuing education for the patient (see Chapter 7).

Education and Training

Much has been documented regarding patients' needs for information concerning treatment or condition. The focus of responsibility for and provision of health care has changed. The public is being encouraged to be more self-reliant and assertive in seeking out knowledge pertinent to them and thus become more in charge of their health (Webb, 1994).

Dialysis is undoubtedly monontonous and demanding and has along with it a spectrum of complications, some potentially life threatening. The period of training a patient undergoes should not be viewed as an isolated event. The need for on-going education for patients and family is essential, as dialysis is for life if the patient is unsuitable for transplantation. As such, the community renal nurse has a vital role in continuing education, updating practical skills, knowledge and technique for dialysis patients, carers and health care professionals.

Accurate nursing assessment is required to establish the patient's current level of knowledge before building on this to increase the understanding of the treatment. Dialysis patients already have to invest much time in treatment and self-care and therefore may not wish to spend 'free time' focusing on the illness and making additional visits to hospital. In this situation, a home visit will update the patient and family education and training in patient's home, using familiar equipment to update dialysis skills, knowledge and technique.

In order to learn, patients need to be actively involved in the process to ensure the best is gained from the experience (Ewles and Simnett, 1985). When teaching, it must be relevant and interesting to the patient (Webb, 1994). Teaching patients requires skill, never more so than when the patient feels ill or threatened (Benner, 1984). In this situation a variety of approaches are required but the main theme of education and retraining will be the promotion of self-care.

District nurses (DN) often require more formal training, such as attendance at renal study days, although much knowledge and practical skills can be gained by the DN during a joint home visit with the community renal nurse and the value of these interactions should not be underestimated. In this scenario the patient has an opportunity to voice their needs, and a plan of care can be formulated that is acceptable to the patient and family.

CULTURAL CONSIDERATIONS IN COMMUNITY CARE

Culture profoundly influences people's lives (Walton Spradley, 1991). That the UK is a multicultural society made up of a range of racial groups is no longer disputed. Within each racial group will be a further division of social classes, language, religious beliefs, education, attitudes, beliefs and values (Elliott, 1994). Although there are broad cultural values shared by those who live in the UK, there is a wealth of subcultures in each society. It is critically important to be sensitive to the needs of each culture (Walton Spradley, 1991). Understanding those cultural influences that affect a person's behaviour is part of the planning of care.

Commencing dialysis requires a change in or modification of behaviour. This can never be achieved by patients from minority ethnic groups unless health care professionals are aware of factors such as family, religion, health and illness and how these shape behaviour.

In order to achieve effective community care the particular needs of patients and families have to be addressed (Elliott, 1994). Co-ordinated information about the people and geographical area served is important. Building up a profile will aid in providing data on population, causes of renal failure,

PATIENT CARE PLAN

SURNAME _MRS X_

FORENAME _Rosie_   M̶R̶/MRS/M̶I̶S̶S̶

ADDRESS _16 Cavendish Street, Oakham_

CENTRE _General Hospital_

Page No. 1/2

KORNER ID _G2716640_

Date	Problem	Overall Aim	Agreed Action with Patient/Carers	Evaluation date	Signature
1-6-97	Anaemia due to chronic renal failure	To increase haemoglobin level to 10–12 g dl⁻¹	1) District nurse to visit twice a week to administer EPO injection	1 monthly	
	Mrs X's exercise tolerance level is poor and she cannot walk further than 150 metres. Short of breath when climbing stairs	For Mrs X to be able to climb stairs and walk without having to stop due to fatigue and weakness	2) DN to check Mrs X's BP prior to injection		
			3) Administer injection into appropriate site ensuring that the sites are used in rotation		
	Baseline/Present State	**Agreed Objectives with Patient/Carers**	4) Dispose of sharps safely		
	Hb 8.4 g dl⁻¹	To have EPO injections twice a week	5) Assess Mrs X's well-being and moniter for improvements in anaemic symptoms		Betty Elliott
	Mrs X has to hold her husband's arm when walking outside the home. Can only walk 150 m without stopping.	To prepare injection equipment on agreed days			

PATIENT CARE PLAN

SURNAME ___MRS X___ FORENAME ___Rosie___ ~~MR/MRS/MISS~~

ADDRESS ___16 Cavendish Street, Oakham___

CENTRE ___General Hospital___

KORNER ID ___G2716640___

Page No. 2/2

Date	Problem	Overall Aim	Agreed Action with Patient/Carers	Evaluation date	Signature
1-6-97	Swelling of ankles due to fluid overload. Mrs X's swollen ankles are uncomfortable and reduce her movement	To reduce oedema and advise Mrs X how to maintain her target weight	1) Mrs X will change her CAPD regimen to: 8 am 2000ml strong bag 1 pm 2000ml weak bag 6 pm 2000ml weak bag 11 pm 2000ml weak bag to aim to lose 3KG	weekly	
			2) Community renal nurse to visit weekly for 3 weeks to moniter Mrs X's fluid		
	Baseline/Present State	**Agreed Objectives with Patient/Carers**	weight loss		
	Ankles swollen and Mrs X has pitting oedema to her mid calf.	To reduce weight to 55KG	3) Advise and encourage Mrs X to adhere to her fluid allowance of 1000ml		Betty Elliott
	Weight 58KG (3KG higher than target weight)	Improve comfort of Mrs X's ankles and promote better ankle movement	4) Encourage Mrs X to eat a low salt diet and reinforce the reason for this. Refer to the renal dietician as necessary		

Fig Care plan 2 (chapter 12)

PATIENT CARE PLAN

SURNAME __MR Z__   FORENAME __George__   MR/~~MRS~~/~~MISS~~   CENTRE __General Hospital__   Page No. __1/1__

ADDRESS __11 The Street, Kingswater__   KORNER ID __G264328__

Date	Problem	Overall Aim	Agreed Action with Patient/Carers	Evaluation date	Signature
1-5-97	Mr Z has chronic renal failure due to polycystic kidney disease.	To ensure Mr Z receives adequate haemodialysis & feels well enough to continue working	1) Community renal nurse to visit monthly		Jane Smith
			2) Discuss any mechanical problems Mr Z may be experiencing eg. difficulty with inserting fistula needles, heparinisation etc.	monthly	Jane Smith
	Requires haemodialysis 3 times a week for 4 hours		3) Discuss any problems with Mr Z & his mother. Offer to relieve Mr Z's mother from the haemodialysis session if possible	monthly	Jane Smith
	Baseline/Present State	**Agreed Objectives with Patient/Carers**	4) Take blood every 2nd month to ensure safe biochemical parameters.	2 monthly	Jane Smith
	Target weight 70 KG	Mr Z will haemodialyse at home 3 times a week for 4 hours			
	Not symptomatic of anaemia or fluid overload				

key health problems and local available services for referral. Roderick *et al.* (1994) argue that ethnic composition is a vital determinant of a population's need. From this study it was concluded that the ethnic composition of a population has an appreciable impact on an area's requirement for renal replacement therapy.

Difficulties with communication and language may be experienced. A family member is often used to help with translation. This situation may not be appropriate as it cannot be assumed that a patient is willing to discuss personal details through family members. Nor can it be assumed that the correct interpretation is given. Accordingly, a local interpreting or linkworker service may be a preferred option. The latter acts as more of an advocate to the patient. Fuller and Toon (1988) state the following are desirable attributes when using a linkworker or interpreter:

- is fluent in both languages;
- has some training in interpretation;
- has some medical knowledge;
- has a good knowledge of how the health service works;
- is available every time the patient is seen;
- is accepted and trusted by the patient and health worker;
- is sensitive to the patient's and health worker's needs;
- will not allow their own beliefs to over-ride those of the patient;
- puts the patient at ease;
- has a good memory and pays attention to detail;
- can translate fine shades of meaning;
- is able to tell the health worker when the patient has problems and why;
- is aware of the cultural expectations of both patients and health workers and can explain them to both;
- is the same sex as the patient;
- is able to carry the responsibility.

PRACTICAL ASPECTS OF CARING IN THE HOME

Safe Disposal of Clinical Waste in the Community

PD and HD generate large amounts of clinical waste and patients need to be aware of the correct disposal methods of the waste in the community. Waste disposal from dialysis treatment at home raises different problems from those in the hospital environment.

Liaison with the patient's local authority environmental services department to reinforce the nature and risks which can arise from unsafe disposal of clinical waste is essential, as it can be hazardous to health or the environment if dealt with incorrectly (DOE, 1990).

Disposal Methods

In the UK, all dialysis waste must be disposed of in a yellow clinical waste bag, sealed with a tie to avoid leakage. Arrangements should be made with the local authority for collection of the waste on a specific day. Until the collection, the waste should be kept inside the patient's home. All waste containers should be left outside for the minimum amount of time possible to reduce any risks of infection to others (DOE, 1990). Local authorities have a duty to collect clinical waste, and there should be no need for nursing staff to transport health care waste.

RISK ASSESSMENT

This is the process of identifying hazards to patients, family and health care workers associated with the patient's treatment and care. Raising the patient's awareness to any specific procedures and protocols of the authority in which the patient lives, and their relationship to the patient, should be highlighted.

The Royal College of Nursing (1994) states that the assessment of risk and subsequent plan of action must be recorded in writing in the patient's care plan. The assessment will be based on information obtained from:

- the patient and any carers involved;
- nursing care plan on discharge from the training programme and into the community;
- medical notes;
- local authority policies.

SUMMARY

With the recognised shift of more technical treatments into the community, patients using home PD and HD can be safely cared for and managed by community renal nurses together with DNs and visits to hospital to the multidisciplinary team.

The community is a complex mixture of health and social care and the nurse needs to have a sound knowledge of treatments available as well as the needs of the patients on dialysis at home. This enables a comprehensive and sensitive service to be available to renal patients, wherever the treatment is carried out.

REFERENCES

BARNES, A. (1987) *Personal and Community Health*, 3rd edn. Baillière Tindall, London.

BEARDSHAW, V. AND ROBINSON, R. (1990) *New for old? Prospects for nursing in the 1990s*. Research Report 8. Kings Fund Institute, London.

BENNER, P. (1984) *From Novice to Expert. Excellence and Power in Clinical Nursing Practice*. Addison-Wesley, Redwood City.

BOOKER, C. AND SIMMONDS, S. (1989) *Community Psychiatric Nursing: A Social Perspective*. Chapman & Hall, London.

BRINDLE, C. AND BROWN, K. (1991) *Community Health Care*. Macmillan Magazines, New York.

BRUNIER, G.M. AND McKEEVER, P.T. (1993) The impact of home dialysis on the family: literature review. *ANNA Journal*, **20**(6): 653–8.

BURGESS, W. AND CHATTERTON RAGLAND, E. (1983) *Community Health Nursing. Philosophy, Process, Practice*. Appleton Century Crofts, Connecticut.

DEPARTMENT OF HEALTH AND SOCIAL SECURITY (1986) Community Nursing: A focus for care (The Cumberlege Report). HMSO, London.

DOE (1990) *Environmental Protection Act 1990. Waste Management. The Duty of Care*. A Code of Practice. HMSO, London.

DOH (1990) *The Health Service. The NHS Reforms and You*. HMSO, London.

DOH (1994) *A Framework for Local Community Care Charters in England*. DOH.

ELLIOTT, O. (1994) Working with black and minority ethnic groups. In *Health Promotion and Patient Education. A Professional's Guide* (ed. P. Webb). Chapman & Hall, London.

EWLES, L. AND SIMNETT, I. (1985) *Promoting Health. A Practical Guide To Health Education*. John Wiley, Chichester.

FULLER, F.H.S. AND TOON, P.D. (1988) *Medical Practice in a Multicultural Society*. Heinemann Medical Press, Oxford.

HEGINBOTHAM, C. (1990) *Return to the Community. The Voluntary Ethic and Community Care*. Bedford Square Press, London.

HULL, R., ELLIS, M. AND SARGENT, V. (1989) *Teamwork in Palliative Care*. Radcliffe Medical Press, Oxford.

HUMPHREY, C. AND MILONE-NUZZO, P. (1991) *Home Care Nursing. An Orientation to Practice*. Appleton & Lange, East Norwalk.

JAFFE, M. AND SKIDMORE-ROTH, L. (1993) *Home Health Nursing Care Plans*, 2nd edn. Mosby, St Louis.

KOHNKE, M.F. (1980) The nurse as advocate. *American Journal of Nursing*, **80**: 2038–40.

MARKS, L. (1991) *Home and hospital care: Redrawing the boundaries*. Research Report No 9. Kings Fund Institute, London.

MILLER, L.A. (1990) At home help for the CAPD patient. *Registered Nurse*, **Aug**: 77–80.

NAYLOR, M. (1992) Home is best. *Nursing Times*, **88**(26): 36–8.

OREOPOULOS, D.G. (1994) Is there a right time to say no to life? Editorial. *International Society for Peritoneal Dialysis*: **14**(3): 205–8.

RIVETTI, M., SERVETTI, L., COTTO, M., FERRERO, R. AND BARACCO, M. (1993) The choice of dialytic treatment. *EDTNA/ERCA Journal*, **19**(3): 25–6.

RODERICK, P.J., JONES, I., RALEIGH, V.S., McGEOWN, M. AND MALLICK, N. (1994) Population need for renal replacement therapy in Thames regions: ethnic dimension. *British Medical Journal*, **309**: 1111–14.

Royal College of Nursing (1994) *Disposal of Health Care Waste in the Community*. RCN Leaflet, Nov, London.

SKIDMORE, D. (1994) *The Ideology of Community Care*. Chapman Hall, London.

STEWART, G. (1991) The renal nurse consultant: perspectives on a new role. Approaches to cost effective, quality care for the renal patient. *EDTNA/ERCA Journal*, **16**(Jan): 2–4.

UKCC (1992) *Code of Professional Conduct*. UKCC, London.

UTTLEY, L. AND PROWANT, B. (1994). Organization of the peritoneal dialysis program – the nurses' role. In *The Textbook of Peritoneal Dialysis* (eds R. Gokal and R. Khanna). Kluwer Academic Publishers, Dordrecht, pp 335–55.

WALTON SPRADLEY, B. (ed.) (1991) *Readings in Community Health Nursing*, 4th ed. J.B. Lippincott, Philadelphia.

WEBB, P. (ed.) (1994) *Health Promotion and Patient Education. A Professional's Guide*. Chapman & Hall, London.

WILSON-BARNETT, J. (1988) Patient teaching or patient counselling. *Journal of Advanced Nursing*, **13**: 215–22.

WILKIE, M. AND BROWN, C. (1994) Sharing the management of patients on CAPD. *Prescriber*, **5**(23): 61–5.

APPENDIX

DRUGS USED IN RENAL FAILURE

DRUG-INDUCED RENAL DISEASE

As most drugs are metabolised in the body and finally excreted via the kidneys, it is no surprise that the use of certain drugs results in the deterioration of kidney function leading to either acute or chronic renal failure. Over 200 drugs have been identified as contributing to renal toxicity, with estimates of up to a quarter of all acute renal failure being drug induced, a figure that is constantly increasing. List of factors that make the kidney vulnerable to drugs is shown on Page 476.

Various forms of drug-induced nephrotoxicity exist and are often categorised into glomerular, tubular, interstitial and vascular. Some drugs may induce multiple renal lesions using a variety of toxic mechanisms, an example being non-steroidal anti-inflammatory drugs (NSAIDs). Some of the sites and type of lesion are shown in Fig. A1.1 together with examples of some of the drugs that may cause them.

Mechanisms of Drug-Induced Damage

Two main mechanisms for drug-induced renal damage exist, namely direct toxic effects and immunological effects.

Direct toxic effect

This affects renal cells and membranes at various sites, resulting in cell damage or changes in the permeability of the membrane to essential electrolytes or enzymes. Toxic or ischaemic insult normally results in an increase in intracellular calcium, causing a reduction in the oxidative and phosphoralative capabilities of cell mitochondria which can lead to cellular damage. In addition, the intracellular metabolism of drugs using the oxidative pathways within the endoplasmic reticulum can result in the production of reactive metabolites and free radicals. Both these species are highly damaging to normal cell function.

Other mechanisms for direct cellular damage have been proposed, for example with antibiotics such as gentamicin and some cephalosporins which have direct toxic effects on mitochondria resulting in cell damage or death. Heavy metals, for example gold compounds, have also been shown to have this effect.

Immunological mechanisms

A number of recognised renal lesions can occur immunologically. Most studies have been undertaken in rat models, using heavy metals as a toxin to induce antibodies. The most commonly found immunological toxicity is acute interstitial nephritis, which results from a hypersensitivity reaction with inflammation affecting the interstitial compartment of the renal cortex and medulla. Secondary involvement of the tubules and eventually the blood vessels can occur.

Examples of drugs that can cause acute interstitial nephritis are penicillins, allopurinol, azathioprine and non-steroidal anti-inflammatory drugs NSAIDs. Interestingly, the withdrawal of the positive toxin, in this case the drug with or without the administration of steroids, is often sufficient to induce recovery although a permanent reduction in renal function may result. Some patients may not recover sufficiently and these patients are classed as having chronic interstitial nephritis.

The most common form of acute interstitial nephritis is that caused by the overuse of NSAIDs. These drugs have a number of effects including the acute prostaglandin effect (see below) on the renal vasculature tubules which contribute further to their toxicity.

Functional Renal Failure

This may occur as a side-effect of drugs used to treat conditions unrelated to the kidneys but which, by various mechanisms including disruption of electrolyte balance and acid–base balance (e.g. diuretics), have profound effects on the way kidneys function.

Hyponatraemia and polyuria are associated with certain drugs, for example opioid analgesics, cyclophosphamide and oral hyperglycaemic

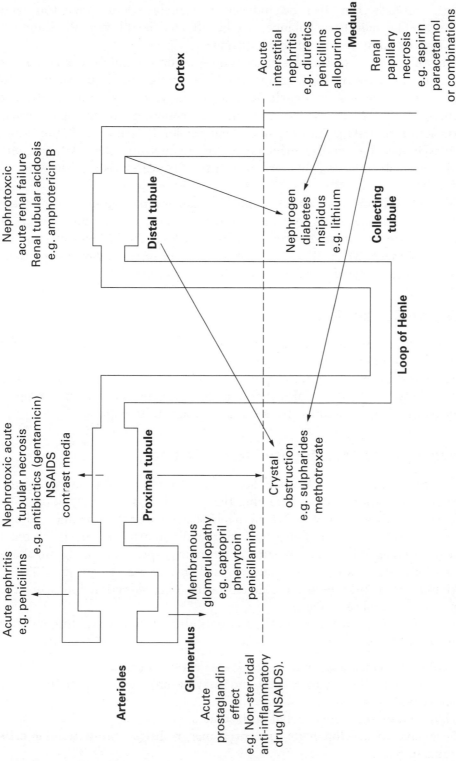

Fig. A.1.1 *Drug nephrotoxicity sites. Reproduced from Nanra RS. Drug-induced renal disease. Medical International 1986, 33: 1367 by kind permission of The Medicine Group (Journals) Ltd.*

drugs. Polyuria can also be induced by amphotericin, phenytoin and lithium. The acid–base balance can be affected by almost all diuretics, making the kidneys susceptible to damage.

One of the most common causes of drug induced renal failure is the use of angiotensin-converting enzyme (ACE) inhibitors used in the main to treat hypertension. Angiotensin II is a potent vasoconstrictor of efferent glomerular arterioles which prevents a reduction in the glomerular filtration rate (GFR). Inhibition of angiotensin II using ACE inhibitors results in the loss of the mechanism for maintaining the GFR; patients with hypovolaemia or dehydration are then at greater risk as the GFR is reduced.

NSAIDs inhibit prostaglandins and thus can reverse the net vasodilatory effect of prostaglandins on the kidney arterioles. The production of prostaglandin is one of the mechanisms by which the kidneys attempt to prevent damage. Thus, this effect can contribute to renal damage, particularly when associated with other renally toxic drugs.

Tubular Obstruction

Formation of microcrystalline stones can occur with some drugs, for example sulphonomides, allopurinol, acetazolamide and aluminium/magnesium hydroxide containing drugs (antacids). This effect is three times more likely to occur in males than females and represents a small proportion of those patients presenting with microcrystalline stones.

Prevention of Drug-Induced Renal Failure

The toxic effects of drugs can in some cases be reduced by improving the patient's hydration and withdrawing the toxic drug at an early stage. The effects of analgesic abuse (analgesic nephropathy) are well documented and this condition is often considered in the differential diagnosis of renal disease. Management and screening of patients suspected of analgesic abuse is an important way of preventing further damage. However, 30% of patients will continue to have deteriorating renal function following the cessation of analgesic abuse.

Some factors contributing to the susceptibility of kidneys to drug-induced damage include:

- kidneys receive approximately 25% of cardiac output;
- the vulnerability of metabolic and enzyme processes, especially in the proximal tubule;
- large glomerular endothelial surface area;
- capacity to develop high concentrations of drugs within tubular cells and lumen;

- the medullary concentration of potential nephrotoxin by the counter-current system;
- liability to immune injury;
- accumulation of drugs and their metabolites due to nephron loss and renal insufficiency.

Drug use in Renal Disease

The kidney is the major excretory organ of many drugs and also of their metabolites. Therefore, the loss of ability of the kidney to regulate body fluid composition due to failure of the excretory function can result in the accumulation of a drug or metabolite. This can have possible toxic consequences due to an alteration in pharmacokinetics.

The factors which need to be considered include:

- *The age of the patient.* Renal dysfunction is common in elderly patients but may not present as overt failure.
- *Polypharmacy.* Complex multiple drug therapy is common due to the nature of the condition and the control of symptoms.
- *The importance of renal excretion as the main route of elimination for a particular drug or its metabolites.* Excretion via the kidney can occur through glomerular filtration, active tubular secretion or a combination of the two. Dose adjustments are not necessary for all drugs but many are prescribed at doses higher than necessary to achieve adequate levels and thus can result in unwanted side-effects being more common.

Renal failure has its main effect on drug excretion; however, all aspects of drug pharmacokinetics such as absorption, distribution and metabolism need to be considered. Alteration in any of these can affect drug concentration at the site of action.

Absorption and Bioavailability

There are several factors that can potentially effect the oral absorption of drugs. The increase in gastric pH in chronic renal failure due to an increase in ammonia production in the stomach will reduce the absorption of drugs that need an acid pH. Drugs affected include iron and some penicillins. Oedema of the gut can also reduce the absorption of some drugs.

Distribution

Drug concentration at receptor sites affects the activity of most drugs. This is directly related to the concentration of the drug in plasma compared to that fraction that is bound to plasma proteins. Any alteration in plasma protein binding can potentially have a profound effect on drug levels. In practice, this is only significant for drugs that are highly plasma protein bound (greater than 80%) and have a narrow therapeutic index.

Metabolism

The liver is the main metabolic organ for drugs. Uraemia may reduce drug metabolism and reduce the non-renal clearance of some drugs, but this effect is minimal. The main effect of the kidney is due to the retention of active metabolites which are normally renally eliminated.

Excretion

The majority of drugs are excreted by the kidney either as the parent compound or water-soluble metabolites after liver metabolism. Excretion occurs mainly by glomerular filtration or tubular secretion. Some excretion also occurs by passive diffusion into the tubules. Any change in renal blood flow will affect these processes. The extent to which renal failure affects the excretion depends on the percentage of the drug that is normally excreted unchanged in the urine.

Extremes of Age

The changes in pharmacokinetics with age makes drug handling more complex at the extremes.

Paediatrics

Standard doses for paediatrics are not just a proportion of the adult dose calculated according to weight. Paediatrics are not mini adults; they handle drugs differently. Dose adjustments that are required when there is no renal impairment present also need to be taken into consideration on top of any adjustment for reduced kidney function other than that due to age.

Kidney function at birth is less than would be expected from a direct comparison with body weight. The functions of the kidney, such as acidification and concentrating effects, become similar to those of the adult shortly after birth. By the time the infant has reached 1 year of age glomerular filtration, urea clearance and tubular secretion are also expected to have reached adult levels.

Absorption   The absorption from the gastrointestinal tract is extended in paediatrics compared to adults. Intramuscular absorption is erratic and percutaneous absorption is often enhanced.

Distribution The total body water is greater compared to adults, often making it necessary to give larger doses of water-soluble drugs to maintain an adequate plasma concentration.

Metabolism and excretion These tend to be slow in the newborn infant, increasing to faster rates than adults during the first few months of life, falling again during adolescence.

Elderly

The elderly are twice as susceptible to adverse drug reactions as younger patients and any reaction tends to be more serious. The elderly are often confused by their medication, whether through confusion or simply the number of medicines they are expected to take and the complex regimes they have to follow.

A reduction in kidney function occurs naturally with increasing age due to a reduction in renal blood flow. This results in a reduction in GFR and hence reduced urea and creatinine clearance. Serum creatinine does not rise to any great extent as a result of this, due to a reduction in muscle mass and creatinine production. The rise in serum urea is also less than expected because of reduced protein intake.

Summary

The dose of potentially toxic drugs, which are normally excreted by the kidney either as active drug or metabolites, needs to be adjusted to avoid toxic effects due to accumulation. Dose adjustment will be by extending the dose interval or by giving a lower dose at the usual interval.

RATIONALE BEHIND DRUG DOSING IN DIALYSIS

Drugs need to be available to be dialysed. The following points can be used to estimate potential for dialysing out a drug if no information is available:

- *Drugs which are renally excreted are likely to be dialysable.*
- *Volume of distribution* (relates the amount of drug in the total body relative to plasma). If this is large then the drug is unlikely to be dialysed (greater than $2 \, l \, kg^{-1}$).
- *If a drug is highly water soluble it is likely to be dialysed.*
- *Protein binding.* Highly protein bound drugs will not be available for dialysis as only unbound drugs can cross dialysis membranes.
- *Molecular weight.* Drugs with a high molecular weight such as protein and peptides will not be dialysable (greater than 500 Da).

● *The type of dialysis being considered.*

In general, Table A1 can be used as a guide.
The loading dose is given the same as for 'normal' renal function. The maintenance dose may require adjustment. Many textbooks are available that give recommendations for dose adjustment to account for renal impairment and dialysis.

Table A1 *Recommendations for drug dosing in renal replacement therapy*

Type	Theoretical GFR	Dose recommendation
HD	150–160 ml min^{-1} during dialysis 0–10 ml min^{-1} between dialysis periods	Severe renal impairment. Supplement doses may be needed post-HD if a drug is significantly removed
CAPD	5–10 ml min^{-1} (4 exchanges per day)	Severe RI
CAVHD CVVHD	15–20 ml min^{-1}	Moderate RI
CAVH CVVH	Ultrafiltration < 15 ml min^{-1} > 15 ml min^{-1}	Severe RI Moderate RI

CAPD, Continuous ambulatory peritoneal dialysis; CAVH, continuous arteriovenous haemofiltration; CAVHD, continuous arterioverous haemodialysis; CVVH, continuous venovenous haemofiltration; CVVHD, continuous venovenous haemodialysis; HD, haemodialysis; GFR, glomerular filtration rate; RI, renal impairment.

GENERAL PRINCIPLES OF DRUG TREATMENT IN RENAL DISEASE

Drugs have the power to help or harm. The drug treatment associated with renal failure is not temporary as it is for many disease states. Renal failure can have an effect on other organs and so this also needs to be taken into account. The treatment of renal failure is aimed at maintaining a relatively normal physiological function:

● *use as few drugs as possible* – avoid multiple therapy;
● *beware of elderly patients* – drug handling is altered;
● *consider the excretion of the drugs;*
● *dose* – is the dose correct or is an adjustment of either the dose or the dose interval needed?
● *if you do not know* – find out;
● *monitor closely* – drug levels as well as the patient. Toxic effects may be apparent and only require a dose adjustment to prevent these.

FURTHER READING

There are numerous texts and references available which give detailed information on drug doses in renal impairment and during renal replacement therapy. The pharmacist is the best source of information in the first instance.

The following texts may be useful:

ABPI Data Sheet Compendium.

BENNETT, W.M., ARONOFF, G.R., GOLPER, T.A. *et al.* (1994) *Drug Prescribing in Renal Failure – Dose Guidelines for Adults*, 3rd ed. American College of Physicians, Philadelphia.

British National Formulary.

BUNN, R., HOUGH, J., McGEE, P. *et al.* (1994) *An A–Z of Drug Use and Guide to Patient Counselling in Renally Impaired Adults ('Renal Drug File').* Renal Pharmacy Group, United Kingdom.

KNOBES, J.E. AND ANDERSON, P.O. *Handbook of Clinical Drug Data*, 7th ed. Drug Intelligence Publications, Hamilton.

SCHRIER, R.W. AND GAMBERTOGLIO, J.G. (1991) *Handbook of Drug Therapy in Liver and Kidney Disease.* Little, Brown, Boston.

SEYFFART, G. *Drug Dosage in Renal Insufficiency.* Kluwer Academic, Dordrecht.

MONOGRAPH SECTION

These contain information on the drugs you would expect to see routinely prescribed for patients with renal failure.

Mode of action and the reasons why a particular drug is used have been included along with common side-effects and any monitoring nurses may be expected to undertake. A monograph also contains information on how to adminster the drug and fluids it is compatible with. Information that may aid patient counselling is included for certain drugs.

The normal doses given are for adults only; however, the dose reduction information may be extrapolated to paediatrics.

ABBREVIATIONS USED IN THE MONOGRAPHS

Formulations

C = capsules	T = tablets
ET = effervescent tablets	P = powder
I – injection	E = enema
L = liquid	S = suppositories

Solutions

NaCl = sodium chloride 0.9%
D5W = dextrose 5%
WFI = water for injection

Dosage

dd = divided doses
OD = once daily
BD = twice daily
TDS = three times daily
QDS = four times daily
prn = as required
q4–6h = every 4–6 hours

Route

SC = subcutaneously
IM = intramuscularly
IV = intravenously
PO = orally
SL = sublingually
TDI = total dose infusion

AV = atrio-ventricular block
N/A = not applicable
GFR = glomerular filtration rate
ESRF = end-stage renal failure
RI = renal impairment

The doses given in the tables are for adults only

CLASS: Anaemia

DRUG GROUPS: Iron overload – chelating agents. Desferrioxamine mesylate (desferral) is the agent used.

SIGNIFICANCE IN RENAL DISEASE: Iron overload is usually associated with repeated blood transfusions. It is also used to chelate aluminium and so reduce the risk of aluminium-related encephalopathy and bone disease in chronic dialysis patients. The use of desferral has diminished since the reduction in the use of aluminium-containing medicines and solutions and the advent of erythro-poietin.

MODE OF ACTION: Desferral chelates free iron (i.e. that not bound to transferrin) resulting in reduced tissue concentrations of the metal. It also chelates aluminium ions, removing them from bone storage sites. The chelates of desferral with either aluminium or iron are eliminated in the urine or through dialysis.

GROUP	CHELATING AGENTS
DRUGS	DESFERRAL
Form	I
Usual adult dose ORAL IV OTHER	N/A for this indication Upto 15 mg kg^{-1} h^{-1}. Max 80 mg kg^{-1} or 2 g 24 h^{-1} S/C 20 mg kg^{-1} Increase to max. of 110 mg kg^{-1} or 3 g 24 h^{-1}. Repeat infusion over 5–6 nights week^{-1}
Dose adjustment in renal failure	N/A
Administration requirements	IV infusion is the most effective route – used for acute poisoning SC infusion is 90% as effective as IV – used for chronic overload e.g. transfusion related
Reconstitution	500 mg desferral with 5 ml WFI. Dilute further with D5W or NaCl 0.9%
Rate of admin.	IV – by infusion over 12 h

SIDE-EFFECTS: Hypotension and tachycardia can occur after large doses (> 14 mg kg^{-1} h^{-1}). Hearing and visual disturbances are common.

PRECAUTIONS: –

CONTRAINDICATIONS: Pregnancy, hypersensitivity and impaired renal function not severe enough to require dialysis.

DRUG INTERACTIONS: Prochlorperazine. Combined use can lead to extrapyramidal effects and in severe cases coma.

NOTES/COUNSELLING POINTS: Oral use is not indicated due to poor absorption from the gastrointestinal tract.

CLASS: Anticoagulant

DRUG GROUPS: Heparin, Epoprostenol.

SIGNIFICANCE IN RENAL DISEASE: These are both used either alone or in combination in dialysis to prevent platelet aggregation and hence maintain the extracorporeal circuit. The main use of epoprostenol is in patients who are at a high risk of bleeding (heparin-sparing effect).

MODE OF ACTION: Heparin inhibits the generation and activity of thrombin (factor IIa). This results in a break in the clotting cascade. Epoprostenol is a naturally occurring prostaglandin and causes an inhibition of platelet aggregation and reduces platelet loss during haemodialysis. It does not prolong the bleeding time.

GROUP	ANTICOAGULANTS	
DRUGS	HEPARIN	EPOPROSTENOL
Form	I	I
Usual adult dose ORAL IV	Refer to local protocols N/A May be a single dose prior to dialysis or a continuous infusion during dialysis	Refer to local protocols N/A 5 ng kg^{-1} min^{-1} IV prior to dialysis then 5 ng kg^{-1} min^{-1} into arterial inlet of machine.
Dose adjustment in renal failure	Reduce dose or avoid in severe RI because of increased risk of bleeding	If DIC present may need to use higher doses (up to 20 ng kg^{-1} min^{-1}).
Administration requirements		500 µg vial gives 10 000 ng ml^{-1} when reconstituted with the 50 ml diluent.This can be given neat or further diluted with NaCl
Reconstitution	N/A	Must use the glycine buffer provided
Rate of admin.	As per protocol	5 ng kg^{-1} min^{-1} depending on blood pressure

SIDE-EFFECTS: The main problem with epoprostenol is that it causes hypotension. Doses need to be adjusted accordingly to prevent this. Other effects related to its vasodilatory properties include headache and flushing. When used alone, clotting can occur in the dialysis circuit. Haemorrhage, especially gastric, is the main problem associated with the use of heparin. It can also cause hypersensitivity reactions and thrombocytopenia.

PRECAUTIONS: Increased risk of bleeding with heparin in patients with severe RI.

CONTRAINDICATIONS: Heparin is contraindicated in patients with haemorrhagic disorders, thrombocytopenia, peptic ulcer and severe liver disease.

DRUG INTERACTIONS: There is an increased anticoagulant effect when heparin is coadministered with aspirin (analgesic and antiplatelet) and dipyridamole (antiplatelet).

NOTES/COUNSELLING POINTS: With patients on epoprostenol, the blood pressure should be monitored.

CLASS: Antiemetics

DRUG GROUPS: Phenothiazines – prochlorperazine; Antihistamines – cyclizine; Metoclopramide and domperidone; 5HT3 (serotonin) antagonists – ondansetron (not first line).

SIGNIFICANCE IN RENAL DISEASE: Nausea and vomiting is a common symptom of chronic renal failure. Uraemia is the usual cause. Dialysis is the best treatment. Effective control with drug therapy is difficult to achieve. Some centres have had success with non-drug treatments such as acupuncture and acupressure. Anaemia can also contribute to nausea and so correction of this may also help.

MODE OF ACTION: Phenothiazines are dopamine antagonists. They act centrally on the chemoreceptor trigger zone. Antihistamines antagonise the effect of histamine and cyclizine also has some anticholinergic action. Metoclopramide and domperidone have an action similar to the phenothiazines. They have an additional peripheral action on the gut which speeds up transit time. Ondansetron is a specific inhibitor of serotonin but should only be used if other agents have failed.

GROUP	PHENOTHIAZINES	ANTIHISTAMINES	
DRUGS	PROCHLORPERAZINE	CYCLIZINE	METOCLOPRAMIDE
Form	I,L,S,T	I,T	I,L,T
Usual adult dose			
ORAL	5–10 mg 2–3 times daily	50 mg up to 3 times daily	10 mg 3 times daily
IV	unlicensed	50 mg up to 3 times daily	10 mg 3 times daily
OTHER	12.5 mg 2–3 times daily	50 mg up to 3 times daily	10 mg 3 times daily
Dose adjustment in renal failure	In severe RI start with small dose. 6.25 mg IM/5 mg PO		Moderate RI – 75% normal dose. Severe RI – 50% normal dose
Administration requirements			
Reconstitution	N/A		
Rate of admin.	Over 3–4 min		Over 1–2 min

SIDE-EFFECTS: All can cause drowsiness. Cyclizine can cause anticholinergic effects such as dry mouth and blurred vision. Prochlorperazine and metoclopramide can induce dystonic reactions. These are more likely in patients with severe renal failure, hence the recommendation to reduce the dose.

PRECAUTIONS: –

CONTRAINDICATIONS: Prochlorperazine and metoclopramide are contraindicated in phaeochromocytoma.

DRUG INTERACTIONS: Increased risk of extrapyramidal effects if metoclopramide is used in combination with an antipsychotic or lithium. The use of anti-arrhythmics, antihistamines or beta-blockers with prochlorperazine can cause ventricular arrhythmias.

NOTES/COUNSELLING POINTS: If one antiemetic is ineffective, then another agent with a different mode of action should be tried.

CLASS: Anti-itch

DRUG GROUPS: Antihistamines – sedating: chlorpheniramine and hydroxyzine; non-sedating: terfenadine. Topical – crotamiton, calamine lotion.

SIGNIFICANCE IN RENAL DISEASE: The pruritis associated with chronic renal failure is thought to be due to the uraemia and high phosphate levels. The use of phosphate binders and dialysis to treat the underlying cause is the most effective treatment. Medication will only provide a relief of symptoms. Itching is often worse at night.

MODE OF ACTION: Antihistamines block histamine H1 receptors and so prevent circulating histamine binding to them and instigating an allergic response.

GROUP	ANTIHISTAMINES	
DRUGS	CHLORPHENIRAMINE (SEDATING)	TERFENADINE (NON-SEDATING)
Form	I,L,T	L,T
Usual adult dose ORAL	4 mg q4–6 h. Max dose 24 mg in 24 h	60–120 mg per day as a single or two dd
IV	10–20 mg	N/A
OTHER	SC or IM 10–20 mg. Max 40 mg in 24 h	N/A
Dose adjustment in renal failure	N/A	N/A
Administration requirements	IV injection should be given straight away Can cause irritation at injection site	
Reconstitution	10–20 mg with 5–10 ml blood, NaCl or WFI	N/A
Rate of admin.	Slow IV bolus over 1 min	N/A

SIDE-EFFECTS: All antihistamines have the potential to cause drowsiness. However, this is usually only a problem with the older agents such as chlorpheniramine. These can also cause headache and antimuscarinic effects such as urinary retention, blurred vision and dry mouth. Palpitations and arrhythmias can occur but these tend to be associated with the newer agents such as terfenadine. Hypersensitivity reactions, convulsions, extrapyramidal effects, blood disorders, sweating, liver dysfunction and depression have also been reported.

PRECAUTIONS: Use with caution in patients with a history of epilepsy, glaucoma, liver dysfunction and prostatic hypertrophy.

DRUG INTERACTIONS: These relate mainly to the non-sedating antihistamines, e.g. terfenadine.
Antiarrhythmics, antipsychotics, tricyclics or beta-blockers (sotalol) – increased risk of ventricular arrhythmias.
Antibacterials – risk of arrhythmias is increased if used with erythromycin due to an inhibition of metabolism.
Antifungals – inhibit metabolism.

NOTES/COUNSELLING POINTS: The sedating antihistamines tend to be more effective at relieving itching than the non-sedating ones. Topical agents tend to be relatively ineffective. Warn patients of the risk of drowsiness. The effects of alcohol may be potentiated. Two antihistamines may be prescribed, with a non-sedating one taken in the morning and a sedating one at night time.

CLASS: Antihypertensives

DRUG GROUPS: Alpha-adrenoceptor-blocking drugs (alpha-blockers). Agents used include terazosin, doxazosin and prazosin.

SIGNIFICANCE IN RENAL DISEASE: Used in the step-wise management of hypertension. Hypertension is common in patients with chronic renal failure. It is the cause of the renal failure in some patients. In others it is caused by the renal failure, usually due to activation of the renin angiotensin system.

MODE OF ACTION: Reduce afterload (arterial vasodilators). They cause post-synaptic blockade of the alpha-adrenoceptors.

GROUP	ALPHA-BLOCKERS		
DRUGS	DOXAZOSIN	PRAZOSIN	TERAZOSIN
Form	T	T	T
Usual adult dose *ORAL*	1 mg OD initially increase slowly to max of 16 mg OD	500 µg BD–TDS increased slowly to max 20 mg daily in dd	1 mg OD initially increased slowly to max of 20 mg OD
OTHER	N/A	N/A	N/A
Dose adjustment in renal failure	N/A	N/A	N/A
Administration requirements			
Reconstitution	N/A	N/A	N/A
Rate of admin.	N/A	N/A	N/A

SIDE-EFFECTS: These are related to the vasodilator properties of this class of drugs and include postural hypotension, dizziness, headache and fatigue. Urinary frequency may also occur. These are all more likely with prazosin.

PRECAUTIONS: It is advisable to start with a low dose and increase gradually to reduce the risk of side-effects occurring. The first dose may cause collapse and should be taken at night before going to bed.

CONTRAINDICATIONS: Congestive cardiac failure that is obstructive in origin.

DRUG INTERACTIONS: There is an enhanced hypertensive effect when given in conjunction with beta-blockers, calcium channel blockers and diuretics.

NOTES/COUNSELLING POINTS: These drugs are usually used in conjunction with a diuretic or beta-blocker. It is advised that they are introduced gradually to reduce the chance of side-effects, but no final dose reduction is necessary due to a mainly hepatic metabolism. Patients should be warned that side-effects such as postural hypotension may re-occur when doses are increased.

CLASS: Antihypertensives

DRUG GROUPS: Angiotensin-converting enzyme (ACE) inhibitors. Agents used include captopril, enalapril, lisinopril and others.

SIGNIFICANCE IN RENAL DISEASE: Used in the step-wise management of hypertension. Hypertension is common in patients with chronic renal failure. It is the cause of the renal failure in some patients. In others it is caused by the renal failure, usually due to activation of the renin–angiotensin system.

MODE OF ACTION: The conversion of angiotensin I to angiotensin II is blocked. This disruption to the renin–angiotensin system results in a vasodilation and hence a reduction in blood pressure. This mode of action makes this class of drug particularly useful in controlling hypertension associated with chronic renal failure (See Figure A1.2).

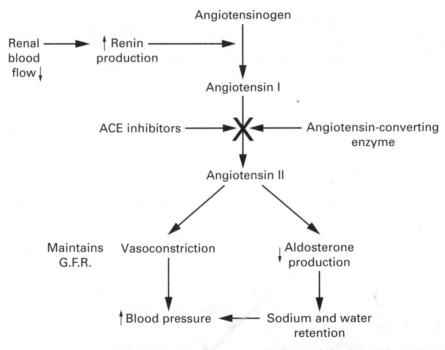

Fig. A.1.2. *Site of action of ACE inhibitors.*

GROUP	ACE INHIBITORS	
DRUGS	CAPTOPRIL	ENALAPRIL
Form	T	T
Usual adult dose ORAL	12.5 mg BD initially. Increased to max 50 mg BD	5 mg OD initially. Increased to max 40 mg OD
IV	N/A	N/A
OTHER	N/A	N/A
Dose adjustment in renal failure	Start with a smaller dose i.e. 6.25 mg BD OD dosing effective in severe renal impairment	Start with a smaller dose i.e. 2.5 mg OD OD dosing effective in severe renal impairment
Administration requirements	2.5 mg given as test dose. BP monitored prior to starting regular therapy	2.5 mg test dose of captopril given as shorter duration of action
Reconstitution	N/A	N/A
Rate of admin.	N/A	N/A

SIDE-EFFECTS: Renal impairment makes side-effects more likely. First-dose hypotension, dizziness, tiredness, headaches, hyperkalaemia, nausea, taste disturbances and dry cough have all been reported. ACE inhibitors can cause or worsen any underlying renal impairment.

PRECAUTIONS: First-dose hypotension is more likely in patients who are taking diuretics or who are dehydrated or have renal impairment.

CONTRAINDICATIONS: Hypersensitivity to ACE inhibitors. Renal artery stenosis.

DRUG INTERACTIONS: Concomitant use of NSAIDs can antagonise the hypotensive effect and increase the risk of hyperkalaemia and a deterioration in renal function. Use with cyclosporin, potassium salts and potassium-sparing diuretics can cause hyperkalaemia.

NOTES/COUNSELLING POINTS: Renal function and electrolytes should be checked before starting treatment and regularly during treatment with ACE inhibitors. Patients should be informed of common side-effects including hypotension, dizziness, taste disturbances and cough.

CLASS: Antihypertensives

DRUG GROUPS: Beta-adrenoceptor-blocking drugs (beta-blockers). Agents used include propranolol, atenolol or metoprolol.

SIGNIFICANCE IN RENAL DISEASE: Used in the step-wise management of hypertension. Hypertension is common in patients with chronic renal failure. It is the cause of the renal failure in some patients. In others it is caused by the renal failure, usually due to activation of the renin–angiotensin system. Patients tend to respond well to beta-blockers.

MODE OF ACTION: Block beta-adrenoceptors in the heart, lungs, peripheral vessels, pancreas and liver. They also reduce cardiac output and some can have an effect on renin release. All beta-blockers will slow the heart rate. Propranolol is non cardioselective and may impair renal blood flow. It has largely been superseded by newer agents. Atenolol is cardioselective in action and is renally excreted but is still widely used. Metoprolol is cardioselective and is hepatically metabolised.

GROUP	BETA-BLOCKERS		
DRUGS	ATENOLOL	METOPROLOL	PROPRANOLOL
Form	I,L,T	I,T	C,I,L,T
Usual adult dose *ORAL* *IV* *OTHER*	50 mg OD Not for this indication	50–100 mg BD–TDS Not for this indication	80–320 mg daily in dd Not for this indication
Dose adjustment in renal failure	Start with small dose Reduce maintenance dose	Start with small dose	Start with small dose
Administration requirements			
Reconstitution	N/A	N/A	N/A
Rate of admin.	N/A	N/A	N/A

SIDE-EFFECTS: All may be associated with tiredness, sleep disturbances, coldness of the extremities and impairment in glucose tolerance. Bronchospasm may be precipated by non-cardiospecific agents.

PRECAUTIONS: Use with caution in diabetics.

CONTRAINDICATIONS: Asthma or a history of obstructive airways disease. Uncontrolled heart failure.

DRUG INTERACTIONS: Increased risk of bradycardia and AV block with calcium channel blockers. There is an increased antihypertensive effect when used in combination with other antihypertensives.

NOTES/COUNSELLING POINTS: Patients may experience tiredness and a reduced exercise tolerance. Cold hands and feet may also be a problem.

CLASS: Antihypertensives

DRUG GROUPS: Calcium channel blockers. Agents used include nifedipine, amlodipine and felodipine (dihydropyridine type) and verapamil. This class of drugs is also used to control angina.

SIGNIFICANCE IN RENAL DISEASE: Used in the step-wise management of hypertension. Hypertension is common in patients with chronic renal failure. It is the cause of the renal failure in some patients. In others it is caused by the renal failure, usually due to activation of the renin–angiotensin system.

MODE OF ACTION: Reduce afterload (arterial vasodilators). Calcium channel blockers interfere with the slow influx of calcium ions into cells. Verapamil reduces cardiac output, slows heart rate and is negatively inotropic. It also has antiarrhythmic activity. The dihydropyridine type relax vascular smooth muscle and cause arteries to dilate.

GROUP	CALCIUM CHANNEL BLOCKERS		
DRUGS	NIFEDIPINE	AMLODIPINE	VERAPAMIL
Form	C,T	T	C,I,T
Usual adult dose ORAL IV OTHER	5–40 mg 2–4 times daily N/A SL = 10 mg per dose	5–10 mg daily N/A	240–480 mg daily in dd N/A for hypertension
Dose adjustment in renal failure	Start with small dose	N/A	N/A
Administration requirements	Take with food Tablets must be swallowed whole		
Reconstitution	N/A	N/A	N/A
Rate of admin.	N/A	N/A	N/A

SIDE-EFFECTS: These tend to be related to vasodilation and include flushing, headaches and swollen ankles. These usually resolve after a few days and are more common with nifedipine. Gastrointestinal disturbances may also occur.

PRECAUTIONS: Should be avoided in heart failure because they can depress cardiac function. Use is cautioned in hepatic failure.

CONTRAINDICATIONS: Severe bradycardia, cardiogenic shock.

DRUG INTERACTIONS: Calcium channel blockers may increase cyclosporin levels and are used to reduce the nephrotoxic effect of cyclosporin in some centres. They may also interact with antiepileptics, beta-blockers and cardiac glycosides.

NOTES/COUNSELLING POINTS: Patients should be advised to swallow modified or slow-release preparations whole. Advice on the vasodilator side-effects should be given. Care should be taken not to confuse the vasodilator side-effects such as swollen ankles with fluid overload.

CLASS: Antihypertensives

DRUG GROUPS: Vasodilators – smooth muscle relaxants. Agents used include hydralazine and minoxidil.

SIGNIFICANCE IN RENAL DISEASE: Used in the step-wise management of hypertension. Hypertension is common in patients with chronic renal failure. It is the cause of the renal failure in some patients. In others, it is caused by the renal failure, usually due to activation of the renin–angiotensin system. These tend to be used as third-line agents.

MODE OF ACTION: Cause vasodilation by relaxing vascular smooth muscle.

GROUP	VASODILATORS	
DRUGS	HYDRALAZINE	MINOXIDIL
Form	I,T	T
Usual adult dose *ORAL*	25 mg BD increased to max of 50 mg BD	5 mg OD in dd increased to max of 50 mg daily
IV	Slow IV – 5–10 mg. Can repeat after 20 min	N/A
OTHER	IV infusion – 200–300 μg min^{-1} initially Maintenance – 50–150 μg min^{-1}	N/A
Dose adjustment in renal failure	Start with small dose	Lower maintenance doses may be effective in patients on HD or PD
Administration requirements		
Reconstitution	With WFI and dilute further with NaCl Suggested volume is 10 ml for injection or 500 ml for infusion. Incompatible with dextrose	N/A
Rate of admin.	Slow IV over 20 min or by infusion	N/A

SIDE-EFFECTS: Hydralazine can cause tachycardia, fluid retention, nausea, headache, rashes and blood abnormalities. Minoxidil can cause sodium and water retention, tachycardia, weight gain and peripheral oedema, increase in urea and creatinine and rashes.

PRECAUTIONS: Angina, after myocardial infarction, pregnancy and breastfeeding.

CONTRAINDICATIONS: Hydralazine is contraindicated in systemic lupus erythematosus, some cardiac conditions and porphyria. Minoxidil is contraindicated in phaeochromocytoma and porphyria.

DRUG INTERACTIONS: Increased antihypertensive effect with anaesthetic agents.

NOTES/COUNSELLING POINTS: Beta-blockers may be prescribed with minoxidil to counteract any reflex tachycardia. Diuretics may also be needed to prevent fluid retention.

CLASS: Antiviral

DRUG GROUPS: Acyclovir, Ganciclovir.

SIGNIFICANCE IN RENAL DISEASE: These agents are used in the field of renal transplantation to reduce the risk of viral infection post transplantation with cytomegalovirus (CMV). Acyclovir is used for CMV prophylaxis and ganciclovir can be used for prophylaxis or treatment. Ganciclovir is more active against CMV than acyclovir but is more toxic.

MODE OF ACTION: Competes with guanosine for DNA polymerase so inhibiting viral replication.

GROUP	ANTIVIRAL	
DRUGS	ACYCLOVIR	GANCICLOVIR
Form	L,I,T	I
Usual dose		
ORAL	800 mg QDS (propylaxis)	N/A
IV	Not for this indication	10 mg kg^{-1} day^{-1} in 2 divided doses (treatment)
OTHER	N/A	N/A
Dose adjustment in renal failure	Adjust dose according to serum creatinine >500 μmol l^{-1} 800 mg OD 250–500 μmol l^{-1} 800 mg BD <250 μmol l^{-1} 800 mg QDS dialysis dependent 800 mg BD (refer to local protocol)	Adjust dose according to creatinine clearance >50 ml min^{-1} 5 mg kg^{-1} BD 25–50 ml min^{-1} 2.5 mg kg^{-1} BD 10–25 ml min^{-1} 2.5 mg kg^{-1} OD <10 ml min^{-1} 1.25 mg kg^{-1} OD
Administration requirements		Centrally or peripherally via fast flowing vein Dose after haemodialysis
Reconstitution	N/A	Dilute with NaCl to give maximum concentration of 10 mg ml
Rate of admin.	N/A	Infuse over at least 1 h.

SIDE-EFFECTS: Occasionally acyclovir can cause rapid rises in urea and creatinine. Liver enzymes and bilirubin may be raised. Neurological effects may be manifested, especially if the dose is too high. These can include tremor, headache, dizziness, confusion, convulsions and coma. Ganciclovir can cause leucopenia and thrombocytopenia. Anaemia can also occur and it may cause fever, rash, abnormal liver function tests and nausea.

PRECAUTIONS: Adequate hydration must be maintained. Acyclovir use during breastfeeding and pregnancy. Ganciclovir use requires monitoring of blood count.

CONTRAINDICATIONS: Ganciclovir is contraindicated during pregnancy and breastfeeding and in neutropenia.

NOTES/COUNSELLING POINTS: Ganciclovir is very irritant and can cause blistering at peripheral injection sites. It is recommended that it is reconstituted in pharmacy rather than on the ward. Prophylaxis with acyclovir is usually for 3 months but local protocols may vary. Ganciclovir prophylaxis would be for 7–14 days and treatment for 14–21 days, but again local protocols may vary.

CLASS: Calcium and phosphate metabolism – phosphate binders

DRUG GROUPS: Calcium carbonate, Calcium acetate, Aluminium hydroxide, Calcium salts used most commonly

SIGNIFICANCE IN RENAL DISEASE: High serum phosphate is a potential complication of renal failure. High serum phosphate is implicated in renal osteodystrophy.

MODE OF ACTION: To bind the phosphate from food in the stomach and therefore reduce serum phosphate levels. Calcium and aluminium ions form an insoluble complex with the phosphate which is then excreted in the faeces.

GROUP	CALCIUM SALTS		ALUMINIUM SALTS
DRUGS	CALCIUM CARBONATE	CALCIUM ACETATE	ALUMINIUM HYDROXIDE
Form	C,ET,T	T	C,L
Usual adult dose *ORAL*	1260–7500 mg day^{-1} in dd	1260–7500 mg day^{-1} in dd	475–9500 mg day^{-1} in dd
IV	N/A	N/A	N/A
OTHER	N/A	N/A	N/A
Dose adjustment in renal failure	N/A	N/A	N/A
Administration requirements	Before or with food	Before or with food	Before or with food
Reconstitution	N/A	N/A	N/A
Rate of admin.	N/A	N/A	N/A

SIDE-EFFECTS: Constipation or diarrhoea.

PRECAUTIONS: Aluminium only used in the short term as it can accumulate during chronic therapy.

CONTRAINDICATIONS: Calcium carbonate/acetate – avoid use if high urinary/serum calcium. Aluminium hydroxide – avoid use if high serum aluminium.

DRUG INTERACTIONS: Reduced absorption of drugs, especially iron and ciprofloxacin if taken within 1 h of each other.

NOTES/COUNSELLING POINTS: Emphasise importance of taking at the correct time.

CLASS: Calcium and phosphate metabolism – vitamin D analogues

DRUG GROUPS: Calcitriol – 1,25-dihydroxycholecalciferol active vitamin D. Alfacalcidol – 1 alpha-hydroxycholecalciferol requires activation in the liver.

SIGNIFICANCE IN RENAL DISEASE: The kidney activates vitamin D (cholecalciferol) from the diet. In renal failure this mechanism is lost. A product that bypasses the renal activation is required.

MODE OF ACTION: Active vitamin D is necessary for the absorption and utilisation of calcium. Reduced serum calcium and increased serum phosphate result in hyperparathyroidism and renal osteodystrophy (see Figure A1.3).

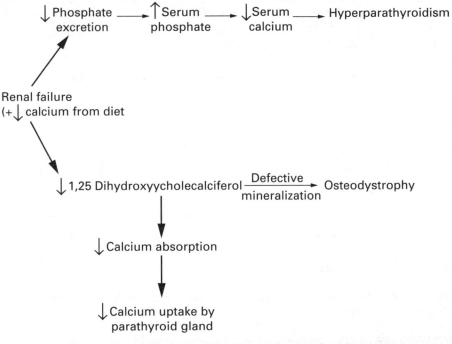

Fig. A1.3 *Mode of action. (See text above.)*

GROUP	VITAMIN D ANALOGUES	
DRUGS	ALFACALCIDOL	CALCITRIOL
Form	C,L,I	C,I
Usual adult dose ORAL IV OTHER	Dependent on serum calcium 0.25–1 μg daily 0.25–1 μg daily N/A	Dependent on serum calcium 0.5–1 μg daily 0.5–3 μg 3 times a week N/A
Dose adjustment in renal failure	N/A	N/A
Administration requirements	Usually given in conjunction with a phosphate binder	Usually given in conjunction with a phosphate binder
Reconstitution	N/A	N/A
Rate of admin.	N/A	N/A

SIDE-EFFECTS: Hypercalcaemia, anorexia, nausea and vomiting, diarrhoea, polyuria, sweating, headache and thirst. All side-effects are rare at therapeutic doses and tend to be related to toxicity.

PRECAUTIONS: –

CONTRAINDICATIONS: Hypercalcaemia.

DRUG INTERACTIONS: Antacids: magnesium containing antacids can result in hypermagnesaemia when given with vitamin D analogues. Digitalis: avoid hypercalcaemia as this can precipitate cardiac arrhythmias.

NOTES/COUNSELLING POINTS: Do not take at the same time as phosphate binders.

CLASS: Correction of anaemia

DRUG GROUPS: Erythropoietin alpha, Erythropoietin beta. Both have similar clinical efficacy such that they are interchangable.

SIGNIFICANCE IN RENAL DISEASE: The kidney is the main producer of erythropoietin (EPO), with a small amount produced in the liver. Hepatic production does not increase to compensate for the lack of renally produced EPO and so the EPO available is reduced. The introduction of genetically engineered EPO as a treatment for and prevention of renal anaemia is highly effective and has revolutionised the management of this condition.

MODE OF ACTION: EPO is a synthetic hormone produced by recombinent DNA technology. It stimulates erythropoiesis. Erythropoiesis is responsible for ensuring an adequate number of red cells are available to provide sufficient oxygenation of tissues. It will cause a response in patients who require dialysis and also in those who do not require dialysis.

GROUP	ERYTHTOPOIETIN	
DRUGS	ERYTHROPOIETIN ALPHA	ERYTHROPOIETIN BETA
Form	I	I
Usual adult dose ORAL	N/A	N/A
IV	Not cost effective. Higher dose needed than SC	Not cost effective. Higher dose needed than SC
OTHER	SC (preferred route) – see local protocol	SC (preferred route) – see local protocol
Dose adjustment in renal failure	N/A	N/A
Administration requirements	SC – Max of 1 ml per injection site IV – Do not dilute. Give over 2 min Store in the fridge. Warm before administration	SC – Max of 1 ml per injection site IV – do not dilute. Give over 2 min Store in the fridge. Warm before administration
Reconstitution	N/A	With the WFI provided
Rate of admin.	N/A	N/A

SIDE-EFFECTS: Allergic reactions can occur. Increased blood pressure, flu-like symptoms, increased potassium, bone pain, sweating.

PRECAUTIONS: –

CONTRAINDICATIONS: Uncontrolled hypertension.

DRUG INTERACTIONS: –

NOTES/COUNSELLING POINTS: Dose recommendations: Correction phase: 50 IU kg^{-1} three times a week. Maintenance phase: 50% of the dose given during the correction phase. Aim for a Hb of 10–12 g dl^{-1}. Iron is usually given concomitantly because of the demand placed on iron stores.

CLASS: Correction of iron deficiency anaemia – iron salts

DRUG GROUPS: Ferrous sulphate is the salt used most widely. Others are available and include ferrous gluconate, fumarate and succinate, which are used orally. Iron dextran is available for parenteral administration.

SIGNIFICANCE IN RENAL DISEASE: Renal patients can be anaemic for several reasons with the lack of endogenous erythropoietin being the major cause. In order for erythropoietin to be effective adequate iron must be available.

MODE OF ACTION: Increase iron stores in the body.

GROUP	IRON SALTS	
DRUGS	FERROUS SULPHATE	IRON DEXTRAN
Form	L,T	I
Usual adult dose		
ORAL	200 mg OD – TDS	N/A
IV	N/A	Depends on Hb for TDI or give 200 mg prn
OTHER	N/A	IM as for IV
Dose adjustment in renal failure	N/A	For TDI the target haemoglobin is reduced to 11 g dl^{-1}
Administration requirements		Available as 100 mg in 2-ml ampoules Can be given as 200 mg IV infusion over 30 min or as TDI (dose calculated from Hb)
Reconstitution	N/A	For IV dilute with NaCl
Rate of admin.	N/A	TDI – use a test dose

SIDE-EFFECTS: All ferrous salts can cause gastric upsets and constipation. Iron can also turn faeces black. If side-effects are a problem then changing to a different salt may help.

PRECAUTIONS: Anaphylactic reactions can occur to iron dextran, so a test dose is recommended.

CONTRAINDICATIONS: –

DRUG INTERACTIONS: Avoid taking at the same time as drugs that can reduce the absorption of oral iron, e.g. tetracyclines, phosphate binders and antacids. Iron can also reduce the absorption of some drugs, e.g. ciprofloxacin and penicillamine.

NOTES/COUNSELLING POINTS: Advise to take with or after food and to avoid taking with milk or at the same time as other drugs. Split the administration by 2 h if possible.

CLASS: Diuretics

DRUG GROUPS: Loop diuretics. Agents used include frusemide and bumetanide.

SIGNIFICANCE IN RENAL DISEASE: Loop diuretics are the most useful in chronic renal failure. They are used to control oedema. In cases of resistant oedema the loop diuretic may be administered with a thiazide such as metolazone or mefruside in order to promote a diuresis.

MODE OF ACTION: Inhibit reabsorption from the ascending loop of Henle in the renal tubule. The oral route is preferred. The intravenous route is useful in those who do not respond. Bumetanide has been reported to have better oral bioavailability in patients who have gut oedema.

GROUP	LOOP DIURETICS	
DRUGS	FRUSEMIDE	BUMETANIDE
Form	I,L,T	I,L,T
Usual adult dose		
ORAL	40–80 mg OD	1–2 mg daily
IV	20–50 mg OD (larger doses by infusion)	1–2 mg (larger doses by infusion)
OTHER	IM inj – 20–50 mg OD	IM inj – 1 mg
Dose adjustment in renal failure	Large doses needed in ESRF or oliguria (up to 2 g day^{-1} orally or 1 g day^{-1} IV)	Large doses needed in ESRF or oliguria (up to 10 mg IV or oral per dose)
Administration requirements		
Reconstitution	250 mg to 50 ml with NaCl or neat via central line	Dilute in dextrose or NaCl
Rate of admin.	250 mg–1 g at a max rate of 4 mg min^{-1}	2–5 mg over 30–60 min

SIDE-EFFECTS: Hypokalaemia (even in renal failure), hyponatraemia, hypomagnesaemia, hypocalcaemia, hypotension, nausea, hyperuricaemia and gout. Too rapid administration of large IV doses can cause tinnitus. Large doses of frusemide have been known to cause blistering of the skin.

PRECAUTIONS: Pregnancy and breastfeeding, hypokalaemia, gout and diabetes mellitus.

CONTRAINDICATIONS: Liver failure – precomatose states.

DRUG INTERACTIONS: Lithium – reduced excretion of lithium. Cardiac toxicity with amiodarone, cardiac glycosides and antihistamines if hypokalaemia occurs. Increased risk of ototoxicity with aminoglycosides and vancomycin.

NOTES/COUNSELLING POINTS: Patients should be warned of the risk of postural hypotension, i.e. dizziness.

CLASS: Diuretics

DRUG GROUPS: Osmotic diuretic. The agent used is mannitol.

SIGNIFICANCE IN RENAL DISEASE: Mannitol is used in the treatment and prevention of acute renal failure. Its use as a prophylactic agent is indicated to protect the kidney during periods of hypoperfusion, e.g major surgery or trauma.

MODE OF ACTION: It acts to produce an increase in urine output. Mannitol inhibits the osmotic transport of water in the proximal tubule and decreases the gradient for the passive absorption of sodium in the ascending limb of the loop of Henle. It also increases glomerular filtration rate.

GROUP	OSMOTIC DIURETIC
DRUGS	MANNITOL
Form	I
Usual adult dose ORAL IV	N/A Anuria – 12.5 g over 5 min as a test dose followed by 50–100 g over 24 h Oedema – 5–10 g h^{-1} (25–50 ml h^{-1} of a 20% solution)
Dose adjustment in renal failure	Discontinue if no response to test dose.
Administration requirements	SC or IM injection must not be used Mannitol is incompatible with blood and blood products Correct hypovolaemia before use
Reconstitution	N/A. Available as 10%, 20% and 25% solutions for infusion
Rate of admin.	50–100 g over 24 h. Adjusted according to urine output

SIDE-EFFECTS: These include congestive cardiac failure, hyper- or hyponatraemia, hyperkalaemia, diarrhoea, and pulmonary oedema. Mannitol can also cause renal failure and allergic type reactions such as fever and chills.

PRECAUTIONS: Care should be taken to avoid extravasation, as this causes inflammation.

CONTRAINDICATIONS: Severe chronic renal failure, pulmonary oedema.

DRUG INTERACTIONS: None of note.

NOTES/COUNSELLING POINTS: A diuresis should occur in 15–30 min after the start of infusion. Solutions greater than 15% can crystallise out at low temperatures. These can be redissolved by warming. The solution should then be allowed to cool to room temperature before use.

CLASS: Electrolyte regulation

DRUG GROUPS: Acidosis – sodium bicarbonate.

SIGNIFICANCE IN RENAL DISEASE: The kidney removes hydrogen ions from the body. In renal failure this mechanism is lost, leading to an accumulation of hydrogen ions. This results in a metabolic acidosis which is seen as a reduction in serum bicarbonate.

MODE OF ACTION: Sodium bicarbonate is given to increase serum bicarbonate and so help to correct the acidosis.

GROUP	CORRECTION OF ACIDOSIS
DRUGS	SODIUM BICARBONATE
Form	C,T
Usual adult dose ORAL IV OTHER	4.8 g or more daily in divided doses. Adjusted according to response Either as 4.2% or 8.4% solution N/A
Dose adjustment in renal failure	Use with caution in severe renal impairment
Administration requirements	Usual route is oral. Given by IV route in severe acidosis
Reconstitution	N/A
Rate of admin.	4.2% at up to 120 ml h^{-1}. 8.4% at 60–120 ml h^{-1}.

SIDE-EFFECTS: Belching is common. An increase in blood pressure and fluid retention may be caused.

PRECAUTIONS: Avoid in respiratory acidosis. Use with caution in those patients where the sodium load may be undesirable, e.g. hypertension.

CONTRAINDICATIONS: None of note.

DRUG INTERACTIONS: None of note.

NOTES/COUNSELLING POINTS: Acidosis is usually corrected by dialysis. 8.4% solution contains 1 mmol of bicarbonate ions and 1 mmol of sodium ions ml^{-1}. Patients should be warned that it can cause belching and a bloated feeling.

CLASS: Electrolyte regulation

DRUG GROUPS: Hyperkalaemia (moderate without ECG changes) – ion exchange resins, e.g. calcium resonium.

SIGNIFICANCE IN RENAL DISEASE: Patients with renal disease lose the ability to excrete potassium when their GFR falls below about 5 ml min^{-1}. This will then accumulate. Ion exchange resins are used to control potassium levels up to about 6.5 mmol l^{-1}. Above this intravenous therapy with other agents or dialysis is necessary.

MODE OF ACTION: Calcium ions are exchanged for potassium ions in the gut. It can be given orally or rectally. Both routes are unpleasant. Large quantities are needed orally and it has an unpleasant and chalky taste. When administered rectally, it needs to be retained for a number of hours.

GROUP	ION EXCHANGE RESINS
DRUGS	CALCIUM RESONIUM
Form	E,P
Usual adult dose ORAL IV OTHER	15 g 3–4 times daily N/A Rectal – 30 g in methylcellulose solution. Retain for 9 h
Dose adjustment in renal failure	
Administration requirements	The powder can be mixed with water or lemonade for oral use. Fruit juices must be avoided as they are high in potassium. It should be given with food
Reconstitution	See above
Rate of admin.	N/A

SIDE-EFFECTS: Oral calcium resonium can cause constipation. A laxative should be coprescribed. Rectal calcium resonium can cause rectal ulceration.

PRECAUTIONS: –

CONTRAINDICATIONS: Hyperparathyroidism, multiple myeloma, sarcoidosis and metastatic carcinoma. There is an increased risk of hypercalcaemia.

DRUG INTERACTIONS: –

NOTES/COUNSELLING POINTS: Some patients will take regular calcium resonium to allow a higher intake of potassium from the diet. Patients should be advised on how to take the powder orally. Many drugs contain potassium, e.g. some antibiotics. In patients with hyperkalaemia any concomitant medication needs to be checked for potassium content.

CLASS: Fibrinolytics

DRUG GROUPS: Streptokinase and urokinase are available, but urokinase is used routinely.

SIGNIFICANCE IN RENAL DISEASE: Fibrinolytics are used to unblock shunts and cannulas. Urokinase is preferred because it is human in origin, unlike strepto-kinase, which is derived from streptococci. This makes the formation of antibodies to urokinase unlikely and so it is suitable for repeated administration if necessary.

MODE OF ACTION: Fibrinolytics cause the breakdown of fibrin and hence the dissolution of the clot by the activation of plasminogen to form plasmin.

GROUP	FIBRINOLYTICS	
DRUGS	UROKINASE	STREPTOKINASE
Form	I	I
Usual dose		
ORAL	N/A	N/A
IV	N/A	N/A
OTHER	5000 IU via shunt/catheter	250 000 IU via shunt/catheter
Dose adjustment in renal failure	N/A	N/A
Administration requirements	Refer to local protocol Slowly inject a volume equal to volume of catheter. Aspirate and then clamp if necessary	Refer to local protocol Slowly inject a volume equal to volume of catheter. Aspirate and then clamp if necessary
Reconstitution	Dissolve in 2–3 ml NaCl. Do not shake.	Dissolve in 2–3 ml NaCl. Do not shake
Rate of admin.	Bolus into affected lumen of catheter	Bolus into affected lumen of catheter

SIDE-EFFECTS: These are rare due to the local action for this indication. Urokinase is less likely than streptokinase to cause allergic reactions. Bleeding complications are the main side-effect.

PRECAUTIONS AND CONTRAINDICATIONS: These tend to be theoretical due to the local action for this indication.

DRUG INTERACTIONS: Anticoagulents – concurrent use may increase the risk of bleeding.

NOTES/COUNSELLING POINTS: Shaking the vial on reconstitution will denature the enzyme. More than one injection of urokinase may be necessary. Once injected into the catheter the solution should be left *in situ* for at least 5 min before an attempt to aspirate the clot is made. These can then be repeated every 5 min until successful. However, if the catheter is not cleared within 30–60 min it is advisable to clamp the catheter and leave the urokinase *in situ* for 1–2 h. The catheter can then be rechecked for patency. Once the catheter is patent a sample should be aspirated to ensure all of the clot and any remaining drug is removed. Some units clamp the catheter as soon as the urokinase is added and make no attempt to aspirate for up to 2 h.

CLASS: Gastric acid inhibitors

DRUG GROUPS: Antacids, H$_2$ antagonists, Proton pump inhibitors.

SIGNIFICANCE IN RENAL DISEASE: Renal disease with associated uraemia increases gastric acid secretion, resulting in a higher incidence of peptic and duodenal ulcer disease.

MODE OF ACTION: Antacids increase gastric pH thereby neutralising gastric pH and preventing irritation. H$_2$ antagonists competitively block histamine receptors on the parietal (acid-secreting) cells. Proton pump inhibitors block energy pathway, preventing release of acidic H$^+$ protons into the stomach.

GROUP	ANTACIDS	CIMETIDINE	H$_2$ ANTAGONISTS			PP INHIBITORS
DRUGS		CIMETIDINE	RANITIDINE	FAMOTIDINE	NIZATIDINE	OMEPRAZOLE
Form	L	L,T,I	L,T,ET,I	T	T,I	C,I*
Usual adult dose ORAL	10–20 ml	400 mg BD	150 mg BD	20–40 mg OD	300 mg OD or 150 mg BD	20–40 mg OD
IV OTHER		200–400 mg	50 mg TDS			
Dose adjustment in renal failure	No	Yes	Yes			No
Administration requirements		Infuse IV doses > 200 mg				Capsules can be opened as administered
Reconstitution		D5W, NaCl				Solution supplied
Rate of admin.		30–60 min	Slow bolus			Slow bolus

SIDE-EFFECTS: Confusion can be a problem with the H$_2$ antagonists. Diarrhoea and headaches are common with omeprazole.

PRECAUTIONS: Antacids have a high electrolyte content. Avoid high doses.

CONTRAINDICATIONS: –

DRUG INTERACTIONS: Cimetidine inhibits cytochrome P450 system. It interacts with a number of other drugs that are also metabolised by this system. See *British National Formulory.*

NOTES/COUNSELLING POINTS: *NAMED PATIENT ONLY.

CLASS: Immunosuppressants

DRUG GROUPS: Azathioprine, Cyclophosphamide.

SIGNIFICANCE IN RENAL DISEASE: These are used in nephritis, systemic vasculitis, and other autoimmune diseases. Azathioprine is also used in immunosuppressive regimes post-transplantation.

MODE OF ACTION: Cyclophosphamide is an alkylating cytotoxic agent. It acts by damaging DNA, interfering with cell replication. It requires metabolism in the liver to the active compound. Azathioprine is a prodrug of 6-mercaptopurine. It is metabolised to this in the liver. 6-Mercaptopurine inhibits purine synthesis so damaging DNA and interfering with cell replication.

GROUP	IMMUNOSUPPRESSANTS	
DRUGS	CYCLOPHOSPHAMIDE (CYTOTOXIC)	AZATHIOPRINE
Form	I,T	I,T
Usual adult dose ORAL	Preferred route 1–2.5 mg kg^{-1} day^{-1} in up to 2 divided doses	Preferred route 1–5 mg kg^{-1} day^{-1}, maintenance 1–3 mg kg^{-1} day^{-1}
IV	As for oral	As for oral
Dose adjustment in renal failure	Give 75% of the normal dose as a single daily dose in severe RI (GFR < 10 ml min^{-1})	Give 75% of the normal dose in severe RI (GFR < 10 ml min^{-1}) .
Administration requirements	Staff administering should avoid skin contact Take after food Can give injection orally if unable to swallow	The injection is very irritant. If IV used flush with NaCl after administration Staff administering should avoid skin contact
Reconstitution	In pharmacy	In pharmacy
Rate of admin.	Over 5–15 min	Over not less than 1 min

SIDE-EFFECTS: Cyclophosphamide can cause bone marrow suppression, a loss of appetite, nausea and vomiting, and can affect fertility. Hair loss occurs in about 25% of patients. Some will experience this as thinning of the hair only. Azathioprine can cause loss of appetite, nausea and vomiting, and diarrhoea and skin rashes. It can also affect liver function and cause a reversible, dose-related bone marrow suppression.

PRECAUTIONS: Full blood counts should be carried out during treatment.

CONTRAINDICATIONS: Pregnancy is a relative contraindication depending on the condition being treated.

DRUG INTERACTIONS: Allopurinol increases the toxicity of cyclophosphamide. Allopurinol enhances the effect of azathioprine, causing an increase in toxicity. If the two are coprescribed the dose of azathioprine should be reduced to one-third of the original dose.

NOTES/COUNSELLING POINTS: Owing to an increased risk of infection, a prophylactic dose of cotrimoxazole is prescribed with cyclophosphamide. Patients should be told to report any signs of infection. Patients should be told to take azathioprine after food.

CLASS: Immunosuppressants

DRUG GROUPS: Cyclosporin – this is a purified metabolite of two strains of fungi. Tacrolimus – This is a macrolide antibiotic produced by a fungus.

SIGNIFICANCE IN RENAL DISEASE: These are used to prevent rejection post-transplantation, i.e. prophylaxis of graft versus host disease.

MODE OF ACTION: Tacrolimus prevents activation of T lymphocytes in response to stimulation by an antigen. It also suppresses T-helper-cell dependent B-cell proliferation and the formation of lymphokines such as interleukin 2 and 3 and gamma interferon. Cyclosporin has its main action on T-helper cells so suppressing the production of lymphokines and hence the maturation of precursor cytotoxic-T cells.

GROUP	IMMUNOSUPPRESSANTS	
DRUGS	CYCLOSPORIN	TACROLIMUS
Form	C,I,L	C,I
Usual adult dose ORAL	Refer to local protocols 10–15 mg kg^{-1} day^{-1} reducing to 2–6 mg kg^{-1} day^{-1}	Refer to local protocols 0.15–0.4 mg kg^{-1} day^{-1} in 2 dd
IV	One-third of oral dose Adjust dose according to levels	0.05–0.1 mg kg^{-1} over 24 h Adjust dose according to levels
Dose adjustment in renal failure	N/A	Dose at lower end of range. Adjust according to levels
Administration requirements	Usually taken in 2 divided doses 12 h apart PVC equipment should be avoided when giving an infusion.	Usually taken in 2 dd 12 h apart PVC equipment should be avoided when giving an infusion
Reconstitution	N/A. Dilute to 50 ml with D5W or NaCl	N/A. Dilute injection with D5W or NaCl
Rate of admin.	Infusion over 2–6 h	Continuous infusion over 24 h

SIDE-EFFECTS: Cyclosporin can cause nephrotoxicity, hypertension, gum hyperplasia, fine muscle tremor, e.g. hands; sickness and hirsuitism. During the first few days of taking this, patients may notice a burning or tingling sensation in their hands or feet. Tacrolimus can cause tremor, hypertension, hyperglycaemia, nephrotoxicity, headache and dizziness. Cardiovascular effects, such as cardiomyopathy, have also been reported. Both will increase susceptibility to infection and lymphoma.

PRECAUTIONS: Can worsen renal function. Any rise in creatinine needs to be investigated to exclude rejection. Blood pressure, liver function, serum potassium and lipids all need to be monitored.

CONTRAINDICATIONS: Any known hypersensitivity to the drug. Cyclosporin and tacrolimus should not be used together. Use in pregnancy is contraindicated.

DRUG INTERACTIONS: Both are extensively hepatically metabolised. In theory any drug that affects the cyctochrome P450 system will interact with these drugs. Others may enhance the nephrotoxicity, e.g. erythromycin, aminoglycosides, calcium-channel blockers, and antiepileptics.

NOTES/COUNSELLING POINTS: The capsules should be stored in their blister pack and only be removed when it is time to take them. Owing to wide interpatient variability in absorption, blood level monitoring is essential. Tacrolimus should not be taken with meals. Patients are advised to take the capsules either 1 h before or 2–3 h after food. There are two formulations of cyclosporin: Sandimmun and Neoral. These are not interchangeable. Patients should be advised to report any signs of infection and counselled on how to avoid infection.

CLASS: Immunosuppressants

DRUG GROUPS: Steroids – prednisolone, methylprednisolone.

SIGNIFICANCE IN RENAL DISEASE: These are used in conditions such as nephritis and systemic vasculitis and as part of immunosuppressive protocols post-transplantation. (Protocols tend to vary from centre to centre.)

MODE OF ACTION: Immunosuppression is mediated through an inhibition of lymphocyte production and suppression of the inflammatory response.

GROUP	IMMUNOSUPPRESSANTS – STEROIDS	
DRUGS	METHYLPREDNISOLONE	PREDNISOLONE
Form	I	ET,S,T
Usual adult dose ORAL IV	Refer to local protocols N/A 500 mg – 1 g per dose Will give for up to 3 days in rejection episodes	Refer to local protocols Up to 60 mg per day N/A
Dose adjustment in renal failure	N/A	N/A
Administration requirements	Rapid injection of large doses can cause cardiovascular collapse	Give in the morning to minimise adrenal suppression. Do not split doses up throughout the day
Reconstitution	With WFI initially then dilute with D5W or NaCl	N/A
Rate of admin.	500 mg or more over at least 20 min	N/A

SIDE-EFFECTS: These include the mineralocorticoid effects such as hypertension, sodium and water retention, and potassium loss (this can present as muscle weakness) and glucocorticoid effects. These include diabetes, osteoporosis and skin atrophy. Steroids can cause hirsuitism and adrenal suppression and increase the susceptibility to infection. Patients may also experience stomach upsets or indigestion.

PRECAUTIONS: Should not be given in infection without the appropriate anti-infective agents being coprescribed. Use is also cautioned during pregnancy, in diabetes, osteoporosis and peptic ulcer disease.

CONTRAINDICATIONS: –

DRUG INTERACTIONS: High-dose methylprednisolone can increase cyclosporin levels. There is an increased risk of hypokalaemia with diuretics such as thiazides, loops and acetazolamide. Antiepileptics increase the metabolism of steroids. There is an increased risk of bleeding when prescribed with non-steroidal anti-inflammatory drugs.

NOTES/COUNSELLING POINTS: In transplant protocols prednisolone is the oral steroid of choice. Methylprednisolone tends to be used by the intravenous route as first-line therapy for acute rejection. For chronic use the lowest effective dose should be used so that the adverse effects relating to long-term use are minimal. Patients are often maintained on alternate day doses to help this. Patients must carry a steroid warning card and not stop taking them abruptly if they are on long-term therapy. They should be warned to report any signs of infection such as a sore throat. They should also be counselled on how to avoid infection. Prednisolone is best taken with food to minimise any gastric irritation. Prophylactic agents such as nystatin are often coprescribed to prevent or treat opportunistic infections such as candida (thrush).

CLASS: Immunosuppressants

DRUG GROUPS: Monoclonal anti T3 antibody serum – OKT3; Antithymocyte globulin – ATG.

SIGNIFICANCE IN RENAL DISEASE: These are all biological agents used to treat steroid-resistant transplant rejection and for prophylaxis of rejection in sensitised patients.

MODE OF ACTION: ATG acts to destroy T lymphocytes. This results in an attenuated immune response. The action of OKT3 is to block the generation and hence the function of T-cytotoxic cells which are responsible for rejection.

GROUP	IMMUNOSUPPRESSANTS	
DRUGS	ATG	OKT3
Form	I	I
Usual adult dose IV	Refer to local protocols 1.25–5 mg kg^{-1} day^{-1} as a single daily dose for 10–14 days, adjusted to provide optimal immunosuppression	Refer to local protocols 5 mg day^{-1} as a single daily dose for 10–14 days
Dose adjustment in renal failure	N/A	N/A
Administration requirements	Given with chlorpheniramine and hydrocortisone to minimise risk of anaphylaxis	First three doses given with paracetamol, methylprednisolone and chlorpheniramine to reduce risk of anaphylaxis
Reconstitution	Dilute with NaCl or D5W. Minimum 25 mg 50 ml^{-1}	N/A
Rate of admin.	By continuous infusion over more than 4 h	As an IV bolus over less than 1 min

SIDE-EFFECTS: These include rigors, marked pyrexia, shivering, chills and tremor. Anaphylactic reactions can occur to the first dose. OKT3 can also cause chest pain, dyspnoea and pulmonary oedema.

PRECAUTIONS: Prophylactic agents should be given to minimise the risk of side-effects (see notes below).

CONTRAINDICATIONS: Pulmonary oedema is a contraindication to the use of OKT3 (patients must not be fluid overloaded). These agents should not be used in patients with acute viral illness.

DRUG INTERACTIONS: These agents can cause an increase in cyclosporin levels. In practice, other immunosuppressants are stopped before a course of ATG or OKT3 is started and then restarted 3 days before the course ends.

NOTES/COUNSELLING POINTS: Prophylactic agents should be coprescribed with the first few doses and given 1 h before the ATG or OKT3.

ATG – Chlorpheniramine 10 mg IV, Hydrocortisone 100 mg IV;
OKT3 – Chlorpheniramine 10 mg IV, Methylprednisolone 500 mg IV, Paracetamol
1 g orally. Patients should be warned about the possible side-effects with the first
few doses. The susceptibility to infection is increased. Prophylactic agents are
often coprescribed. These include nystatin for fungal infection, acyclovir for
cytomegalovirus and cotrimoxazole for pneumocystis carinii pneumonia (PCP).

CLASS: Skeletal muscle relaxants

DRUG GROUPS: Quinine salts, e.g. quinine sulphate.

SIGNIFICANCE IN RENAL DISEASE: Cramp is a common symptom associated with chronic renal failure. The cause is not completely understood but it is mainly due to uraemia and electrolyte imbalances. It often occurs following haemodialysis sessions. Many patients will take quinine; however, they often do not respond.

MODE OF ACTION: Quinine increases the refractory period of the muscle and reduces excitability at the neuromuscular junction. This results in a decrease in activity of the muscle. Its efficacy for this indication has not been firmly established.

GROUP	SKELETAL MUSCLE RELAXANTS
DRUGS	QUININE SULPHATE
Form	T
Usual adult dose	
ORAL	200–300 mg at night and when required
IV	May be used in extreme cases
OTHER	N/A
Dose adjustment in renal failure	N/A
Administration requirements	
Reconstitution	Available as the dihydrochloride at a concentration of 300 mg ml^{-1} Dilute with NaCl
Rate of admin.	Infuse over 4 h

SIDE-EFFECTS: These are unusual at the doses used but can include nausea, headache, tinnitus, visual disturbances, abdominal pain and confusion. Hypoglycaemia can occur after parenteral administration.

PRECAUTIONS: Atrial fibrillation and conduction defects.

CONTRAINDICATIONS: –

DRUG INTERACTIONS: Cardiac glycosides–increased plasma concentration of digoxin. Cyclosporin–decreased plasma levels.

NOTES/COUNSELLING POINTS: –

CLASS: Sympathomimetic

DRUG GROUPS: Dopamine is used.

SIGNIFICANCE IN RENAL DISEASE: At low dose (up to $5\,\mu g\,kg^{-1}\,min^{-1}$ it is used to increase renal perfusion. The effects of dopamine are dose dependent. The other inotropic sympathomimetics do not have the same effect on renal blood flow. At low doses, dopamine does not increase heart rate or raise systemic arterial pressure, i.e. does not provide inotropic support.

MODE OF ACTION: Dopamine dilates renal and mesenteric blood vessels by stimulation of dopaminergic receptors. The resultant increase in renal blood flow increases the GFR and hence urine output.

GROUP	SYMPATHOMIMETIC
DRUGS	DOPAMINE
Form	I
Usual adult dose ORAL IV OTHER	N/A Renal support – 2–$5\,\mu g\,kg^{-1}\,min^{-1}$. Adjusted according to response N/A
Dose adjustment in renal failure	N/A
Administration requirements	Must be diluted before use. Minimum dilution is 200 mg in 50 ml Local nomograms available for easy calculation of rates
Reconstitution	Dilute with NaCl 0.9%, D5W or sodium lactate. Incompatible with bicarbonate
Rate of admin	2–$5\,\mu g\,kg^{-1}\,min^{-1}$.

SIDE-EFFECTS: Causes nausea and vomiting, hypo- or hypertension, peripheral vasoconstriction and tachycardia. Stopping the infusion will bring side-effects under control quickly as dopamine has a half-life of approximately 2 min.

PRECAUTIONS: Hypovolaemia should be corrected before use.

CONTRAINDICATIONS: Phaeochromocytoma and tachyarrhythmias.

DRUG INTERACTIONS: Antidepressants. Risk of hypertensive crisis with monoamine oxidase inhibitors.

NOTES/COUNSELLING POINTS: Dopamine will cause renal vasoconstriction at inotropic doses.

DOSE CALCULATION: For 200 mg dopamine per 100 ml the following may be used: Rate of infusion $(ml\,h^{-1})$ = weight (kg) × dose $(\mu g\,kg^{-1}\,min^{-1})$ × 0.03.

INDEX

Page numbers in *italic* refer to illustrations and tables; **bold** page numbers indicate a main discussion.